# Experiential Anatomy

## Therapeutic Applications of Embodied Movement and Awareness

# EXPERIENTIAL ANATOMY

## THERAPEUTIC APPLICATIONS OF EMBODIED MOVEMENT AND AWARENESS

### Leila Stuart, BA, LLB, RMT (ret.), C-IAYT

Foreword by Carol Davis

Illustrated by Bruce Hogarth

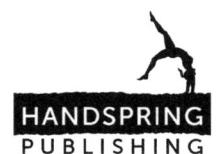

HANDSPRING
PUBLISHING

First published in Great Britain in 2024 by Jessica Kingsley Publishers
An imprint of Hodder & Stoughton Ltd
An Hachette Company

I

There are supplementary materials which can be accessed via https://www.youtube.com/
playlist?list=PL3j_YuMBqigE1Pih3KnUtycHGV2MEKFCE for personal use with this program, but may
not be reproduced for any other purposes without the permission of the publisher. In the text, an 🔊
indicates the practice has accompanying audio, while 📹 indicates the practice has accompanying video.

A photo of human fascia taken with an endoscopic camera is reproduced in Chapter 4 with the kind
permission of Endovivo productions and J. C. Guimberteau MD. Four photos of tensegrity structures are
reproduced with permission of Fernando Tejero: 2 views of a tensegrity icosahedron (simplex Juliana and
simplex Juliana perfil) and 2 views of a tensegrity spine (columna Adriana and columna AdrianaTorcida).

A CIP catalogue record for this title is available from the British Library and the Library of Congress

ISBN 978 1 91342 621 7
eISBN 978 1 83997 629 2

Printed and bound in Great Britain by CPI Group

Jessica Kingsley Publishers' policy is to use papers that are natural, renewable and recyclable
products and made from wood grown in sustainable forests. The logging and manufacturing
processes are expected to conform to the environmental regulations of the country of origin.

Handspring Publishing
Carmelite House
50 Victoria Embankment
London EC4Y 0DZ

www.handspringpublishing.com

John Murray Press
Part of Hodder & Stoughton Limited
An Hachette UK Company

This book is dedicated to my beloved teacher Judith Koltai (1937–2024)

*"Teaching people to be in their bodies is a radical political act because people who are embodied cannot be controlled."—Judith Koltai*

Without her graceful modeling of presence and intelligence in action, this book would not exist.

# Foreword

*Getting from Where We Are to Where We Need to Be*

Let me begin by saying that this is an outstanding teaching manual, one of the most interesting and well written I've read. It is in a league of its own in terms of extensiveness, expertise, and excellence in educating clients', patients', and teachers' inner awareness through experiential anatomy. It includes the latest science of fascia, biotensegrity, and complex systems theory, and explains these new sciences with lived experience, illustrating the research by translating it into meaningful lessons that combine yoga, somatic inquiry, breath, alignment, and movement repatterning. In the words of the author: "This book is a guide to embodying and teaching experiential anatomy as a pathway to self-knowledge and self-healing."

As an academic teacher, researcher, and writer and as a physical therapist clinician practicing myofascial release and exercise for soft-tissue-related pain, I am devoted to the process of reading, understanding, and translating the latest discoveries in the sciences of soft tissue and movement practices that will benefit my patients, my students, and my colleagues in the professions of pain management and rehabilitation.

When Leila asked me to read her chapter drafts, I readily agreed for I had sensed her expertise after experiencing the benefit of her teaching me embodied awareness. From the very first reading of Leila's work, I was delighted and amazed at her ability to write so visibly and to translate her work onto the page with clarity for

the benefit of students and teachers alike, for all who are interested in translating intellectual information into an inner experience that can be understood and embodied in ways that facilitate healing and integration from within.

What do we mean by "embodied"? Dutch phenomenologist and embryological anatomist Jaap Van der Wal teaches that there are two realities when we speak of our bodies: the "lived" body and the "studied" body.[1] In German, there are two different words for these two bodies: "Korper" for the studied body, and "Lieb" for the lived body.

The studied body is the body that is observed and dissected, the anatomical body, the body we "think" exists. In truth, this is a secondary reality to the lived body. The lived body is our "felt" reality, reality as experienced. It is the body of participation, the body we are, the body we sense, the body we feel inside ourselves with our eyes closed. And it is through experiencing the lived body that true self-awareness is developed, which is suggested as a pathway to healing. Until we can locate the self within the lived body, we cannot truly know who we are.

This book has been expertly designed to facilitate growth and deepening awareness of the lived experience of your body—embodiment—and this experience is deepened with an integration of the five koshas from yoga: the physical body, the

---

1    Van der Wal, J. (2020, May 27) Personal communication.

energy body, the mental body, the wisdom body, and the innermost sheath. Each chapter explores different anatomical areas of the body, but their relationship to the irreducible whole is always an underlying principle. Read and followed with mindful focus, this book can transform teachers' and students' practice from where it is, to where it needs to be to facilitate systemic balance and healing. I believe it is a book you will keep and refer to again and again for yourself and for your patients and clients. Enjoy it!

*Carol M Davis, DPT, EdD, MS*
*Scarborough, Maine, USA*

# Preface

During the 16 years I was sick with debilitating chronic fatigue and inflammatory arthritis, I somehow managed to create and teach the yoga therapy training that ultimately formed the foundation of this book. I still don't know how I did it when I was so physically, emotionally, and mentally challenged, but my type A personality probably had something to do with it. Even after I was no longer "sick", I felt challenged to regain my mojo or the confidence to venture back into the world after being housebound for so many years.

During the process of writing this book I got myself back little by little, chapter by chapter. I realized that all those years, like many people in severe chronic pain, I had been living "a short distance" from my body. As I did the practices repeatedly, they helped me develop agency and become more fully embodied. By the end of the book, I had regained my confidence, sparkle, and, most importantly, my Self.

May this book assist you in reclaiming all parts of your wellness and Wholeness.

Leila Stuart, July 2023

# Acknowledgments

I am in deep gratitude to the many people who supported me on the journey of writing this book.

My students over the last 35 years. This book evolved from your contributions in public classes and in the Anatomy of Yoga Therapy training I taught for 15 years. Thank you for your curiosity, enthusiastic exploration, and nuanced feedback as we journeyed together through the body. The names associated with quotations from my students have been changed to protect their privacy and ensure their confidentiality.

My teachers. I have been blessed to study with many influential teachers in the body-mind tradition. Judith Koltai, my movement teacher since 1989, thank you for introducing me to the phenomenological approach of Charlotte Selver and Sensory Awareness, to the work of Therese Bertherat, and for your gentle insistence on precision and economy in words and movement. Your teachings inform all my work. Sandra Sammartino, for over 30 years of witnessing your passion for an experiential approach to the multi-dimensionality of yoga and your fearlessness in teaching deep yogic wisdom. Donna Farhi, for the depth of your teaching methodology and unique way of teaching yoga from inside out. Jane Ellison, for introducing me to experiential anatomy decades ago. Bonnie Bainbridge Cohen and the all-encompassing work of Body-Mind Centering. Although I've studied very little directly with Bonnie, I have absorbed the work through her and her students' books.

My advance readers Jane Hardcastle, Sharon Abondanza, Lisa Peterson, Carol Davis, Libbie Nelson, Susan Turtletaub, my sister Patty Stuart Macadam, Jill Massengill, and Terry Anderson. Each of you brought a unique perspective, and your insightful comments and suggestions clarified and streamlined the book. Patty, thank you for our weekly phone calls and your bony revelations.

Additional readers who reviewed chapters in their area of expertise—Joanne Avison (a special thank you Joanne for encouraging me to write this book), John Sharkey, Matthew Taylor, Robin Rothenberg, Cherie Dostal Ryba, Susan Lowell de Solorzano, and Chris Clancy.

My writing coach, Aggie Stewart. Your compassion and skill with embodied practices and co-meditation guided me through this challenging writing journey. You saved me.

The Handspring publishing team. Sarena Wolfaard for wanting this book to be written, Claire Wilson for her calm wonderfulness and patience, and everyone on the production team.

My husband Michael Weiner. Thank you, sweetheart, for your loving support and patience, periodic editorial comments, and title suggestion that perfectly embraces the essence of these teachings.

To my unseen writerly "team" for your inspiration, whispered words, and supportive presence. Mom and Dad, I am so grateful that you instilled in us a love of physical activity, knowledge, and well written words. I have felt your loving support every step of the way.

Some of the material for Chapter 7 has been drawn from *Pathways to a Centered Body*, co-authored by Leila Stuart and Donna Farhi, 2022 (Embodied Wisdom) and used with permission.

*A Sanskrit-English Dictionary*, Revised Edition, 1992 (Oxford University Press), was consulted for the meaning of Sanskrit words cited in this text.

*Oxford Latin Desk Dictionary*, Bilingual Edition, 2005 (Oxford University Press), was consulted for the meaning of Latin words cited in this text.

The digital edition of the Merriam-Webster dictionary was consulted for English word etymologies cited in this text.

# Contents

# Introduction

## MY STORY

When asked what I do, the short answer is I teach awareness. The fuller answer is that I empower people to become active participants in their own healing process using experiential anatomy to access their deeper self.

Experiential anatomy (EA) transformed my life and clinical work. My passion ignited when I discovered that abstract intellectual information could be understood somatically and embodied in healing ways. Inspired to share this revelation with yoga students and massage therapy clients, I developed workshops combining yoga with EA, somatic inquiry, and breath, alignment, and movement repatterning. I opened a yoga therapy studio in 1999, offering these gentle practices to people experiencing pain or disability not generally addressed in regular yoga classes. As students explored their anatomy with inner sensing, something magical happened. Physically, maladaptive patterns changed, pain decreased, and function improved. And, to my astonishment, the awareness fine-tuned in physical inquiry translated into reports of positive changes in other aspects of their lives. After consistently hearing about these transformational shifts, I realized that the body is a rich well of personal wisdom and resources, and that these integrative somatic practices could open a door to the deeper Self.

I was heartened to observe that students organically shifted the narrative with their bodies from judgment, forcing, and rejection to one of friendliness, self-compassion, and agency in their own healing. They were enthusiastic about the therapeutic process and more likely to adhere to daily practice knowing they could transfer new learning to daily activities like sitting at a desk, standing, walking, and reaching into a cupboard. As students learned to sense into and differentiate anatomical structures experientially, they connected with their own wisdom and inherent wholeness. Consequently, they experienced greater ability to access inner resources, self-regulate, and connect with themselves, others, and the cosmos. Many related feeling more vital, embodied, and responsive to the truth of each moment rather than reacting from conditioned patterns. New sources of support were discovered as they shed habits of bracing against or "muscling" through life. "Doing" less and "being" more meant living with added ease and flow. My own experience mirrored that of my students.

> After the foot workshop I found I could "stand up" for myself more when interacting with my partner.
>
> *Lynn*

In workshops and clinical practice, I noticed that students whose health issues resolved faster were open to learning about their body and willing to participate in their own healing process. I began screening prospective patients by explaining my approach and asking if they were willing to work collaboratively. In honesty, I had become weary of "doing" something "to" a passive someone who expected me to take responsibility for their healing. Neuroscience and motivational research reflected my experience, confirming that active rehabilitation and patient empowerment are crucial keys to long-term resolution of pain and biomechanical dysfunction (Chen 2006; Small et al., 2013).

> I was shattered after witnessing my son's suicide. As I learned to compassionately attend to my body, every class I felt like I "got more of myself back" and could reintegrate my dissociated parts.
>
> *Nadine*

Nadine's experience is not uncommon. Students commonly compare EA practices to saying a "warm hello" to each body part, and that this simple act of acknowledgment helped them accept themselves and experience the inherently healing quality of compassion for their own suffering.

I began using movement as therapy when I suffered a severe back injury as a young adult. A friend recommended yoga, but since classes were scarce in 1974, I began with a yoga book and diligent practice. For almost 20 years, I managed my back pain with morning yoga and movement breaks throughout the day. When the long-standing condition resolved during my first yoga teacher training, I understood the vast healing potential of yoga. This realization subsequently deepened as I relied heavily on physical and subtle practices throughout 16 years of suffering debilitating chronic fatigue and crippling inflammatory arthritis. Every morning, I would painfully stagger downstairs one step at a time to my studio, hanging on to the railing. After 45 minutes of yoga and somatic practice I could enter my day with more tolerable pain levels. The subtle practices calmed my nervous system and helped me accept the reality of my illness and devastating loss of my former life and career. My practice became my lifeline.

During that first yoga teacher training, I was introduced to the ancient model of the koshas as different densities of consciousness describing human experience (see Chapter 1). This multidimensional understanding was further validated in postgraduate studies in neuromuscular and craniosacral therapy, which taught me the wisdom of viewing each person as a whole being. Working with individual parts was necessary, but always in the context of the whole. The physical body became a doorway for students to access their more subtle dimensions and understand themselves as unified consciousness.

As I learned to assess structure and function globally, I could identify local and distal forces likely contributing to presenting symptoms. Without this approach, I was chasing symptoms, not underlying causes, and headaches or backaches wouldn't resolve. The impact of contributory nonphysical factors, such as high job stress or trauma history, on therapeutic outcomes also emerged as important.

> This makes so much sense. Why didn't we learn it in school?
>
> *Dorothy*

My passion for teaching mindfulness and EA as a doorway to the deeper Self culminated in The Anatomy of Yoga Therapy, a comprehensive 300-hour training that I taught for 15 years locally before expanding the work in international workshops. This book distills some of the key principles and practices evolved over three decades of ongoing experimentation and collaboration with colleagues and students, to whom I am eternally grateful.

## HOW TO USE THIS BOOK

This book is a guide to embodying and teaching EA as a pathway to self-knowledge and self-healing. While it uses yoga therapy as a framework and underlying methodology, the practices are equally applicable to other manual and movement therapies, somatic therapies, and modalities such as personal training, physiotherapy, and kinesiology. EA offers an accessible entry point for the process of developing self-awareness, the first step to self-healing in all modalities. The practices are simple, easily understood, and relevant to anyone experiencing dis-ease, regardless of yoga experience. The learned self-awareness is functional in all activities of daily living.

Extensive knowledge of anatomy is not necessary to teach EA. The true value of knowing anatomy lies not with proficiency in naming structures, but in cultivating a felt sense of those structures to help you move with ease, establish right relationship with yourself and the earth, and live with more equanimity. This book provides sufficient information to enable you to use EA as an organizing principle for personal exploration and therapeutic practice (although an anatomy text may be helpful).

Each chapter covers different body parts, yet the underlying premise is that everything is connected, and that each part reflects the whole. Individual parts are differentiated to appreciate their uniqueness and multidimensional effect on the whole organism. The practices provide opportunities for you to develop self-compassionate awareness of habitual breath, alignment, movement, and mental patterns, then register qualitative differences in felt experience following each exploration and in your lived experience of integrating new learning in daily life on both physical and nonphysical levels.

Many practices have accompanying audio or video that can be accessed via https://www.youtube.com/playlist?list=PL3j_YuMBqigE1Pih3KnUtycHGV2MEKFCE 🔊)) indicates the practice has accompanying audio, while 🎥 indicates the practice has accompanying video.

The *how* of the practices is infinitely more important than the form or movement; process-oriented exploration of structure and movement through the senses takes precedence over accomplishing a particular endpoint. Cultivating an attitude of open-minded curiosity while doing explorations with subtlety and awareness leads to a felt sense of anatomical structures and healthy respect for their capabilities and limitations. This deepening of functional interoceptive awareness (see Chapter 1) is the main aim of EA and this book. The second aim is to simplify complex anatomical information into digestible bites and embody them to repattern unhelpful habits. The third aim is to offer a toolkit of simple body-mind practices that are accessible to the average person attending a class or private session with a health professional and that will make a functional difference in their everyday life.

The first three chapters establish conceptual and educational frameworks for learning and teaching EA as therapy. In this Introduction, EA is defined and expanded as a therapeutic practice, while Chapter 1 introduces key concepts that will enrich reader experience in subsequent chapters. The ABCs of the kosha model, interoception, neuroplasticity, and pain science explain *why* EA is therapeutic. Chapter 2 details the model and principles of teaching EA and offers guidelines to deepen the learning experience. As the first experiential chapter, Chapter 3 explores foundational practices to liberate the breath and establish it as the link between body and mind. Chapter 4 sets the stage for experiencing the wholeness of the body through fascia before exploring individual parts in subsequent chapters. Chapter 5 explores organs as a source of inner support that can minimize excessive muscular tension and habitual overeffort. The remaining chapters delve into individual anatomical parts that are typically addressed in therapy. Each experiential chapter contains foundational practices to equip a self-healing toolkit. The EA explorations, self-palpation, somatic inquiries, yoga asana, and imagery in this book are by no means exhaustive, but have been selected from my practice, experience, and student and colleague feedback over decades of teaching. The experience of some explorations is deepened with use of yoga props and easily accessible balls.

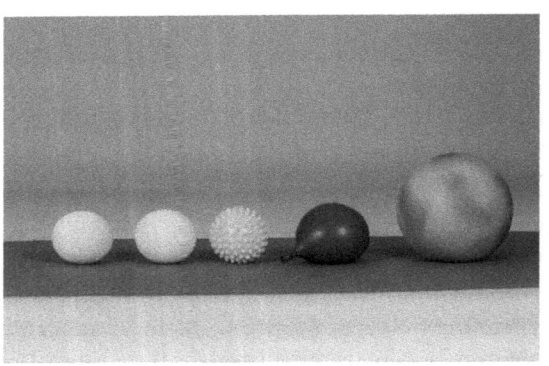

This book presents a roadmap of self-discovery and self-healing on philosophical, physical, energetic, mental, and spiritual levels. It is designed to be read and experienced as a logical, cumulative progression of material from beginning to end. I encourage readers (both professional and others) to digest the intellectual information and layer it into the physical practices to experience the greatest benefit. You may want to periodically return to this Introduction and teaching methodology in Chapters 1 and 2 as you refine progressive levels of self-awareness and evolution. Cultivating your own felt sense experience is crucial to effectively articulate the fullness and depth of EA explorations to others. By embodying the practices, you will develop awareness and discernment to spiral you, over time, into new and deeper levels of understanding in your own body and how you teach.

This expanded awareness refines self-knowledge and strengthens self-compassion, leading to deeper embodiment, self-evolution, and a radical shift in experiencing wholeness. In the wise words of Jaap van der Wal, "[w]e never stop birthing ourselves" (2019). The practices in this book can assist in this process of constantly becoming ourselves.

> Note: Although some practices are available as recordings, I suggest that you personally record others to consolidate your learning experience.

## WHAT IS EXPERIENTIAL ANATOMY?

Learning anatomy is useful but often dry and boring, requiring rote learning of anatomical structures. In contrast, EA is a rich, embodied method of learning, combining interoceptive awareness (IA) and mindful movement to foster whole-person healing and integration. Interoception is the process of registering sensations

of internal physical and emotional states, then processing and integrating that information to generate self-regulatory responses (see Chapter 1). EA begins with an intellectual, two-dimensional understanding of anatomical structures and forces in the living body, then expands into direct personal experience that is ultimately transformative. As we mindfully explore the "laboratory" of our own body, we become curious about the vast world inside and how our physical body, emotions, and personal and cultural conditioning influence each other. Through guided explorations, anatomical parts are differentiated in the neural landscape while their relationships with other structures are simultaneously highlighted. I liken the process to family systems therapy; repatterning work with individual members can change dynamics of the whole family. In this way of working, anatomical structures and systems are viewed as possessing awareness, intelligence, and the capacity to initiate movement. As intelligence awakens in each structure, cells can better communicate with each other, the nervous system can register the presence of each part, and all parts can function as a harmonious "family of the body."

EA is a learning approach based on the indivisibility of the body-mind; it involves all of who we are. When we learn that bones are part of our internal supportive scaffolding and establish felt sense that we are standing in our bones, we use our body laboratory to explore how to establish structural, mental, and emotional integrity. We then sense and compare the sensations of habitual patterns of standing and moving with new understanding gleaned from EA explorations. We choose which way feels just right and form an intention to repattern and integrate the new habit. We learn that the skill of cultivating awareness of physical habits is easily transferred to habits in all levels of life.

> Our body is our self... It is not opposed to our intelligence, to our feelings, to our soul. It includes them and shelters them. By becoming aware of our body we give ourselves access to our entire being—for body and spirit, mental and physical, and even strength and weakness represent not our duality but our unity.
>
> *Therese Bertherat (Bertherat and Bernstein 1989, p. xi)*

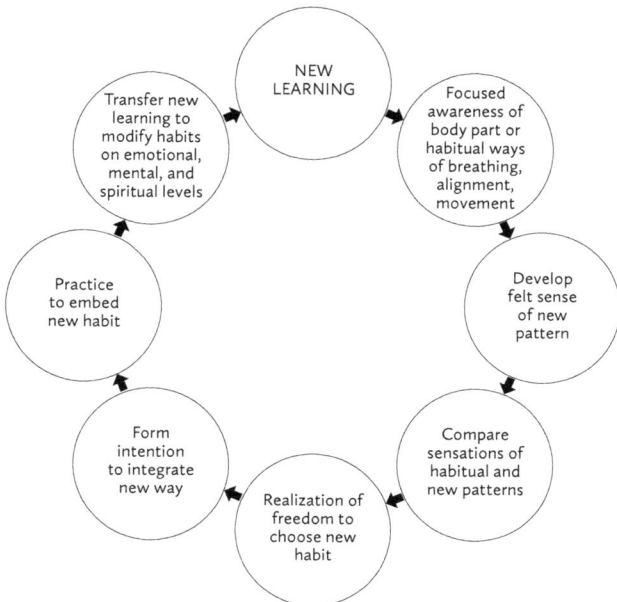

Flowchart 0.1 Repatterning Habits

## Experiential Anatomy Is Therapy

Many of us are uneducated about our bodies, what we look like inside, how things work, or the possibilities of our magnificent structure. We may have a distant relationship with our body and consider it primarily a vehicle for transporting our all-important energy and attention-demanding mind. This disconnected relationship can manifest in limited, inefficient ways of moving and being in our bodies. Sages for centuries have counselled "know thyself," and the body can be an accessible entry point to the self-knowledge necessary for healing. When we center our mind in our body, it slows down to body time and we become present and aware, setting the stage for healing.

> In an age of speed, I began to think, nothing could be more invigorating than going slow. In an age of distraction, nothing could feel more luxurious than paying attention.
>
> *Pico Iyer (2014, p. 66)*

The English word *health* originates from the same Old Norse root as *whole* and *holy*. The Sanskrit word for health is *svastha*, which means "self-abiding or seated in the self." The word *therapy* originates from a Greek word meaning "to attend, to serve, take care of." When EA is used therapeutically, we are attending to ourselves in ways that unearth inner resources. Through a process of self-inquiry, we access tools that help us move, breathe, and "be" in healthy, self-actualized ways. This process can shift perception and experience in ways that invoke our innate capacity for self-healing and uncover worlds of untapped potential. We learn to trust ourselves, the wisdom of our body, and our capacity to heal. The paradox of this practice is that working with distinct parts leads us to experience the whole.

## EA Is a Nonintellectual, Somatic Experience

EA practices can calm the thinking, storytelling mind and move us into the feeling body. Instead of evaluating, judging, or rejecting, we use direct sensory perception to connect to something palpable, solid, and an endless source of captivating sensations—our own body. Intellectual anatomical concepts are transformed into felt experience, making structures tangible and real. Brain maps are differentiated and clarified as we pay attention to anatomical structures, and the nervous system then expands participation of those parts in future movement. Direct experience allows us to feel ourselves, to be centered within the breath and within the movement rather than merely thinking about it. Movement becomes full and potent rather than rote and mechanical.

EA inquiries often uncover distant underlying causes of dysfunction; we may think the shoulder itself is causing pain, but a pelvic EA exploration may resolve the shoulder pain, increase function, and initiate systemwide changes. This somatic awareness of anatomical structures moves beyond ideas of alignment, strengthening, and core stability. Simply experiencing one's own structure through EA can pattern these concepts in an organic, self-generated way.

EA invites us to identify touchstones, structures within our bodies that help attain certain states, access inner resources, or self-regulate. For example, when one student of mine needs to self-soothe, he visualizes his lungs squeezing and tenderly "hugging" his heart with each inhalation. His visualization not only slows his breathing rate but helps him access self-compassion. Touchstones like this reliably reproduce significant physical and nonphysical sensations and effects that we can access whenever needed.

## EA Develops Interoceptive Skills

Anatomical structures are tangible; many can be felt, seen, or sensed. EA practices stimulate interoceptive (sensing inner processes) and proprioceptive (perception of position and movement of body parts: see Chapter 1) awareness. We register the state of our body-mind through sensing and feeling ourselves *throughout* a practice. As we track sensations or the way force sequences through structures, we become conscious participants in feedback loops that refine and alter our responses and lead to embodied learning. After cultivating these mindfulness skills, students often eagerly tune into their body wisdom and learn more about themselves to better understand their pain, challenges, and possibilities. Interoception can be viewed as the underlying mechanism of mindfulness. Linda Graham, revered for her work on resilience, characterizes mindfulness as a practice that strengthens structures of the brain used to focus attention, reflect on experience, shift perspective, discern options, and ultimately choose wise actions (Graham 2018).

Neuroscience continues to clarify the neural networks associated with interoception and how the quality of neural inputs influences output. Slow, subtle, and mindful EA practices fine-tune interoceptive skills and send high-quality sensory inputs to the brain. Mindful movement, done with conscious awareness of associated sensations, is foundational to learning; neural networks involved in sensory experience and movement are also involved in higher-level intellectual processing (Clark 2015). As we refine felt sense of body structures through EA, we are cultivating inner resources and building our capacity for social and emotional intelligence. We develop the fluidity to respond and move in ways appropriate to the moment.

Thomas Hanna coined the term *sensory motor amnesia* to describe how the nervous system habituates to unconscious patterns of muscular activation (1988, p. xiii). We may perpetuate inefficient and potentially harmful patterns because sensations of movement or posture register as "normal." When a structure is explored, palpated, and moved precisely with anatomical awareness, the brain receives higher-quality information that clarifies sensorimotor maps and eases sensory motor amnesia. Once a structure is registered in the nervous system and experienced in the body as felt sense, the direct experience can be deliberately replicated. The more frequently anatomical structures are notated in the neural landscape with intention, attention, and practice, the more integrated they become. The family of the body can then work together as an integrated whole.

## EA Uses the Physical Body as a Doorway to Other Aspects of Self

For most people, the body is accessible; we sense and feel it through sensation, breath, and movement. Even though we may breathe suboptimally or have limited movement repertoires, focusing attention on body structures is usually an achievable exploration. Yet, to focus solely on the physicality of explorations hinders realization of true health, or svastha. The body is the doorway: awareness in the physical realm kindles awareness of our energetic, emotional, mental, and spiritual selves.

> Attention slowly brings us into the shelter of intimacy, the tangled nest of conversation between body, heart, soul, and world.
>
> *Francis Weller (2015, p. 96)*

EA helps us attune to subtle inner experiences of slight shifts in balance, cadence of breath, flow of emotions, and physiological messages. As sensitivity increases, we become aware of our natural responses to internal and external environments. For example, after practicing EA we may be sensitized to somatic clues indicating intuition or recognize a particular sensation arising when someone trespasses our boundaries. As we establish an interoceptive experience of being seated in ourselves, we feel more comfortable in our own skin and deepen trust in ourselves and in life. Without this trust, we may feel unstable, disconnected from support, and living from a place of control and *doing*, rather than the ease and flow of allowing *being* to unfold. With this trust, it can be easier to access inner stillness and intentionally return to it. Students consistently report less emotional reactivity; more connection to self, others, and the environment; and awareness of their inherent wholeness. They find self-regulation easier when feeling more empowered and internally resourced.

## EA Encourages Embodiment

In his short story, "A Painful Case," James Joyce (1914, p. 134) depicts the protagonist, Mr. Duffy, as living "a short distance from his body," which eloquently describes the typical experience of people living disconnected from their body, emotions, and sensations. Most people I see clinically exhibit some degree of dissociation. This makes sense; it's challenging to live in a painful, traumatized, or dysfunctional body, or hear its messages and respect its limitations. Some people view painful parts as "objects" needing "fixing" rather than aspects of themselves requiring kind attention. Chronically painful parts are sometimes not considered "self" or belonging to one's body (Osborn and Smith 2006). Dissociation may also result from *muscle armoring*, the physical holding patterns resulting from unexpressed emotions. These states can increase stress and cause physiological consequences, including diminished circulation, movement deficits, and excessive tension. EA offers one pathway to embodiment.

EA explorations can uncover buried memories and emotions in safe, gentle ways that initiate self-healing through potentially reclaiming disowned parts and processing embedded trauma. As a tenuous sense of embodied Self is strengthened through interoceptive inquiry, perception and behavior can alter. EA is an inquiry into Self, offering a way to connect to what is present, how it feels, and what is an appropriate response. As we develop felt sense of anatomical structures, connections, and interrelationships, we can wholeheartedly inhabit our body and live from the fullness of our embodied Self, moving from feeling disempowered to empowered, from "I can't" to agency, and from fear to courage. In this embodied state, we are less likely to override body signals, disregard our own needs, or look for external validation. With growing trust in our own body and perceptions, self-support and self-regulation arise naturally, providing a powerful base from which to respond to changing circumstances. One student described it as a process of befriending each body part and understanding its needs, how to support it, and how to move in healing ways. Disconnection, rejection, and judgment often transform into a relationship of compassionate care. Others describe the process as "coming home" to themselves and report more ease in connecting with their innate wisdom. We become more skilled at observing when we are disconnected and can more easily choose to return to ourselves; we learn to live with one eye in and one eye out.

I grew up in an unstable, unpredictable, abusive household. My dissociative defenses continued into adulthood. I never understood the concepts of "safe," "centered," or "grounded" until experiential anatomy allowed me to experience and understand them in my body. I realized that slowing down and going within could heal my past trauma. I could count on my femur to always be my femur, and to move in predictable ways. Combining knowledge with felt sense of my body was a game-changer for me.

*Jenny*

## EA Is Safe Movement

We all "muscle" through movements (and life) at times, expending more effort than required, and sometimes hurting ourselves in the process. When we know what we look like inside, we learn to respect our limitations and capitalize on the possibilities of our anatomical structures. While exploring safe, restorative movements, we learn to access different sources of support and recognize sensations indicating qualities like steadiness, **Right Effort**, and ease. We develop direct understanding of the interplay between structure and safe function. When movement is deliberately initiated from specific structures, done slowly, and with moment-to-moment awareness of each point in the arc of movement, safe range of motion is easier to sense. As we discover pleasurable, attainable movements that decrease pain, fear of movement lessens and we develop competence and confidence to move more. The motivational element of hope arises as our pain levels diminish (Or *et al.*, 2021).

Injury potential increases when physical injury and/or mental or emotional distress inhibits proprioception and interoception (Lephart 1997). When discernment skills are internalized through EA practices, we can clearly register sensations and learn to trust our own bodies. As trust and self-knowledge build, unconscious repetition of unhelpful habits is curbed and movements can be tailored in ways that feel safe, integrated, and that honor structural capacity. These interoceptive and proprioceptive sensations associated with safety and comfort are an integral part of trauma-informed therapy (Payne, Levine, and Crane-Goddreau 2015). Feeling the feet on the ground or breathing from deep within the pelvis, for example, can evoke the sense of safety in the nervous system that is necessary for clear perception and relearning supportive patterns.

## EA Is Accessible and Practical

EA is an accessible, reproducible way of experiencing the body-mind to build kinesthetic intelligence, encourage self-regulation and resilience, and deepen sense of self. EA explorations can be considered preliminary movements or "preyoga" that provide a foundation for any movement practice. By generating an internal felt sense of the body, movement is shaped in a self-directed way from the inside out, rather than conforming to idealized shapes and patterns. It's counterproductive asking students to move in certain ways when their bodies lack the physical capacity, their mental body maps are fuzzy or distorted, or they are afraid to move.

EA is available to a wide range of students, from those with severe disability to elite athletes; even those with limited movement capacity can focus on a specific structure, breathe into it, use visual imagery, and imagine initiating movement from it. The nervous system doesn't differentiate between imagined and actual movement, therefore mental practice can activate the same neural networks and create similar benefits (Pasqual-Leone *et al.*, 1995). Basic EA practices involve accessible slow, low-load, low-amplitude movements with an emphasis on awareness and process rather than performance. Integrative movements incorporating the new awareness can be tailored and incrementally progressed according to students' ability.

EA is practical; the explorations are not specific to defined movements but can be easily applied to any movement or gesture one might perform during activities of daily living, whether work, household tasks, or leisure. Reaching into a cupboard for a cup or reaching an arm through water while swimming can both benefit from enhanced body awareness and application of EA principles. For some, EA explorations may provide transformational healing, while others may use the practices as a foundation for accomplishing more complex, challenging movements.

As self-awareness deepens through EA self-inquiry, we feel empowered to make sustainable, healthy choices. Self-regulation is mobilized through cultivating awareness of habitual ways of standing, breathing, and moving, and directly experiencing effects of these patterns on body, health, and self. Inner resources become accessible as embodied awareness of anatomical structures is established; the feet provide reliable grounding, the psoas contributes spinal support and connection, and organs offer inner support and buoyancy. Over time we forge a friendly and dynamic relationship with the body-mind that results in deeper integration and balance. Based on personal and clinical experience, I know that EA can transform lives. With this book I welcome you into this powerful, profound journey of self-exploration and transformation.

> We do not have bodies: we are bodies... I am smart precisely because I am a body. I don't own it or inhabit it; from it: I arise.
>
> *Guy Claxton (2015, p. 3).*

## KEY CONCEPTS

- Experiential anatomy is a way to access inner resources and self-regulate.
- Direct sensory perception moves us from the thinking mind into the feeling body.
- EA practices stimulate interoceptive and proprioceptive awareness.
- The physical body is a doorway to energetic, emotional, mental, and spiritual selves.
- EA practices help us fully inhabit our bodies and live from the fullness of our embodied selves.
- EA helps us respect limitations and capitalize on possibilities of our anatomical structures.
- EA is an accessible, reproducible way of experiencing the body-mind to build kinesthetic intelligence, encourage resilience, and deepen sense of self.

## CHAPTER 1

# The Groundwork

Experiential anatomy is better understood when viewed in context with the foundational concepts presented in this chapter. Extensive research in the last few decades on interoception, neuroplasticity, and pain science confirms the multidimensional, integrated, body-mind perspective of ancient yogic knowledge and its emphasis on the power of the mind. These yogic concepts interweave all three avenues of research and underpin the fundamental kosha model forming the framework of this book. This chapter describes the model and reviews interoception, neuroplasticity, and pain science from a koshic perspective.

## THE KOSHA MODEL

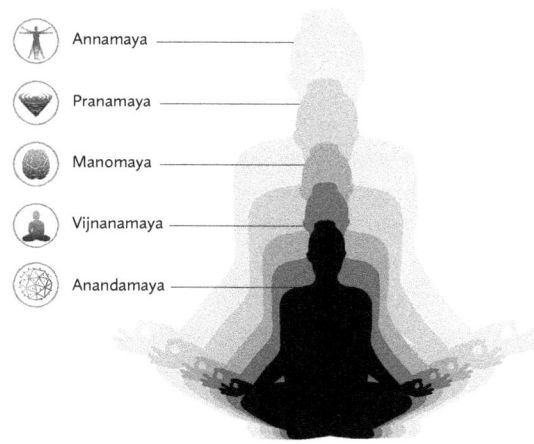

Annamaya

Pranamaya

Manomaya

Vijnanamaya

Anandamaya

This ancient model of human development was described over 2500 years ago in the *Taittiriya Upanishad*, an early yogic scripture. The underlying assumption of the model is that we are souls in a body; the physical body is one of five interpenetrating and interdependent koshas, or sheaths, of consciousness enveloping the soul (in Sanskrit, *atman*, the pure, eternal self). The model encompasses the full scope of human experience from physical to spiritual and offers a map for navigating the human task of clarifying each kosha to reveal the luminous light of the soul and to live from that soulful place—from the inside out. The five koshas manifest on a continuum of densities from physical structures like bones to more subtle dimensions of breath, habitual patterns of emotional expression and thinking, and refined spiritual awareness. We can tune into individual koshas to clearly see, feel, and be guided by their unique qualities and contents.

Each kosha affects and is affected by the others. This awareness helps students understand how "physical" EA practices can produce transformative therapeutic effects on other levels, including experiencing a heightened sense of self. The model explains how tracking diaphragmatic movement can reduce pain, or why establishing felt sense of grounding through the feet can moderate emotional reactivity. For some students, physical restoration may be unachievable, but the healing journey can prompt meaningful relief on other levels. The koshas offer pathways to explore five different aspects of consciousness that can initiate deeper healing, self-knowledge, and the ability to self-regulate. Interoception is the way in, and each kosha can be known through the distinctive sensations it generates. Although changes on any koshic level will affect other levels, for most students, the physical body is an accessible starting point for realizing their own healing capacity.

### Annamaya Kosha (Physical Body) ⊕

In *annamaya kosha*, we meet our flesh and blood body. The densest, grossest kosha manifests as anatomical structures and includes *subkoshas*, including bones and joints, fluids, muscles, fascia, nerve and vascular tissue, organs, and glands. We come to know our physical body as a living process providing us with valuable information and a vehicle for action. When we access this kosha through EA explorations, our physical function improves through deeper body awareness, optimal skeletal alignment, and functional movement patterns. The intelligence of each anatomical structure awakens as we cultivate its felt sense and encourage its efficient participation in movement. For example, annamaya kosha is highlighted when we decrease hip pain by redistributing weight equally over our feet or breathe into our back to calm asthmatic shortness of breath.

> Sarah discovered felt sense of her midline through somatic exploration—an embodied touchstone she consistently used to find physical balance and center herself psychologically when caught in old habits of giving away her power.

We feed this kosha with movement and food; the quality of our movement and the food we eat affects each kosha. We perceive annamaya kosha through physical sensations such as compression, tension, temperature, pleasure, and pain.

### Pranamaya Kosha (Energy Body) ⬙

The pranic or energy body permeates the physical body but is less dense or tangible. We recognize this kosha as life-force energy that animates and moves us and enlivens all life forms. It is prana that keeps us alive. Also known as *chi* or *ki* in Oriental medicine, prana circulates through and links the koshas. In yogic wisdom, prana is the interface between mind and body. As the vital, orchestrating movement force behind all physiological processes, prana, among other things, causes blood and lymph to circulate, thoughts, emotions, and nervous impulses to flow, and digestion to proceed. When prana is abundant and flowing freely through thousands of *nadis*, or energy channels in the body, it bestows vibrant aliveness, lustrous skin, bright eyes, and optimal metabolic function. When our prana is diminished or blocked, we experience suffering on all koshic levels.

In the yoga tradition, prana is carried by breath (where breath goes, prana flows). EA explorations and breath practices can liberate breath and connect us to the power of *pranamaya kosha*. Prana can also be moved or liberated with mindful intention (where thought goes, prana flows), like visualizing ground force energy streaming up from the earth through specific pathways in the body. We also access our energy body as we attentively track force during movement.

Students commonly report that subtle, mindful EA explorations liberate prana, which they experience as increased vitality and sensations like effervescence, streaming, and spaciousness. Feeding this kosha with breathing practices or absorbing nature can balance energy levels and improve physiological and psychological functions.

## Manamaya Kosha (Mental Body) ⬤

*Manomaya kosha*, or the mental body, expresses; through the five senses, our thinking conscious mind, and the subconscious. The mind, or *manas* in Sanskrit, is considered an organ that receives and processes information, communicating sensation and experience to the intellectual kosha (vijnanamaya), and transmitting influences of subtle koshas to other koshas. It's the part that senses through directing and sustaining attention, learns by gathering information from the internal and external world, and forms memories. We experience this kosha as sensations, thoughts, emotions, and reflexive action, each with its unique sensory signature.

EA explorations refine and focus our attention to heighten perception of sensory information and develop somatic memories that can transform neuromuscular patterns. As we patiently cultivate sensory awareness of structures and hone the ability to deliberately shift awareness, we are also learning strategies to calm a busy mind and manage difficult emotions. Without this awareness, we may not register our clenched jaw and shallow breath when angry or notice that our mind calms with balanced weight distribution in our feet. We may struggle to notice habits of breath, alignment, and movement, or recognize sensations that distinguish dysfunctional physical or emotional habits from healthier, more supportive responses learned through EA practices.

The sensory awareness skills developed through EA can help us self-regulate when sensations, feelings, and emotions arise during practice and everyday life. With an attitude of open attention, we learn to meet sensory information, including emotions, with a mindset of *Oh, isn't this interesting*. We feed manomaya kosha with beautiful sensory impressions, mindfulness, *mantra* (repetition of sacred words), and paradoxically, the yogic practice of *pratyahara* (withdrawal of the senses from the outer world).

> For every thought supported by feeling, there is a muscle change. Primary muscle patterns being the biological heritage of man, man's whole body records his emotional thinking.
>
> *Mabel Todd (1937, p. 1)*

## Vijnanamaya Kosha (Intellectual Body) ⬤

*Vijnanamaya kosha* lies beneath the thinking mind and includes the ego, the underlayer of personality, and the conditioning that generates our thoughts, emotions, and intentions. As the core of individual identity, the ego colors the lens through which we perceive sensation and experience, weighs and assigns value to that experience, and generates an impulse to take action reflecting our values, beliefs, and nature. It shapes who we are, how we make meaning, and how we express ourselves in the world.

Vijnanamaya kosha also includes cultural archetypes and metaphors that mold body and behavior. Someone expressing a military archetype may have rigid posture and charge through life, while a victim archetype may manifest as collapsed posture and inability to stand up for oneself. We understand ourselves and the world through metaphor, and the body is a source of metaphors in our everyday language (Lakoff and Johnson 1980). Each part of the body metaphorically reflects characteristic aspects of being human, and, like archetypes, body metaphors can shape us. For example, the feet reflect our foundation and how we move in the world. Compare the posture of someone who "steps up to the plate" with another who "digs in their heels." Body metaphors and imagery can be used as healing tools to transform movement patterns. Introducing metaphors in this way can also shift pain behaviors, including pain-related catastrophizing (Gallagher, McAuley, and Moseley 2013). The way we stand and move is often influenced by deep-seated unconscious patterns originating from survival responses to past events and environments.

Even though ancient sages didn't use contemporary terms like *valence network* or *insula*, they clearly understood the power of the mind to control physical and nonphysical states and influence healing. Underlying our conditioned mind is *buddhi*, a wise discerning consciousness that can transcend past conditioning to access inner resources and choose to live by higher values and principles. Buddhi is the inner awareness of ourselves feeling, thinking, and experiencing. We are aware of being aware. As EA practices awaken cellular intelligence, we more easily access this deep inner wisdom. Buddhi, also known as the **Witness**, is key to developing nonjudgmental awareness of conditioned patterns and transcending them by consistently choosing wiser and healthier ways of being. As Thich Nhat Hanh counsels, "the seeds we water are the seeds that grow" (Hanh and Anh-Huong 2006, p. 22). When fed with self-study (*svadhyaya*), meditation (*dhyana*), and selfless service (*seva*), this kosha can guide us toward a soul-infused, rather than an ego-infused, life.

EA builds on the innate capacity of the nervous system to form energy-efficient patterns as we compassionately witness and identify habits on any level that arise during explorations, such as noticing a tendency to hold the breath or over-effort during movement practice. From here, we seek to understand the commonly subconscious genesis of the habits and their multidimensional effects. For example, childhood admonitions to "hold your tongue" may generate a lifelong habit of jaw tension and breath restriction. With newfound awareness, we can set intentions to transcend conditioning by committing to helpful practices and expanding our perspective. Buddhi makes vows to have patience or treat ourselves with kindness and compassion as we travel the path toward health and well-being. We may discover that working on this level has consequential physical effects, as it did for one student with fibromyalgia who found that a consistent forgiveness practice relieved her pain more than movement practices.

Awareness and self-knowledge in this kosha can arise through intuition, healing dreams, or flashes of insight stimulated by EA practices. With this inner guidance, we can repattern lifetimes of conditioning and significantly elevate our sense of self and how we perceive and express ourselves in the world.

## Anandamaya Kosha (Spiritual Body)

*Anandamay kosha*, the most subtle sheath, signifies our soulful Self connected to the cosmos, the world, and other beings. It reflects the reality of oneness and enables us to form relationships and act from the perspective that we are all one. This highest level of human consciousness knows that *I am much bigger than my body, mind, or medical condition. Ananda* refers to the inherent blissful nature of our essential Self, an abiding joy independent of circumstances. We access this deeper dimension by cultivating a relationship with the Divine, however we name it.

In anandamaya kosha, we move beyond worldly duality and attachment to experience a sense of wholeness, connection, and oneness with all creation, even when we are suffering. We may have a transformative experience of stillness in meditation or a moment of profound wonder and gratitude for our ability to heal. Lack of acknowledgment of this deepest part can lead to feelings of meaninglessness and hopelessness, manifesting as depressed body posture, shallow breathing, digestive issues, and other related physiological dis-ease. Knowing that we can access this part provides a wider context of meaning and purpose that somehow makes pain or suffering easier to bear—I have a body, but I am not my body. This awareness can accelerate an inner knowing that we are already whole, that joy, peace, and unity are inherent, and that we can intentionally shift focus from suffering to a transcendent place beyond suffering.

The way we relate to our physical or mental

conditions can influence therapeutic outcomes. When we frame our condition as one part within the context of our greater Self, this relationship can transform from resistance, rejection, or dissociation to one promoting healing. This is the emergence of unconditional love. The evolving felt sense of connectedness within us can overflow into relationships with others and the external world. As EA practices reveal sensations generated by right relationship between structures, we can strengthen our ability to establish right relationship with ourselves, others, the environment, and the Divine. This is one way to understand the word *yoga*—a harmonious union of all parts.

Profound changes in anandamaya kosha can result from physical EA practices. Working with anatomical parts can paradoxically evoke an experience of wholeness. A lifetime of self-condemnation can transform into tenderness and embracing of oneself, or organ sensing can touch a deeper sense of self. We nurture this kosha in daily life with prayer, ritual, and practicing gratitude and reverence for ourselves, others, and the environment.

## The Map Is Not the Territory

The koshas are interdependent and multifaceted, and it's not always possible, or necessary, to identify specific ones evoked in EA practices. For example, sensory receptors registering physical sensation represent the physical kosha, nerve impulses generated are transmitted by the energy kosha, registered in the mental kosha, interpreted, given meaning, and assigned further action in the intellectual kosha, while the spiritual kosha provides the greater context of meaning and wholeness and promotes gratitude. Ultimately, what matters is *how* the practices heighten awareness and help us identify and transform physical and mental habits with self-compassion. The kosha model acknowledges that we are continuously evolving and self-creating organisms and provides five unique but interrelated pathways of self-awareness supporting our journey toward integration and wholeness.

## INTEROCEPTION

Interoception is the foundation of therapeutic applications of EA. We need to feel what we want to heal and felt sense of anatomical structures is developed through interoception. Although traditionally restricted to visceral sensations, recent expanded definitions refer to the process by which awareness of body sensations and states build a subjective sense of self, inform physiological and emotional self-regulation, and confer meaning to experience (Schmitt and Schoen 2022). A succinct definition is "the processes by which an organism senses, interprets, integrates and regulates signals originating from within itself" (Chen *et al.*, 2021). This definition acknowledges that the interoceptive process involves data received from various sensory processes: *exteroception* (the traditional five senses), *proprioception* (awareness of body position and movement arising from receptors in fascia, muscles, and joints), *visceroception* (conscious and unconscious signals from inner organs), and *vestibular awareness* (sense of body velocity and head position in gravity).

Sensory data is received, organized, and integrated in brain structures related to emotion, memory, motivation, and cognition. The result is a gestalt of a feeling, knowing self motivated to take self-regulatory action. *Gestalt* is "an experience that, when considered as a whole, has qualities that are more than the total of its parts" (Cambridge University Press n.d ). In simple terms, interoception is the perception, processing, and integration of sensations arising from the body that informs perceptual felt sense and emotional feeling states and motivates self-regulatory behavior. Through interoception we can map emotions in our body, like feeling love in our heart or butterflies in our stomach.

Most interoception is unconscious; the nervous system registers sensory information primarily from organs to regulate physiological homeostasis. We're unaware of our kidneys balancing electrolytes, or the release of digestive enzymes. The conscious aspect of interoception has generated a surge of research over the last decade with the discovery of associations between interoception and numerous medical and psychological conditions, and even our feeling of *this is me* (Monti *et al.*, 2022). In this conscious sense, interoception is how our bodies talk to us; signals from organs tell us we've overeaten, are sexually aroused, or need to nap. Interoceptive signals from our skin direct us to dress warmly in response to cold temperatures, while signals in fascia, muscles, and joints help us register qualities and effects of movement and any emotional responses evoked. An EA foot practice may generate feelings of groundedness and confidence, or an organ exploration may lead to noticing inner fullness and support. The cumulative effect of these signals creates a subjective representation of our bodies. Conscious interoception is a skill that can be strengthened in body-mind practices, including EA.

Purposely registering sensations can build body ownership and agency and can motivate healthy habits as we learn to respect messages from the body. Body ownership describes the sense of *this is my arm and I feel tingling sensations in it*, while body agency refers to an experience of intentionally initiating action, as in *I am moving my arm in a circle* (Gallagher 2000). This ability to perceive and register sensory information is termed *interoceptive awareness* (IA) (Herbert and Pollatos 2012). When we intentionally deepen IA through EA practices, we are more likely to pay attention to body signals and take self-regulatory action based on them. Interoception may even establish "a felt sense of psychological

and physiological safety that is foundational to meaningful participation in life" (Schmitt and Schoen 2022).

Table 1.2 summarizes benefits of IA as reported by students over three decades of teaching.

**Table 1.1 Benefits of Interoceptive Awareness**

| Benefit | Skill |
|---|---|
| Enhanced emotional intelligence | Ability to identify emotions and respond appropriately |
| Self-regulation | Capacity to notice and respond to physiological messages |
| Stronger sense of self | Knowing one's habits of perception and response and changing inputs to alter maladaptive patterns |
| Sense of safety | Connecting more easily, having empathy and compassion, making good decisions, learning |
| Presence | Ability to focus attention on the here and now |

Please note: Although body awareness and attending to present moment experience has well-documented benefits, self-focused rumination may be counterproductive in those with complex trauma, anxiety disorders, or other mental health challenges (Mehling *et al.*, 2009). Some students and clients with these conditions might find interoceptive practices exacerbate their condition and may benefit from a referral to a trauma-informed or mental health therapist who can appropriately guide them to connect with their bodies in a safe, therapeutic way.

Increasingly, interoceptive processing is perceived as a key factor in health and well-being. Numerous physical and mental health conditions have been associated with decreased interoceptive abilities, and therapeutic interventions that increase IA have produced positive outcomes

(Farb *et al.*, 2015). Conditions including sickness behaviors and fatigue, anxiety, depression, eating disorders, and autism have been related to interoceptive impairment (Quadt, Critchley, and Garfinkel 2018). Those with other mental health conditions such as PTSD, mood, and addictive and somatic disorders also exhibit dysfunctional interoception, as do people with chronic pain (Di Lernia *et al.*, 2020; Khalsa *et al.*, 2018).

## The Koshas and Interoception

Interoception can be considered through the lens of the kosha model. Although ancient yogis didn't have sophisticated laboratories or scientific vocabularies, they used this model to describe how reception and integration of sensations contribute to a stable sense of self; the ego knows itself as an "I" because of perceived sensations. Centuries before science established an association between interoception and medical and psychological conditions, *ayurveda*, the sister science of yoga, counselled that misuse of the senses (overstimulation or deficiency of sensory activity) is one of the main causes of disease.

The physical annamaya kosha contains structural hardware of the interoceptive process. The physiological network for interoception includes sensory receptors, spinal cord pathways, and brain structures, including the insula, cingulate cortex, prefrontal cortex, and somatosensory and sensorimotor cortexes. Interoceptive signals are processed in this complex functional brain network of structures that assesses the importance (salience) and value (valence) of interoceptive signals in terms of safety or threat, adds personal and emotional content, compares prior experience, and then orchestrates appropriate changes in behavior and cognition (Weiner 2022). The insula plays a key role in integrating and translating sensory input from multiple sources into subjective feelings, self-awareness, and motivation (Craig 2009). For example, you feel a heaviness in your heart, know that it's grief over your cat's death, and are motivated to ask for a comforting hug.

In yogic wisdom, the prana in pranamaya kosha links mind and body. As the vital force animating movement in the body, prana carries sensory input to the brain for processing, and motor output to orchestrate action. Prana can be viewed as the energy firing the process of interoception.

Manomaya kosha is the sensing part of us that receives information through interoception and the five external senses and relays it to vijnanamaya kosha for processing. From manomaya kosha, we make decisions about where to place and sustain attention, and learn by gathering sensory information from internal and external worlds. This kosha colors experience with emotional tone and generates reflexive impulses to act. On the emotional level of manomaya kosha, skillful interoception has been associated with improved emotional regulation (Pinna and Edwards 2020).

Interoceptive practices situate the mind in the body, slowing it down to body time. This builds presence. Physical bodies exist in time and space, while the mind ranges to other times, places, and experiences. When we focus the mind on body sensations, we are *with* the experience and less likely to ruminate or create stories *about* our experience. Focusing on this kosha hones our interoceptive awareness.

The ego aspect of vijnanamaya kosha imprints our perception, gives meaning to sensory experience, and generates a sense of self—*I feel therefore I am*. The wise buddhi receives sensations from manomaya kosha and assigns value to sensory experiences (like the valence network in the insula), then generates an action impulse reflecting our conditioning and beliefs (like the cortical input to interoception). Buddhi helps us understand conditioned patterns of interoception and transcend them by adopting healthier choices and applying higher principles like self-compassion. As we refine our sense of self with interoceptive practices, we more easily access the **Witness** and connect with our deeper Self.

In anandamaya kosha, interoceptive clarity can help us realize a felt sense of unity and wholeness. As sense of self is refined, we may also access deeper meaning and purpose in our lives, or even experience a transcendent gestalt.

## Experiential Anatomy

In EA practices, IA includes the registration of felt sense of an anatomical structure's size, weight, and blood flow, and sensations like lightness or tingling. We come to know the "is-ness" of the structure, like the "arm-ness" of the arm. This gives direct experience of having a body with differentiated anatomical structures and provides personal meaning to that experience. We become curious about the quality of our breath, energy level, and how a movement feels. We realize that our thoughts and emotions can be experienced as physical sensations guiding us toward appropriate action. As we attune to sensations on every level, we can use that vast array of information to change not only our movement but also our experience. As we unite our thinking mind and feeling body, we know who we are and what we need.

As an organizing principle, IA reveals ways of arranging our bodies efficiently and harmoniously. Rather than blindly obeying external instructions, we use interoception to find an internal sense of "rightness" as we seek qualities like stability, strength, ease, balance, and clear force transmission. Over time this exploration can repattern the motor control system to make better choices and change brain mapping at the sensorimotor level, which incrementally transforms alignment and movement strategies. Ultimately, IA builds trust and confidence in one's own body and sensations.

## Interoception and Proprioception

Although proprioception involves different receptors, spinal pathways, and brain structures, it's connected both functionally and anatomically to interoception. Both interoception and proprioception (from *proprius* in Latin, meaning "one's own") arise from the somatosensory system. Proprioceptors in joints, muscles, skin, and fascia register body position and movement, and sense tension, force, and direction. Most of us can lightly touch a finger to our nose with eyes closed or successfully walk down a staircase. With good proprioceptive abilities, we coordinate alignment and refine motor control to organize and stabilize ourselves in movement and stillness.

Interoception gives information about qualities and effects of movement: how it feels to move in a particular way, what meaning it has, and how to respond to it. Thoughts, images, or beliefs may arise while tracking sensations, informing our choices about how to move. We may alter variables like quality, timing, speed, intensity, and amplitude, or decide to pause.

Proprioceptive signals meet interoceptive signals in the insula where they are assigned valences of important or unimportant, pleasant or unpleasant, then both are integrated with information from the five senses, vestibular system, and other brain areas to manufacture emotional feelings. Proprioception informs us that we are raising an arm overhead, while interoception tells us *I have an arm*, that the movement is easier when sensing fascial connections to the midline, and that a feeling of competence is evoked.

> If you don't feel at home in your body, you will never feel at home in the world.
>
> *Y. Harari (2019, p. 60)*

## EXPLORATION: INTEROCEPTIVE AWARENESS OF THE KOSHAS 🔊

### Learning Objective

- Build interoceptive awareness.

### Instructions

Stand comfortably with bare feet. Take a few moments to notice your body and surroundings. Throughout the practice intend to receive incoming sensory information as raw data, without judgment or storyline.

- Shift attention to your senses.

    - *What can you see? Do certain objects, shapes, or colors attract you?*
    - *What sounds can you hear? Outside the room? Inside the room? Can you hear your breath?*
    - *What can you feel? The floor beneath you? Weight and texture of your clothing? Room temperature?*
    - *What can you smell? Food aromas? Shampoo?*
    - *What can you taste? Coffee? Toothpaste?*

- Turn your attention inward. If comfortable, close your eyes, or turn them downward. Become aware of your feet and their interface with the floor.

    - *Where is there more pressure?*
    - *What parts aren't touching the floor?*
    - *What is the outline of your feet?*
    - *Is floor contact the same on both sides?*

- Alternate lifting each foot a few inches off the floor.

    - *How does your body accommodate the weight shift?*
    - *Can you track the movement of your foot in space?*

    - *What sensations indicate that your foot is moving?*
    - *Are there sensations of ease? Of tension? Discomfort?*
    - *How is your body arranged?*

- Turn your attention to your breath.

    - *What do you feel in your nostrils?*
    - *Where else can you feel your breath?*
    - *Is your breath shallow or deep? Slow or fast? Nourishing?*
    - *What is your energy level? Do you feel tired? Full of energy? Somewhere in between?*
    - *Can you sense your inner aliveness?*

- Notice your emotional tone.

    - *What emotions have you experienced lately, both positive and negative?*
    - *Do you have an emotional "hangover"?*

- What is the quality of your mind?

    - *Is it clear? Foggy? Sharp? Dull?*
    - *Do you feel calm? Anxious? Depressed? On alert?*

- How present are you in your body?

    - *How connected do you feel to yourself?*
    - *How have you related to yourself lately? With judgment? Kindness? Compassion?*

- Pause and notice whether your self-perception is different after deliberately shifting your attention to specific types of sensory information.

    - *How could you integrate IA into your everyday life?*

## NEUROPLASTICITY

We are a collection of habits encoded in the nervous system. The ways we breathe, move, align, perceive, and respond are neural patterns formed by networks of neurons repeatedly firing together. Butler and Moseley suggest *neurotag* as a descriptive term for these unique patterns of neuronal firing (2013). *Hebb's law* describes how patterns are ingrained: The more frequently a set of neural impulses travel a pathway, the more *facilitated* the pathway becomes, enabling easier occurrence of the pattern. The brain continually creates efficiencies for itself. Habits are formed because when neurons fire together, they wire together.

Neural patterns underlying habits are mostly reflexive, usually beyond conscious control. They are the best option the nervous system strategized to keep us erect, moving, functional, and safe. However, sometimes the best option in the moment turns maladaptive. The nervous system may devise compensatory patterns that eventually contribute to physical and physiological disharmony. For example, limping with a sprained ankle is a protective compensation, preventing potentially harmful movements and pressure. The limping pattern is encoded in neural circuitry and, long after the ankle heals, an almost imperceptible limp may linger and perhaps contribute to future back pain.

The ability of the nervous system to change its structure and function according to thought, experience, and activity is called neuroplasticity. Our daily routines and practices continually repattern neural circuitry. We deepen patterns the more attentive we are to their sensory signature and how we intentionally modify them. In his fascinating book, *The Brain That Changes Itself*, Dr. Norman Doidge reports that paying close attention is essential to long-term plastic change in the brain (2007). Movement and neuroplasticity are inextricably connected. Every movement habit is reflected in sensorimotor maps in the brain indicating sensing and usage of body parts. These maps are dynamic, and frequently sensed or used body parts occupy more map space. Doidge also suggests that many movement problems arise from underrepresentation of body parts in brain maps and that sensory input from mindful movement may help the nervous system refine movement patterns (2015).

EA practices may reconfigure neural maps and neurotags by offering sensory and motor experiences encouraging neuroplastic changes. The quality of neural maps determines quality of future movements. As we attentively and repeatedly explore practices and integrate the learning, our capacity to sense and refine movement increases. Interoception is how the nervous system receives, processes, and integrates sensory information, while neuroplasticity is the result of interoceptive impulses to create or repattern habits of perception, integration, and action.

Neuroplastic changes manifest from bidirectional communication pathways between mind (top-down) and body (bottom-up). EA practices such as setting an intention, directing attention, or using imagery are top-down cognitive approaches. Intending to move mindfully, consciously restraining a movement habit, or visualizing the shape of the shoulder joint during flexion gradually alter entrenched physical, emotional, and mental habits through a top-down approach. Bottom-up processes are body-based activities like breath and movement that provide sensory feedback to the nervous system. As we move slowly and mindfully while paying exquisite attention to fluctuating sensations, the nervous system is supplied with high-quality sensory input to use in its continuous quest to predict, compare, and adjust movement. As we refine IA and increase the quality of inputs through repetition, variation, and novelty, the brain discovers optimal movement efficiencies and self-corrections. Body-mind practices like yoga and EA combine both top-down and bottom-up approaches. We learn about anatomy, embody the learning by developing felt sense, then practice repatterning breathing, alignment, and movements. As we mindfully attend to sensations generated during EA explorations then compare sensations after the practice, the bidirectional communication flow encourages self-regulation through neuroplastic changes. This process of neuroplasticity takes time, patience, and dedicated practice. Both top-down and bottom-up mechanisms can alter physiology, immune function, and emotional well-being (Taylor *et al.*, 2010).

The process of neuroplasticity involves all five koshas. The physical structure of our brain (annamaya kosha) alters as it receives repeated sensory feedback (manomaya kosha) from our breath (pranamaya kosha) and body (annamaya kosha). We intentionally change what we do and how we do it according to our personality, values, and beliefs (vijnanamaya kosha), and the result is a deeper sense of wholeness (anandamaya kosha).

## PAIN SCIENCE

My movement teacher, Judith Koltai, often said that pain is a message from our bodies to *try another way*.

Current pain science is informed by interoception, neuroplasticity, and the biopsychosocial model increasingly underpinning rehabilitation and treatment principles. In this model, pain and dysfunction are viewed as outputs of the nervous system after processing varied bio (body), psycho (mind), and social (family, work, culture, environmental) inputs, assigning importance and threat value to each one, then deciding that we are in danger and need protection. In the same way the brain sees and hears after processing sensory inputs from eyes and ears, it generates pain after processing nociceptive sensations (extreme temperature, mechanical forces, and chemicals). Contrary to popular belief, pain is not dependent on tissue damage (Butler and Moseley 2013). Numerous multidimensional factors influence pain perception, including beliefs, expectations, emotional state, past experience, socioeconomic status, spiritual meaning, loneliness, nutrition, and sleep patterns. A stressful work environment, several days of fast food, and a trauma history that leaves us feeling generally unsafe can all heighten the lived pain experience. Disordered interoceptive processing also affects perception and modulation of pain and contributes to persistent pain (Di Lernia *et al.*, 2020).

### The Koshas and Pain Science

The ancient kosha model is more encompassing than the biopsychosocial model. Terminology may differ, but modern science confirms yogic understanding that movement, breath, environmental factors, and mental processing interact to affect emotions, well-being, and even sense of self. These variables are different for everyone, so each pathology or case of pain must be viewed in the unique context of the person experiencing it. A key difference between the models is that koshas are meant to be embodied. Yogic practices teach how to consciously inhabit and navigate the koshas. We learn to recognize which ones are imbalanced or need nourishment. EA practices also reflect and promote this koshic perspective by developing awareness of sensory signatures of different koshas.

Applying the kosha model to pain management offers a multifaceted approach, acknowledging that pain affects every aspect of self and that addressing one kosha affects the others. In annamaya kosha, students discover how pain affects alignment, flexibility, strength, and movement patterns. They explore gentle, restorative practices enabling them to stand, sit, and move in ways they previously thought unattainable. As excessive tension levels reduce, they may realize how tension perpetuated their pain.

Exploring different breathing techniques in pranamaya kosha may help students understand how breath affects their nervous system and experience. They may discover, like research participants, that mindful breathing decreases pain and induces calm, peaceful mental states (Hu et al., 2021).

Pain is a sensation registered by the organ of the mind in manomaya kosha, then referred to vijnanamaya kosha for processing. In manomaya kosha, we use our attention to observe habits of movement and thought affecting our pain experience and develop the skill of staying present with pain sensations. Pain is an emotional experience. Interoceptive processing of nociceptive stimuli assigns emotional qualities to pain. We may recognize a familiar pain and panic when remembering the life disruption we previously experienced. Therapeutically, we can use top-down approaches of cultivating emotions, such as empathy, to change the way we experience pain (Bushnell, Ceko, and Low 2013).

Pain is an experience confirming existence of Self in vijnanamaya kosha, although it can also cause distortions in body awareness and body image. The content of this kosha will affect pain experience. Our personality, beliefs, experiences, and expectations can either modulate or intensify the pain experience. We can use buddhi mind to "befriend" our pain, cultivate self-compassion, and shift perspective to acceptance, hope, and confidence. Buddhi recognizes that pain is changeable and that we can take proactive self-regulatory action.

On the anandamaya kosha level, pain can lead to feelings of disconnection with self, others, and the Divine. Addressing spiritual needs can improve physical, functional, and emotional outcomes. Spiritual practices can help us find meaning and alter our interpretation and experience of pain (Garschagen et al., 2015). During the process of making meaning through spiritual practices, our pain may reduce, and we may be inspired to new levels of self-love and care.

## Sensitization

Pain is an interoceptive experience. Unmyelinated nerve endings register both interoceptive and nociceptive inputs that travel through the same neural pathways to the interoceptive neural network that integrates and translates sensory and motor stimuli into motivations and behaviors. Acute pain may become persistent as the brain "learns" chronicity through neuroplasticity. Pain neurotags are strengthened the more frequently nociceptive signals travel through them. The nervous system becomes "sensitized," and processing of nociceptive signals is distorted. This neuroplastic pain may be influenced by increased densities of free nerve endings in affected tissues that alter pain generation and perception (Suarez-Rodriguez et al., 2022). Sensitization makes the nervous system overprotective. It magnifies and misinterprets otherwise benign movement and sensory stimuli, especially in stressful situations (Mansour et al., 2014). Over time, patients may experience more intense pain, more frequently, and over a larger area.

> At a lecture I attended with clinical pain neuroscientist Lorimer Moseley, he humorously quipped that he tells patients "neuroplasticity got you into this mess... and neuroplasticity can get you out of this mess."

Harnessing the positive aspect of neuroplasticity can desensitize the nervous system through repatterning. Dr. Moseley suggests that if neurons in the pain neurotag can be decoupled by engaging them in other neural circuits that generate safety signals, the pain experience will modulate (2018). For example, mindfulness practices and interoceptive movement can generate pleasant sensations influencing the brain to register safety and decide that pain is unnecessary.

Body-mind techniques like yoga and meditation are increasingly used for controlling pain (Di Lernia et al., 2020). By paying attention to ourselves, pain modulation systems in the brain can be activated, effectively diminishing pain perception and experience (Bushnell et al., 2013). As a body-mind practice, EA teaches that pain is a valuable messenger asking students to *try another way* and that pain can be modulated. We gain agency and self-efficacy by discovering how our pain experience transforms by calming the breath, moving with awareness and self-compassion, or challenging beliefs about pain like *that movement will hurt*, or *I will always have pain*. As compromised interoceptive abilities of those with chronic pain are improved through mindful practices, they develop the capacity to stay present with uncomfortable sensations, which has been shown to reduce pain. (Riegner et al., 2022).

Understanding anatomical structures and their capabilities and functions builds confidence and trust in the resilience and healing capacity of our bodies, and this "resourcing" can influence our lived pain experience. With EA practices that generate feeling tones of safety, stability, and connection, we feel empowered to gradually return to activities that give our lives purpose and meaning.

## EASE AND EFFORT

EA practices are most beneficial when done in a state of ease. Almost everyone is surprised to realize how much unnecessary effort they expend to accomplish simple daily tasks. Overeffort is common, right effort or ease, less so. Grandmother of body-mind practices Charlotte Selver suggested that all tension arises from either overeffort or withholding (Koltai, personal communication, 1994). Excessive physical tension results whether we habitually overeffort daily tasks, withhold tears, or brace against criticism, pain, or life in general. For example, one student tried so hard to make herself heal that she lived in a state of sympathetic arousal, ultimately hindering her healing process. When overeffort and withholding are compassionately identified and dissolved, ease or right effort can arise.

Overeffort is a mental phenomenon manifesting physically in the body. Neurotags for habitual effort levels are reinforced by past experience, societal and parental programming, and beliefs. We are conditioned to accept myths like "if I don't try hard, I won't progress," or "no pain, no gain." In truth, awareness and presence are more readily accessed with ease, not effort. When ease, or *sukha* in Sanskrit, is the primary directive, right effort emerges as we stay present with needs of the immediate moment.

Overeffort, withholding, or bracing in fear of movement (kinesiophobia) cause muscular tension that compromises our ability to discern subtle changes in sensation and movement, making it difficult to know when we go too far, too long, or too hard. It's harder to sense ourselves through the sensory overload of excessive tension. The Fechner-Weber law describes this phenomenon: If a sensory stimulus, like muscle tension, is strong, we notice only extreme variations in stimulus levels. When sensory input is minimized by reducing muscular effort and creating ease, the nervous system can register and integrate subtle differences into future movements. As we explore right effort, we discern precisely how much energy is required to do a movement and consciously inhibit unnecessary effort. The resulting movement is usually more easeful, graceful, and integrated. As we realize that right effort is a choice, we can repattern it in other areas of our lives. On the nonphysical level, right effort helps us stay in touch with ourselves and our needs.

## FOUNDATIONAL PRACTICE: RIGHT EFFORT 📖

This practice is adapted from a practice developed by Judith Koltai.

### Learning Objectives

- Explore habits of effort.
- Discern sensations indicating task-specific effort level.

### Props

- 1–1.5 m (4–5 ft.) bamboo pole, wooden dowel, broom, or mop handle

### Instructions

- Begin in a standing position holding the pole vertically in your dominant hand. Close your eyes or turn your gaze downward.

- Sense your usual way of holding the pole.
  - *How much force are you using?*
  - *What are the sensations in your fingers, hand, forearm, upper arm, shoulder, neck?*
  - *Is tension associated with your habitual grip?*
  - *What is the quality of your mind? Your breath?*

- Sense the weight of the pole. Exaggerate your effort level by squeezing harder.

  - *What are the sensations in your fingers, hand, forearm, upper arm, shoulder, neck?*
  - *What is the quality of your mind? Your breath?*

- Gradually and incrementally release your grip until the pole slides through your fingers. Do this several times, tracking sensations as you exaggerate then lighten your grip.

  - *What is the felt sense of overeffort?*
  - *Are these sensations familiar?*

- During repetitions, notice the effort level just prior to dropping the pole, where your grip precisely meets the pull of gravity. Call this right effort.

  - *What is your felt sense of right effort?*
  - *What are the sensations in your fingers, hand, forearm, upper arm, shoulder, neck as you approach right effort?*
  - *Any change in your breath or quality of mind?*

- With right effort, hold the pole in front of you with one hand, then move hand over hand up the pole, finding right effort with each change of position. When you reach the top, start the downward journey to the bottom. Repeat this up-and-down practice several times, first slowly then faster.

  - *Does your effort level increase with speed?*

- Repeat the practice on the other side.

  - *How does the experience differ?*

- Incorporate awareness of right effort into your daily life. Notice habits of overeffort, like gripping your toothbrush or steering wheel or using excessive effort during sport or movement. Choose one habit to play with for a week. Observe yourself repeating the pattern, then replace it with right effort.

  - *How does the practice of right effort affect your body, mind, breath?*
  - *Are you surprised at your habitual levels of effort?*
  - *Can you have compassion for yourself?*

## KEY CONCEPTS

- The ancient kosha model of interpenetrating and interdependent levels of human experience is foundational to therapeutic applications of EA.
- The kosha model provides five pathways of self-awareness supporting the journey toward integration.
- Interoception is the process of perception, processing, and integration of sensations arising from the body that motivates self-regulatory behavior.
- Proprioception and interoception are functionally related.

- Neuroplasticity is the ability of the nervous system to change structure and function according to thought, experience, and activity.
- Application of the kosha model to pain management offers a multifaceted approach, acknowledging that pain affects every aspect of self.
- Overeffort is a mental phenomenon manifesting physically in the body and can be repatterned into "right effort."

## CHAPTER 2

# The Teaching Model

*This is common sense. Why don't we learn it in school, like having an owner's manual for the body?*

DALE, A STUDENT

Adults are motivated to learn when they can generate personal meaning from events in ways that transform their experience and understanding (Mezirow 1991). EA inspires us to learn about our bodies when we realize how our lives could be enriched. Reducing pain, moving with ease, or sleeping better are persuasive motivations. As an embodied educational approach, EA interweaves intellectual learning and safe somatic inquiry that ignites curiosity by making it personal. Engaging both body and mind shifts perspective and encourages application of new learning to everyday life and activities. When teaching EA, we guide students in practices that ground them squarely in physical presence, while simultaneously connecting them to deeper presence and inner resources. If we articulate the practices in terms of enhanced mindfulness and building skills rather than achieving an endpoint position or state, then the stage is set for lifelong exploration. When we stimulate wonder and curiosity in students, they learn to explore their anatomy like a baby discovering its toes for the first time: *Aren't I interesting? Oh, look what happens when I do this!*

The transformational possibilities of EA are experienced when taught in an integrated, multidimensional way. Learning about a structure, exploring it somatically with sensitive attention, and reflecting on the experience both during and afterward builds skills that synergistically transform the way we live and move. This approach to teaching and learning involves designing a context for the learner to experience, reflect, and access inner resources that motivate choices for health and well-being.

Embodied learning is an educational approach in which "the whole person is treated as a whole being, permitting the person to experience... self as a holistic and synthesised acting, feeling, thinking being-in-the-world, rather than as separate physical and mental qualities which bear no relation to each other.

*Steven Stolz (2015)*

Embodied learning is "the deliberate use and recognition of multimoda body-mind activities and strategies to facilitate shifts in perspectives, perceptions, paradigms, behavior and actions."

*Marth Munro (2018)*

Leading students through an embodied experience of their anatomy involves three distinct steps:

1. **Learn It**

First, we learn about an anatomical structure cognitively. Through spoken word (auditory, linguistic), anatomy books (visual), videos (auditory, visual, and spatial), and skeleton models (visual, spatial, kinesthetic), we learn its location; shape and size; structure and function; movement and stability possibilities; and relationship to other structures. Evoking a mental picture of an anatomical structure makes it more real for the body. Anatomical knowledge helps us appreciate possibilities and respect limitations of the structure. It also aids understanding of inefficient or maladaptive alignment, breath, and movement patterns by comparing anatomical and physiological information with lived experience.

My anatomy instructor often acknowledged the Celestial Design Committee when marvelling at the intelligent design of the human body.

2. **Feel It**

*If you feel it, you can heal it.*

In the second step, students are encouraged to embody intellectual understanding using interoceptive awareness to cultivate direct subjective experience of structures, a felt sense based on their unique personal experience, observation, and reflection. They ask themselves, *How do I know I have hands? How do I know I am breathing? What are the sensations?* Buddha used the term *ehipassiko* to encourage his followers to "come and see for yourself" (Palmo 2002), and likewise this step urges students to dive into direct experience. They first establish a sensory baseline of usual, habitual awareness in stillness or movement, then explore a movement or structure while paying attention to feelings and sensations that arise. After explorations, students return to baseline to register any changes in their body, breath, and mind. Developing a clear mental picture and somatic felt sense of a structure can update and refine brain maps and alter future movements both consciously, as learned awareness is applied, and unconsciously, as modified neural maps are integrated.

EA invites students to focus on specific structures and differentiate them from surrounding structures by discerning their unique sensations. Through explorations that include somatic inquiry, touch, breath, sound, and movement, students gradually develop felt sense of each structure and its relationship to others. They may shift focus to different aspects of the structure during movement, use imagery, do micro-movements, move in nonhabitual ways, or use their hands to palpate. Palpating and moving a partner's body helps to awaken awareness of those structures in the student's own body. During explorations, students aspire to remain in open, neutral awareness of sensations while acknowledging thoughts and feelings that arise. Sensing and feeling in this way can lead to restful present moment awareness and slower, more subtle and mindful movement.

This type of attentiveness can awaken the intelligence of the structure and reconfigure somatosensory maps in the brain. Through feeling and sensing we initiate a "dialogue" with our anatomy that can impact posture and function, leading to therapeutic transformation as new awareness is incorporated into more complex movements. Norman Doidge writes that "[s]ensation's purpose is to orient, guide, help, control, coordinate, and assess the success of a movement" (2015, p.170).

Zoe had the most rigid pelvis I'd encountered in clinical practice. During yoga therapy sessions, I discovered she mentally pictured her pelvis as one solid bone, which was reflected in the way she walked and moved. As she developed felt sense of pelvic structure and movement possibilities, her back pain resolved and her movement became more fluid. As a bonus, her mental rigidity also relaxed.

Differentiation is a necessary first step to integration; each part retains autonomy and informs the whole. At first, structures may feel like undifferentiated masses moving in automatic, disconnected ways. As structures are highlighted through EA practices, sensations are refined and parts can be accessed with more specificity and precision as neural maps are clarified. Even though we isolate one part for contemplation, that part is always known and moves in relationship to the matrix of the whole. Through exploration, we learn about locations and relationships between structures. For example, when movement is initiated from a structure, we track how the rest of the body follows, supports, and responds. With practice, we identify and make meaning of a recognizable and reproducible set of sensations indicating qualities such as ease, clear force transmission, balance, and stability. Consequences of habitual patterns become conscious when we compare our felt experience post-inquiry to initial baseline. Consistent practice of attending to sensations and qualities of movement creates an inner referencing system that cultivates adaptability and choice.

The whole is greater than the sum of its parts.

*Aristotle*

3.  **Heal It**

Elsa Gindler, another grandmother of body-mind therapies, proposed that "[l]ife is the playground for our work" (Koltai 1999). If learning is to be integrated, IA must be applied to therapeutic movement practices and everyday activities involving both specific and whole-body movement. After an exploration we ask, *Now what?* and *What can I do to support my body to integrate this learning in future movement?* The overarching purpose of EA practice is for each person to become more functional, adaptable, and integrated as previously unconscious alignment, breath, and movement habits are brought into consciousness and repatterned. As the nervous system learns different responses that are safer and more functional, future stresses can be better managed. We need to know what we are doing to know where to go next.

Once I recognized my unconscious habit of locking my knees when emotionally triggered, I could shift to a more grounded, responsive state when I centered my weight through my knee joints.

*David*

With compassion and consistent practice, students refine their sensory perception. This may catalyze transformative changes in response and state of mind, inspiring informed ways of moving and being that bring more ease, or sukha, and steadiness, or sthira. Structural coherence becomes a self-generated state arising from EA explorations, and alignment, balance, and movement become self-directed dynamic processes supporting self-regulation. Rather than trying to remember and impose alignment instructions, students can use felt sense of their own anatomy as an organizing principle. The awareness cultivated in physical explorations translates to other koshic levels as upgraded emotional and mental self-regulation.

In EA practices, movement is explored with the intention of increasing awareness. In this step we ask, How do I do that? from mental, emotional, and physical perspectives. The form or movement itself is not the endpoint but merely a vehicle for gaining awareness and exploring new skills. The goal is embodied participation in the process rather than how far, how big, or how much it looks like the photo in the book. Instead of aiming to achieve specific physical outcomes, our intention is to seek the qualities of healing movement: steadiness, balance, ease, connection, safety, and comfort. Students discover ways to reproduce these qualities by first doing a movement habitually, then contrasting the experience of moving in a "new" or "informed" way. Pausing during explorations is a necessary element in this process as it enables the nervous system to register effects of the practice.

Over time, neuroplasticity alters both structure and function of the nervous system. Awareness gained in EA practices can challenge entrenched neural patterns of perception and action and inhibit unconscious repetition of unhelpful habits while new habits are integrated. Physically, functional movement patterns, refined motor control, and balanced tension and compression forces evolve through EA practices.

> I don't experience any pain now when I imagine my arm radiating from my navel.
>
> *Anne*
>
> My hockey playing drastically improved when I practised skating from my psoas.
>
> *Sam*

Mindful repetition builds competence. The more frequently an awareness arises and is acknowledged, the sooner the new pattern of breath, alignment, or movement will be integrated. In this key integration step, students notice how their daily experience transforms when awareness, perception, and comfort levels are altered through EA practices.

## TEACHING PRINCIPLES

The "how" of learning can either ignite curiosity and exploration or relegate potentially helpful practices to obscurity. Our effectiveness as teachers depends on how we relate to students and the communication principles we use. The following principles support effective teaching of EA as therapy and set the stage for enthusiastic learning and active participation of students in their own healing process.

### Principles not Prescriptions

Applying principles and avoiding "fix it" solutions allows EA practices to become meaningful, embodied experiences. Rather than performing an exercise to correct something that is "wrong," students explore anatomical structures to discover alignment and movement possibilities that create greater safety, ease, and efficacy. They recognize and respect that imbalances and dysfunctional patterns are the best possible adaptations their body has discovered to remain upright and move in functional ways. Self-compassion arises with the understanding that pain and dysfunction are messages from the body advising *try another way*. Becoming aware of patterns and understanding that choice is possible, students are empowered to make conscious decisions to transform habitual behaviors. When we create opportunities to see what is functional and "right" and focus on growth and learning, we help students become more responsive and adaptive human beings. Real learning starts with basic skill building, which creates a foundation for future innovation and improvisation. Table 2.1 contrasts experiential and prescriptive teaching methodologies.

**Table 2.1 Comparison of Experiential and Prescriptive Methodologies**

*Adapted from Koltai (2018) and Farhi (1997)*

| Experiential Methodologies | Prescriptive Methodologies |
|---|---|
| Assumption that people are innately capable of self-balancing and self-healing | Assumption that people require external intervention to heal |
| Focus on growth and skill development | Focus on fixing something that is "wrong" |
| Values awareness, attention, and direct experience | Values empirical measurements |
| Encourages exploration and numerous attempts to discover best choices | Encourages correct performance |
| Student cocreates therapeutic process guided by internal sense of rightness | Teacher chooses therapeutic interventions |
| Development of awareness as a skill generates self-correction, dynamic response, and evolution | Symptomatic relief or correction |
| Active participation of student in own healing process | Student as passive receiver of instructions |
| Inside out, bottom-up approach | Outside in, top-down approach |
| Development of IA and motor control | Performance of movement |
| Creation of environment where student can learn, respond, and adapt | Methodology of information, exercises, and prescription |
| Focus on wholeness | Focus on fixing parts |
| Teacher as guide or mentor with ongoing relationship and communication | Teacher as authority |
| Process-oriented | Performance-oriented |
| Student experiences increased sense of agency, self-trust, and empowerment | Problem is "fixed" |

## Role of Teacher or Therapist

When teaching EA, the teacher or therapist functions as a guide or facilitator instead of perpetuating the power differential often experienced in more traditional teacher/student relationships. Our role as teachers is to educate in the original Latin meaning of the word *educere*, which means "to bring out, lead forth." We meet and interact with students in the space of respectful inquiry. Students actively discover and develop their own resources and capacity for discernment rather than passively receiving information. When the intention is to encourage skill building rather than imparting knowledge, students learn which skills best serve them through direct experience. The teacher is less directive and seeks to create learning environments that encourage IA and result in more student autonomy. Students explore the "laboratory" of their own body with self-discovery, enhanced self-awareness, and conscious choice as intended destinations. The process of exploring structure and movement through the senses takes priority over a predetermined outcome. As teachers, we must thoroughly explore and integrate EA practices in our own bodies before teaching them to others.

## Empowerment and Agency

When we explicitly value the wisdom and authority of students, self-autonomy flowers. By validating their subjective experience of perceptions, feelings, and sensations, we guide them toward independence and empowerment. Students develop an inner referencing system that enables them to discern the state of their body and mind, connect with their innate body wisdom, and make more skillful choices. Rather than following directions toward specific solutions, students are empowered to discover their own answers and to replicate learned, positive outcomes. Form, alignment, and movement patterns are important, but striving for them may override the ability to discern which subtle sensations offer more connection, safety, stability, and strength.

As empowered, active participants in the therapeutic process, students are more likely to realize their personal capabilities and to stay motivated. As agents of their own healing process, they can choose from a bag of self-healing tools whenever pain or discomfort arises. The ability to accurately discern the state of their body and mind can translate into interactions with the outer world and help students respond to daily challenges with insight and skillful agency.

## Encouragement of Self-Realization

When students are encouraged to cultivate felt sense of their body while exploring possibilities and respecting limitations of their anatomy, they learn how to release old patterns and access new options. By reframing "problems" as a courageous attempt by the body at self-healing, students are often able to discover clues for healing. They are empowered to generate possible solutions by proactively asking themselves, *What do I need to relieve my suffering?* This process of compassionate self-study is called svadhyaya in yoga. Inquiry into the vast world of sensations in the body can be a doorway to self-discovery that ultimately leads to understanding the unity of body, breath, mind, and spirit. Connecting directly to bodily experience can help us discover this truth.

> The cure for pain is in the pain.
> Good and bad are mixed.
> If you don't have both, you don't belong with us.
>
> *Rumi (Barks 1995, p. 205)*

## Focus on Wholeness

Although EA focuses on individual anatomical structures, the part is always viewed in the context of inherent wholeness. To assist healing, we must view each person in their totality rather than as a collection of separate symptoms and honour the interdependent functioning of all components. Rather than viewing dysfunction of individual parts as barriers to experiencing wholeness, they can be viewed from the context of wholeness. Initially, we do this by remembering the physical context of the part and its relationship and connection with the rest of the body. Then, we consider subtle koshic connections to emotions, mental patterning, and spiritual Self. By expanding perspective to the experience of Self as wholeness, students can know themselves as a whole person that may include a physical challenge. This can lead to deepened self-compassion and appreciation for the sacredness of life.

> I had a life-altering epiphany when I realized *I am Sherry and I have MS.* I felt liberated when I no longer defined myself by my illness.
>
> *Sherry*

## Contemplations for Teachers

- *Where is my teaching style on the principles/prescription continuum?*
- *How can my teaching style motivate development of students' internal reference systems?*
- *How can I empower students to develop agency?*
- *How can I encourage compassionate self-sensing in students?*
- *How can I affirm inherent wholeness in my teaching?*
- *How can I inspire students to trust their inherent ability to self-heal?*

# HOW TO TEACH EXPERIENTIAL ANATOMY

In our externally focused world, learning usually relies on visual and auditory senses. This learning style bypasses IA and the potential to learn through somatic experience. Learning to focus attention inwardly can be difficult and frustrating at times as it challenges our dominant approach to contemporary life. Yet, the process of refining sensitivity and cultivating IA is hugely rewarding. It allows discernment of subtle distinctions between sensations that help to self-correct, self-regulate, and make better decisions.

The key question is: *How do I do that?* The *how*, that is, the process of exploring structure and movement through the senses, is much more important than *what* you do. Pondering this question encompasses more than simply noticing movement initiation and muscular action. It involves tuning into all koshic levels to notice the participation of your whole self: how you breathe, how much energy you expend, the quality of movement, your attitude or mental focus, the thoughts and emotions that arise, whether you are moving with self-criticism or self-compassion, and your sense of wholeness or disconnection. While the voluntary nervous system is satisfied with accomplishing a movement, the interoceptive network is busy with sensing, connections, context, and implications.

The principles below offer guidelines for enriching EA practices.

## Dial Down Sensory Input

The simple, basic interoceptive practice of sensing is the foundation of EA. To absorb new information and clarify sensory awareness, the nervous system must be receptive. You learn best in the calmer, parasympathetic state. The process of learning awareness requires simple, clear neural input. When background "noise" is decreased, the nervous system becomes available for the important work of conscious sensing. Getting out of our head with its looping storylines and into our body enables the possibility of direct, felt experience.

This process of pratyahara (withdrawing the senses from the busy outer environment) allows sensory refinement and recalibration, which can be deeply restorative.

> Where you put your mind matters. When you deliberately turn inward, the mind can slow to body time and attune to subtle sensations.

### HOW DO I DO THAT?

*Establish a Sensory Baseline*

Baseline can be positions like supine, sitting, or standing, or a movement done in a habitual way that highlights breath and sensations associated with established patterns. Baselines capture a snapshot of present sensations and experience. After EA explorations, returning to baseline allows the nervous system to register and compare sensations and effects of habitual and informed movement, or heightened awareness of structures. At first, you may not feel much but your sensitivity will refine with practice.

### Keep it Simple

When IA is initially patterned in positions or movements that give the nervous system a simplified focus, integration into more complex positions and movements will be easier. You must learn to walk before you run. Engage the brain in simple patterns and build from there.

- Start in non-weight-bearing positions that quiet postural muscles and allow the body to attune to gravity. Once new awareness is integrated in a position that minimizes muscular engagement, it can be explored in progressively complex positions.
- Begin with movements involving one joint, one limb, one side of the body, one plane of movement, only upper or lower body, or one aspect of an anatomical structure.
- Start with dynamic movements, consciously moving in and out of postures before sustaining them. Repetition establishes and strengthens efficient neuromuscular pathways and builds understanding of interrelationships between anatomical structures.
- Deconstruct movements into component parts and practice each component before consolidating into more complex movements.

### Slow Down

Although the unconscious mind can process 11 million bits of information per second, the conscious mind can process only approximately 50 bits per second (Markowsky 2023). Moving slowly gives the conscious mind fewer inputs to process and anchors them in the body, allowing you to register nuances of the movement. Slowing down allows you to attune to any sensations, thoughts, and feelings arising during explorations.

- Move slowly to observe yourself and differentiate sensations and qualities of movements.
- Couple movement with breath rhythm to encourage slowing down. Breath can be used as a metronome to calibrate the mind to body time.
- Allow adequate time for the practices so you can move in a calm, relaxed way. Learning something new requires time, both during the initial practice and with subsequent repetition.
- Take short pauses throughout the practice to give the nervous system an opportunity to reset and recalibrate. Remain in open attention to register effects of the practice.

> Slower movement leads to more subtle observation and map differentiation, so that more change is possible.
>
> *Norman Doidge (2015, p.170)*

### Minimize Effort (see Chapter 1)

Excessive effort can cause sensory overload that interferes with the nervous system's ability to sense and differentiate sensations. A nervous system busy orchestrating excessive muscular tone is less available for sensing and organizing subtle movement. Muscle tension can also compress nerve endings and diminish sensory sensitivity.

- As you move, become aware of unnecessary effort in parts that are trying to "help." Scan your body, asking yourself:

- What is the minimum effort required to do this movement?
- What nonessential effort can I undo so my movement is pure and efficient?
- How can I make this movement more subtle?

## Tune In

The term *felt sense* originated with Eugene Gendlin, developer of the body-mind practice called "focusing" to describe a nonlinear, wordless, inner body sensation beyond thoughts and feelings that encompasses everything we know and feel about an experience. He advocated working with felt sense by focusing on it with curiosity and welcoming its messages (Gendlin n.d.). Felt sense can be deepened with pratyahara, by deliberately withdrawing your attention from the outer world and directing it to specific body structures, linking mind to body. As you maintain a steady focus on the structure, you can become aware of its qualities and responses, initiate movement from it, and sense connections to other structures. Remember, you are befriending and building relationships with your parts so you can receive helpful information to repattern unhelpful habits and, perhaps more importantly, sense your wholeness.

### HOW DO I DO THAT?

- In open attention, allow sensations to register. Stay with the direct experience of a structure, movement, or bodily process rather than going into storyline or commentary.
- Continually refine your sensitivity by tracking, registering, and contrasting sensation.
- Breathe calmly and slowly to attune to subtle sensation.

- Imagine that each cell has eyes, ears, and feelers. Consciously activate them.
- Imagine the moving part as the main actor and the rest of the body as a supportive, attentive audience.
- Be curious and compassionate. Instead of judging, try saying to yourself, *Isn't this interesting?*
- Track each point along an arc of movement or a pathway of force. Notice sensations indicating qualities like stability, safe range of motion, integration, and ease.
- Use feedback from your body to modify what you are doing.
  - What is activated, moving, supporting, connected?
  - What thoughts, feelings, and observations arise?
  - Are old habits intruding?
  - Which way feels stronger, more stable, easier, connected, or whatever quality you are intending?

## Explore

From an EA perspective, yoga poses and other movements offer a starting point or vehicle to explore new information and awareness. Through self-directed exploration, you can find your way to desired qualities or states of being. At times you may feel awkward or inept. Welcome this state of uncertainty because it means you are learning. The form or shape of a movement can change according to your avenue of exploration; it need not resemble the textbook photo. A repeated movement may look the same to an observer, but your inner experience can fluctuate dramatically by shifting focus. Your experience and response will differ from that of other people. After doing the same practice, you may feel weighted in your feet while they feel light and more upright.

**HOW DO I DO THAT?**

*Variation*

The nervous system thrives on novelty and differences and pays attention when you try something new or move in nonhabitual ways. The brain doesn't have established neural networks for performing the variation so must create new synapses that will ultimately promote learning more adaptive movement patterns. Recall that movement-related discomfort can be viewed as a message from the body to *try another way*, an invitation to explore movement variations that may provide relief. In any position or movement, you can intuitively play with elements like jiggling, moving in different angles or planes, and other nonhabitual ways of moving.

Giving the nervous system information in slightly different ways can clarify neural maps. Experimenting with variations presents opportunities to experience nuances in sensation that reveal ways to move with greater ease and integration. Variations in angle, tempo, and load cause a response in the fascial system that can improve fascial health by increasing remodeling and elasticity (Huijing 2007).

Variation may include:

- Intensity: Strong effort or intensity can overwhelm the nervous system with too many sensory inputs, while subtle movement allows greater distinctions to be registered.
- Speed: While exploring speed variations, you may discover habitual patterns and subtle differences that go unnoticed when moving at your usual speed.
- Breath: You can alter breathing patterns by adjusting locus, rate or intensity of breath. Inhaling during a movement gives you a different experience than exhaling doing the same movement.
- Quality of movement: While moving, you can explore movement qualities, including sustained, oscillatory, smooth, fluid, heavy, or percussive.
- Angle of movement: You can vary directionality by changing the angle of an anatomical part or movement. For example, a standing forward bend can be done with feet in neutral, internal rotation, and external rotation.
- Locus of initiation: You can initiate movement from specific anatomical structures, or experiment with initiating proximally (closer to the midsection) and distally (distant from the midsection).
- Restraint: You can deliberately restrain extraneous habitual movement or isolate movement in specific structures by restraining adjacent structures. For example, a habit of thrusting the ribs forward during arm elevation can be restrained to discover uncompensated shoulder range of motion.
- Visual imagery: Working with different images changes quality of movement. For example, imagining your arm attached to your navel with an elastic might feel stronger than visualizing your arms supported by your heart and lungs.

*Shift awareness*

EA explorations can wake up disused or underutilized brain areas. Shifting your awareness between structures, or from interoceptive to proprioceptive or exteroceptive focus will vary your experience as your brain processes different sensory inputs. When repeating movements, experiment with shifting awareness to determine what gives you reliable and desirable outcomes. Notice what happens as you expand focus from specific structures to whole-body movements involving the "family" of the body. As you practice shifting perspective, notice effects on your capacity to shift mental perspective in everyday life.

*Circle the Dragon*
In Chinese medicine, the principle of circling the dragon advises initially working peripherally to the "problem" area. Increasing awareness and exploring movement in adjacent or distant structures can stimulate circulation, wake up neuromuscular connections, and strengthen feelings of safety and mastery. Proximal or distal joint dysfunction may be a contributing factor. Initially working there may lighten maladaptive load and decrease pain in the problem area. For example, EA exploration of the feet may reveal that unbalanced weight distribution patterns contribute to low back pain.

*Connections*
As you practice EA, notice connections between structures. Even if you isolate movement in one part of your body, every structure in the body-wide fascial network participates in some way. Notice both functional and nonfunctional relationships between structures. As you initiate movement from a structure ask yourself:

- How does the rest of my body respond to the movement?
- What parts support the movement?
- What parts resist or obstruct the movement?
- Are some structures "glued" together?

*Discernment*
Sensing subtle distinctions offers useful feedback and may reveal more helpful ways of moving. As you play with variations or shifting awareness, notice how your experience changes. Comparing your habitual way of moving to the "informed" way can highlight previously unconscious habits contributing to discomfort. Doing a movement in your habitual way before and after an exploration can underline differences and help you choose more functional movement patterns.

*Safe Range of Motion*
Differentiating sensations or qualities that signal healing, comfort, and ease results in safe, restorative movement. Gently explore pain-free range of motion by tracking point-by-point through the arc of movement and notice when you approach discomfort or activate unhelpful compensatory patterns. Your range of safe movement may increase as you experiment with variations. Notice whether specific variations are *helpful, neutral, or unhelpful*. Use your inner reference system to determine whether you need to decrease a variable such as intensity, range, number of repetitions, or effort level.

## Summary: Guidelines for Learning EA

- Limit sensory input
- Simplify
- Slow down
- Minimize effort
- Tune in
- Explore variations
- Shift awareness
- Pause
- Discern

## KEY CONCEPTS

- Students are inspired to learn EA when they realize how it enriches their lives and transforms their experience and understanding.
- Experiential anatomy can be effectively taught by following an embodied learning educational model of "learn it, feel it, heal it."
- EA is best taught through principles, not prescriptions, and by creating

- opportunities for an empowering, cocreative therapeutic process.
- The EA teacher or therapist functions as a guide or facilitator, interacting with students in a space of respectful inquiry.

- EA can be a doorway to self-discovery that ultimately leads to self-realization.
- In the EA teaching model, dysfunction is viewed from the context of wholeness.

## CHAPTER 3

# Opening to Breath

*I can breathe easy now.*
*She waited with bated breath.*
*Don't breathe a word of this to anyone.*
*The sunset took my breath away.*

"We live in a breathless society," wrote Carola Speads almost a century ago (Speads, 1992). Little did she know that the average adult breath rate would increase from nine breaths per minute then to 12–20 per minute now (Chourpiliadis and Bhardwaj 2022). We breathe more, but less efficiently. Our cells are starved for oxygen, contributing to the current tidal wave of chronic health conditions. Breath is a superpower we can use to improve digestion and cardiovascular health, decrease pain and lift depression. Realizing that breath is the link between mind, body, and spirit, sages thousands of years ago evolved an array of breath practices to shift mood, enter meditative states, and improve physiology. Ample research confirms this ancient knowledge of the link between good breathing and improved physical and mental health.

Disordered breathing is a common feature of many acute disorders and may play a pathogenic role in the development of systemic diseases (Laffey and Kavanagh 2002). Conditions including chronic pain, cardiovascular disease, premenstrual tension, and anxiety have been clinically associated with disordered breathing. Breathing patterns change automatically to accommodate varying metabolic needs of posture, activity, state of mind, and emotions. For example, a chronically collapsed posture and depressed state of mind can entrench shallow, upper chest breathing patterns.

My students have reported countless ways breath practices have dramatically changed their lives, from helping one breathe through the agony of her husband's death to another who used conscious breathing to control blood pressure. One client, after learning a simple breath practice for her frequent panic attacks, burst into my clinic the following week exclaiming: "It's the breath! The breath is the key."

Although remedial breathing practices may be indicated, we first need to master the foundational practice of restoring easy, natural breath. This *integral breath* is relaxed, adaptable, calm, and emanates naturally from a responsive body. When EA is used as a preliminary practice to awaken and free breath structures, subsequent breathing practices are more effective. Without this preparation, practices are often *imposed* and can reinforce physical or psychological patterns initially contributing to disordered breathing.

Breath is a multifaceted event, involving structural elements including bones, muscles, fascia, and organs. Interoceptive EA practices can optimize the function of each element, freeing the respiratory system to play its rightful role in wellness. Interoception is the foundational skill in EA and has been proposed as one of the mechanisms underlying positive health benefits of slow breathing (Zaccaro *et al.*, 2018)

> In my early teaching days more than one student confessed to struggling with my remedial breath instructions.

## KOSHIC PERSPECTIVES: ALCHEMY OF THE BREATH

Quality of breathing has profound effects on every aspect of our life from muscular tension to mood, heart function, and ability to focus. Since lack of integral breath will be uniquely reflected on each koshic level, an EA approach can result in multidimensional healing effects. Healing is encouraged when we access the ease and efficiency of the integral breath. For example, Sarah, a client with scoliosis, diligently practiced to realign and repattern her musculoskeletal structure and maximize her lung capacity. Her pain decreased and movement was easier, but she was delighted with the bonus of renewed vitality, mental stability, and ability to flow with life. When the primary therapeutic intention is to free the original, integral breath, effects are experienced on each koshic level.

> I once observed the face of a first-time client soften and change color from pasty white to rosy pink as circulation increased during a simple breath-focused yoga therapy session.

Freedom of breath is intimately tied to ease and mobility of annamaya kosha structures. When breathing is constricted, the sternum, clavicles, ribs, and numerous joints between ribs and spine can become immobilized. Absence of rhythmical breath movement causes overlying myofascia to contract and tightly shrink-wrap the breath container, hampering diaphragmatic movement. A vicious cycle may evolve: breathing dysfunction constrains breathing structures, which further limits the breath, and so on. Hyperventilation, characterized, in part, by shallow, upper chest breathing may result, which overstimulates the sympathetic nervous system and, if sustained, generates a second vicious cycle that ultimately results in systemic myofascial tension and decreased cerebral blood flow.

When physical structures are optimally balanced and freed to participate in breath movement through EA practices, integral breath is liberated and the body is more capable of flexibly adapting to breath demands. As one student expressed it: "Now there's more room for me."

The prana in pranamaya kosha refers to life-force energy (from *pra* to bring forth and *na* the eternal cosmic vibration). The yoga tradition teaches that breath carries prana and *where breath goes, prana flows*. Liberating integral breath frees prana to circulate and function as an internal source of support. When breath is constricted or breathing patterns are disordered, we may feel unsupported or experience life as a struggle. Doing, controlling, and manipulating may predominate over being. Freely circulating prana is often experienced as feelings of vitality, inner aliveness, and enhanced ability to flow with life. Many students report effortless increased breath capacity and more energy along with improved sleep and digestion after EA breath practices. When integral breath is accessed, movement efficiencies minimize energy expenditure, liberating energy for other uses.

Dysfunctional breathing has a critical impact on emotional states, clarity of thinking, and the ability to make good decisions in manomaya kosha. It's impossible to be anxious and breathe freely. The bidirectional link between emotions and breathing was demonstrated in a 2010 study in which participants induced emotional states by consciously reproducing breath signatures of selected emotions (Philippot, Chapelle, and Blairy 2002). Breath affects emotions, and we have all experienced how emotions affect breath, like holding our breath when feeling anxious. Conscious regulation of breath influences interoceptive communication, which in turn affects state of mind, emotions, and emotional volatility. Learning to free the breath and breathe consciously into difficult emotions can build self-regulation skills and create more mental and physical spaciousness.

Disordered breathing patterns change brain chemistry and initiate a cascade of physical and mental events. Reduced blood flow to the brain can cause mental fogginess, disconnection, and irritability that prevent awareness and skillful expression of emotions. EA breath repatterning practices increase felt sense of breathing structures and movement and enable us to discover newfound emotional steadiness; breathing becomes a barometer for inner experience and a welcomed resource for self-regulation.

A lack of sensory awareness of dysfunctional breathing patterns and their associated physiological effects can lead to musculoskeletal pain, and over time to long-term stress-related health consequences (Lin and Peper 2009). In this study, researchers noted symptoms of sympathetic arousal, including body tension and increased respiration and heart rate, as participants texted on mobile phones. The 83 percent of subjects observed holding their breath were mostly unaware of doing so, as are most of us when occupied with many daily breath-holding opportunities besides texting. Lin recommended breath awareness and relaxation training as an antidote, validating my clinical observations that EA practices can increase self-awareness of breath structures

and movements and help us consciously shift physical and emotional states.

As the link between mind and body, breath serves as a tool of self-inquiry and self-regulation in vijnanamaya kosha. The Celestial Design Committee kindly appointed respiration the only autonomic function under conscious control; we can use breath to change our perspective and generate other desired effects. The yoga tradition teaches *where thought goes, prana flows*, so where you put your mind matters. This interplay between breath and thought is employed in EA practices like using visualization and breath to soften tension or pain in specific body parts.

By observing how the quality of our breath reflects the interplay between our inner and outer worlds, breath represents a metaphor for how we live. Breath clues us into habitual patterns of expansion and resistance, love and fear, effort and ease, and can be used consciously to shift into more life-enhancing responses.

Focusing on breath also draws us into the present moment. EA practices can help us breathe into what we cannot control, and into pain or difficult emotions to cultivate the acknowledgment and spaciousness needed to become more present. Other nonphysical outcomes reported by students include more presence, and ability to self-regulate and respond to needs of the moment rather than reacting from old patterns. As the integral breath is freed, we gain resilience and skillfulness in allowing life to happen and giving ourselves permission to express our whole self in the world.

On anandamaya kosha level, breathing practices have been used throughout history to induce spiritual awareness and achieve heightened states of consciousness. In Latin, Hebrew, and other languages, breath is synonymous with spirit. Breath is seen as the connection to life itself, and the cosmos. Historically, before the word *inspiration* was used for breath, it referred to Divine influence (Merriam-Webster n.d.). With each inspiration, we literally "draw in spirit." We are inspired by a beautiful poem or inspired to create.

Conscious breathing can generate experiences of feeling part of the cosmos, connected to and supported by the universe. The degree to which we acknowledge and strengthen this connection can influence the quality of our participation with the outer world. Breath can be a reliable and accessible gauge of the degree of openness and enthusiasm (or resistance) with which we experience the mystery of life. When the integral breath is patterned through EA practices, it can encourage a relationship of reverence with ourselves, others, the environment, and the entire universe.

## LEARN IT

The bony container of softer respiratory contents is formed by thoracic vertebrae, clavicles, sternum, and rib "basket," and knitted together by myofascia and ligaments. The Celestial Design Committee intended these elements to form an integrated tension and compression system facilitating continuous breath throughout life with minimal effort. The state and quality of the container's bony compression elements affects tensile soft tissue elements of the contents and vice versa. Rigidity, misalignment, or excessive tension in bony structures or associated soft tissue can imbalance tension and compression forces, decreasing breath capacity and producing far-reaching effects on all koshas. Felt sense of breathing structures is cultivated to awaken cellular intelligence and deepen cellular participation in breath and movement.

### Sternum and Clavicles

The bony "blade" of the sternum protects the tender heart and articulates with the upper seven ribs at sternocostal joints. It rises and falls vertically with each breath. The sternum has three parts: the wider manubrium articulating with clavicles at sternoclavicular joints, the long, narrow sternal body, and the xiphoid process, a cartilaginous structure which is often ossified in adults, and absent in over half the population.

The fibrous joint between the sternal body and manubrium is designed to move with breath. As the body rises on inhalation, the joint hinges slightly (Beyer *et al.*, 2017). Freedom of breath, regular movement in multiple planes, and balanced posture may prevent this hinge joint from ossifying with age.

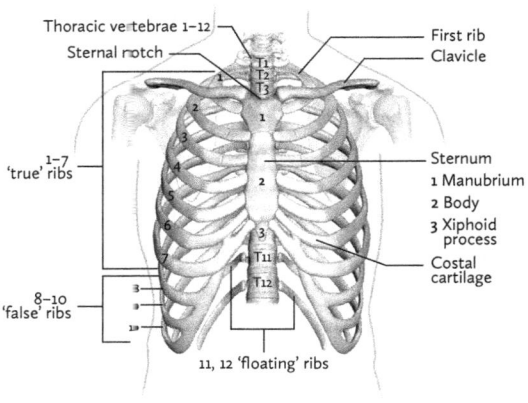

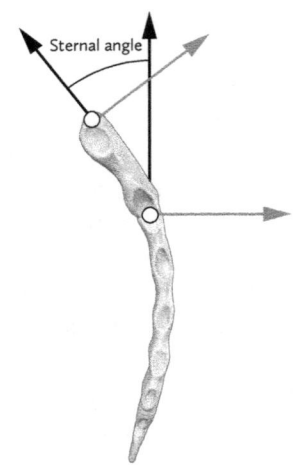

The clavicles (Latin for *key*), linking sternum and arms, transfer waves of breath movement into the arms. These S-shaped bones spread and spiral laterally as the manubrium rises and hinges on inhalation. If the shoulders are habitually elevated or hunched, this movement is restricted, and the clavicles are unable to contribute to maximum respiratory capacity (Ljunggren 1979).

## Rib Basket

The rib basket (I use this term instead of rib cage, which implies rigidity and restriction) protects the vulnerable heart and lungs and changes shape to expand or decrease available space in the torso. It is cone-shaped, narrow superiorly, wider inferiorly, and significantly convex posteriorly, forming a heart shape in cross section. Most people underutilize the potential breathing space provided by this convexity.

The basket is formed by 12 pairs of curved spiralic ribs slanting diagonally upward from anterior to posterior. The upper seven "true" rib pairs join the sternum directly through individual cartilage at sternocostal joints and with the spine at costovertebral joints. The eighth to tenth pairs attach indirectly to the sternum through the seventh rib cartilage, and the lowest two pairs of floating ribs connect only posteriorly to thoracic vertebrae. Ribs are both plastic—they can bend—and elastic—they return to their original shape. The flexible cartilage contributes to the rib basket's ability to change shape.

The ribs contain approximately 100 connections to spinal vertebrae. Each rib connects to the body of the vertebra above and below, the disc in between, and the transverse process on the vertebra of the same number. So many movement possibilities!

Costovertebral joints (*costo* is Latin for *rib*), with the spine, are hinged joints designed to rotate and fan open on inhalation. These movements are essential to full and unobstructed integral breath. Three layers of intercostal muscles occupy the space between the ribs.

Freely moving ribs encourage both physical and nonphysical effects:

- Organ function: Healthy breathing optimizes organ physiology in two ways. As the rib basket changes shape, organs have more space to function and are rhythmically massaged. Both are key to heart health. Shallow, upper chest breathing has been associated with heart disease (Abidov *et al.*, 2005).
- Spinal resiliency: The spine and associated soft tissue are also rhythmically massaged by healthy breath movement, promoting hydration and elasticity. Tension in paraspinal soft tissue restricts costovertebral joint movement and compromises breath freedom.
- Base of support for head and neck: As the ribs expand and move freely, increased dimensionality creates a wider foundation of support for the cervical spine and neck, which can relax into the support from below.
- Allowing life: When rib movement is unrestrained and breath moves freely in and out, an experience of liberation and uninhibited participation in life is more accessible.

## Spine (see Chapter 9)

The 24 spinal vertebrae are designed to move with breath. When the spine is healthy and mobile, breathing initiates ripples of spinal extension and flexion. Breath movement hampered anywhere in the bony breath container can compromise both spinal stability and sequential movement. Without breath freedom, spinal movement is compromised, affecting movement patterns throughout the rest of the body. The container and contents affect each other: restricted spinal movement diminishes breath capacity, and compromised breath hampers freedom of spinal movement.

## Breathing Muscles

Lungs are *passive* structures inflated and deflated through the work of respiratory muscles and shape changes in the rib basket. Although the diaphragm does the lion's share of work, internal and external intercostal muscles between the ribs are also considered primary breathing muscles. The diaphragm contains slow-twitch, fatigue-resistant fibers functioning continuously from our first to last breath. When breathing muscles are relaxed and pliable, breath naturally occurs lower in the torso and contributes to a calm, grounded state.

When metabolic need for oxygen increases, like when mountain climbing or running to catch a bus, additional accessory muscles are recruited. These include the scalenes, sternocleidomastoid, upper trapezius, levator scapula, serratus anterior and posterior, subclavius, ileocostalis thoracis, omohyoid, and pectoralis minor. When accessory muscles chronically function as primary breathing muscles, breath occurs higher in the torso, causing muscular overdevelopment and sympathetic nervous system stimulation. Most people don't realize that breathing this way may underlie their unclear thinking, anxiety, or chronic digestive problems.

All torso myofascia could potentially facilitate or inhibit the act of breathing. For example, a student with postural imbalances and excessively tensioned paraspinal muscles will likely have trouble breathing fully. Prevented from moving in full range of motion, the diaphragm may become dense and unyielding, further obstructing breath movement and triggering a vicious cycle of cumulative diaphragmatic restriction and diminished breathing.

When we voluntarily control our breath, we can override the autonomic control that we trust to keep us breathing while asleep. By consciously recruiting specific respiratory muscles, we can alter breathing patterns to do the practices in this book.

## Diaphragm

The diaphragm is arguably the most important myofascial structure in the body. It affects physiology, alignment, and emotional experience, and if it stops working, life ceases. It's a large, thin, double-dome-shaped muscle forming an elastic boundary between thoracic and abdominal cavities. Shaped like a mushroom or parachute draped over abdominal organs, the dome attaches to the inner rib circumference. When the diaphragm contracts, the vertical dimension of the thoracic cavity increases approximately 1.5 cm (0.6 in.) during quiet breathing and an impressive 6–10 cm (2.5–4 in.) during deep breathing (Gatzoulis 2008). The diaphragm presses *down* on abdominal organs during inhalation and presses *up* on heart and lungs during active exhalation.

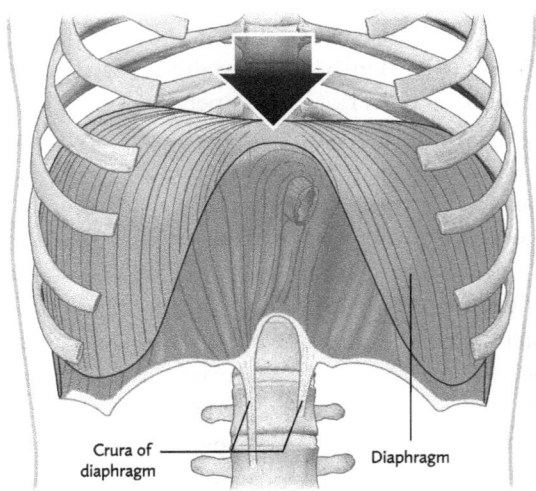

Crura of diaphragm     Diaphragm

This hard-working, horizontally oriented myofascial structure does double duty as the main breathing muscle and major stabilizer of the trunk (Kolar *et al.*, 2012). The considerable fascial component has extensive connections to multiple organs, the base of the tongue, cervical spine, and all four limbs (Bordoni and Zanier 2013). These pervasive fascial relationships suggest that tension anywhere in the body can potentially inhibit diaphragmatic movement. Without rhythmical massage provided by full diaphragmatic movement, organ health may suffer. One student was able to connect the dots between his digestive troubles, unconscious breath holding, and a habit of toe clenching.

The diaphragm has three parts: the central tendon, multiple rib attachments, and two crura.

The top of the "mushroom" is the central tendon, the only tendon in the body unattached to bone. It is continuous with the pericardium of the heart which sits on the dome, indicating the symbiotic relationship between the cardiovascular and respiratory systems. The heart is both embraced by the lungs with each inhalation and massaged as it rides up and down with rhythmical breath movement. This intimate connection suggests that restricted diaphragmatic movement can have profound consequences for heart health; without rhythmical massage, heart physiology suffers.

Rib attachments arise from the inner sternum and surfaces of the lower six ribs. Diaphragmatic muscle fibers radiate from the central tendon to the circumference of inner ribs where they interdigitate with transversus abduminus fibres, highlighting the role both myofascial structures play in spinal stability. The mushroom "stem," or tendinous pair of crura, anchors the diaphragm posteriorly to the bodies and discs of the twelfth thoracic to third lumbar vertebrae. The crural fibres interdigitate with the quadratus lumborum posteriorly and psoas major anteriorly at T12. The inseparable relationship of these muscles explains why slow, conscious breathing can be helpful in relieving back pain. Three openings in the central tendon allow passage for the esophagus, blood vessels, and nerves. No wonder the circulatory, digestive, and respiratory systems affect and are affected by each other (Bordoni and Morabito 2018).

## Intercostal Muscles

The external intercostals are superficial, angling diagonally down and forward from the lower border of one rib to the upper border of the rib below. On inhalations, they activate to elevate the ribs and widen and deepen the thoracic cavity. The two layers of internal intercostals are continuous with inner ribs. The fibers angle diagonally up and forward from the upper border of one rib to the lower border of the rib above. They draw the ribs closer together and narrow the rib basket with forceful exhalation. The intercostals are active in both inspiration and expiration to control the size of the intercostal spaces between the ribs.

## Pelvic Floor Muscles

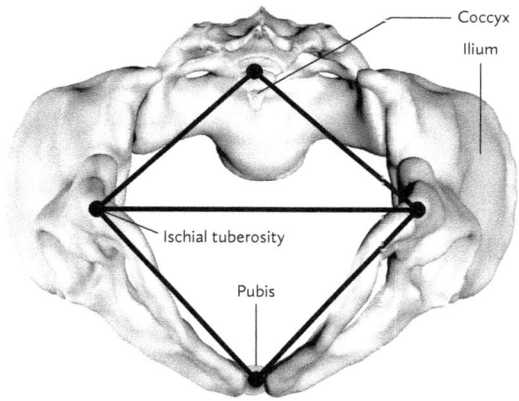

The pelvic floor muscles are contained within a bony pelvic diamond formed by the ischial tuberosities, pubic bone, and coccyx. Superficial and deep layers support the pelvic organs and are responsive to breath. The superficial perineum is a horizontal layer of fibrous muscles, while the deeper pelvic diaphragm, composed of larger, thicker muscles, forms a muscular funnel emanating upward from the pelvic diamond. These muscles radiate from the coccyx like a fan, attaching to the inner surfaces of pelvic bones. Movement of the pelvic floor and respiratory diaphragm is coordinated during breathing; both move in the same direction, although when one is engaged, the other is relaxed. Pelvic floor muscles relax and mimic the downward movement of the diaphragm on relaxed inhalation, while on exhalation the pelvic floor slightly activates. A toned pelvic floor offers slight resistance to the downward movement of inhalations. These muscles can be consciously activated to produce desired effects, including modulating intra-abdominal pressure.

## Core Cylinder

The core cylinder of support is formed by transversus abdominus anteriorly, multifidus and quadratus lumborum posteriorly, with the respiratory and pelvic diaphragms forming the roof and floor. I also include the psoas muscles because of the additional diagonal stability they provide. When all these muscles cocontract, the increase in intra-abdominal pressure and consequent regulation of fluid pressures contributes to both spinal and pelvic stabilization. During breathing, abdominal muscles are active in forceful exhalation. However, habitual excessive activation can ultimately compromise core stability and interfere with freedom of breath.

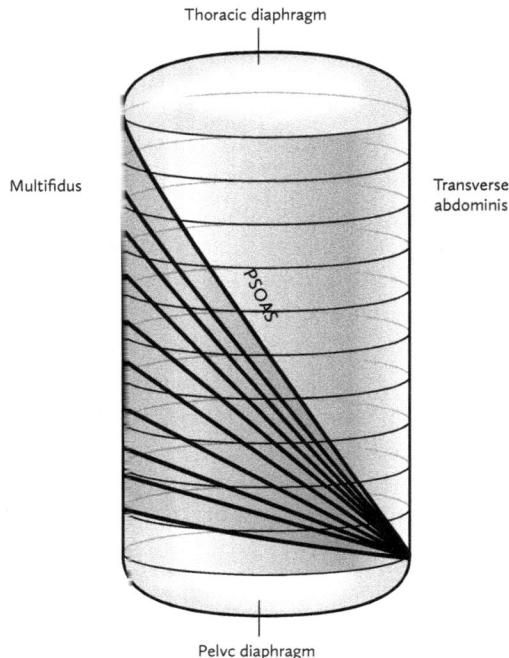

Thoracic diaphragm

Multifidus

Transverse abdominis

PSOAS

Pelvic diaphragm

## Contents of the Breath Container

The heart and lungs sit atop the diaphragm and are fascially continuous with its upper surface; they ride up and down with the breath. The intimate proximity of heart and lungs interweaves the health and function of circulatory and respiratory systems. The right lung has three lobes, while the two lobes of the left lung yield more room for the heart. Lung structure mimics an upside-down tree; at the level of the fourth thoracic rib (T4), the trachea branches into two bronchi, which then branch multiple times into smaller bronchioles, finally ending in clusters of tiny air sacs called *alveoli*. If the 480 million alveoli were laid flat, the surface area would cover half a tennis court! Each alveolus is closely surrounded by a capillary system for oxygen and carbon dioxide exchange. A sticky substance called *surfactant* coats the inner alveolar surfaces, reducing surface tension so alveoli expand more easily and don't collapse on exhalations.

Blood and blood vessels account for over 50 percent of lung volume. Gravity causes their weight to settle into lower lungs, providing greater opportunity for efficient gas exchange. Unfortunately, the average person doesn't normally breathe into lower lobes, so this opportunity is often underutilized unless consciously practiced.

The lungs are large. They occupy almost the whole rib basket from front to back, side to side, extending from clavicles to lower ribs where they rest atop abdominal organs.

The lungs are passive. They contain elastic fibres that expand and recoil; lung inflation and deflation depend on elastic forces in the rib cartilage, diaphragm, and abdominal wall.

The spongy lungs are covered in two layers of connective tissue called *pleura*. Visceral pleura outlines lung surfaces while parietal pleura borders the chest cavity and is continuous with the diaphragm. The pleural space between the two layers is a vacuum lubricated by pleural fluid, allowing the lungs to fill and empty without friction.

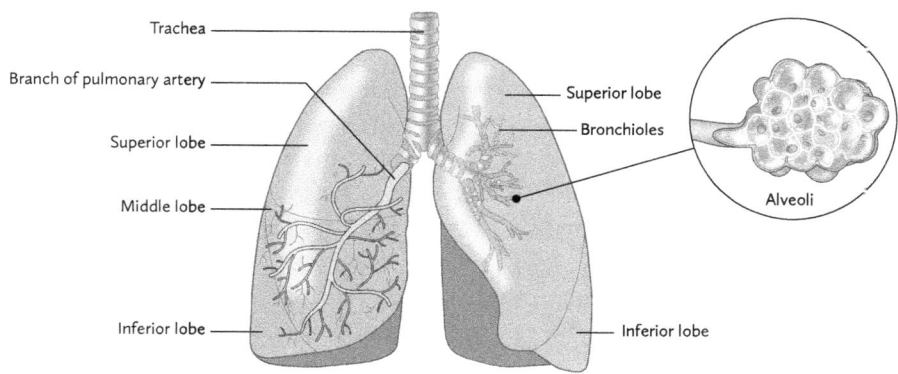

## FEEL IT

## SETTING A BREATH BASELINE 🔊

### Learning Objective

- Establish a breathing baseline for comparative purposes.

### Instructions

Like the red dot on a shopping center map indicating your location, you need to know your starting place so you can sense and register changes post-exploration and gauge which practices are most accessible and effective for you. Before and after breath explorations, repeat this baseline reading, or a brief version of it, to register differences in felt sense of your structure, breath, energy level, and state of mind.

- Lie in supine with support under your knees and head, if required. Alternatively, find a comfortable seated position. Take time to become aware of the floor beneath you and how your back body presses into it.

- With open and nonjudgmental attention, tune into your breath. The act of observation often stimulates change, but, as much as possible, allow your breath to remain as usual.

  - *What do you notice about your breath?*
  - *Is it audible?*
  - *How do you know you are breathing in, breathing out? What sensations indicate this?*
  - *Where do you feel the resonance or echo of your breath?*
  - *What parts of your body move with breath? Notice your belly, chest, sacrum, head, shoulder blades, arms, legs.*
  - *Is inhalation or exhalation longer?*
  - *Do you pause after inhalations and exhalations?*
  - *What is the amplitude of inhalations and exhalations? Are they deep or shallow? If successive breaths were plotted on a graph, what would the breath waves look like?*
  - *How much effort are you using?*
  - *What is the quality of your breath? How would you describe it: velvety, jerky, fluid, uneven, laboured, weak?*
  - *Is a feeling tone associated with the quality of breath?*
  - *What is your state of mind?*

- When you feel ready, open your eyes.

## EXPLORATION: DISCOVER YOUR STERNUM AND CLAVICLES

### Learning Objectives

- Deepen felt sense of the sternum and clavicles.

- Explore movement possibilities of the sternum and clavicles.

### Instructions

- Sit in a comfortable position, then do a brief breath check-in. Move your head slowly from side to side and notice the sensations and quality of movement.

    - *How do your sternum and clavicles move with breath? How easy and comfortable are neck rotations?*

### Palpation

- Use the fingertips of both hands to lightly tap and vibrate the sternum and clavicles. Breathe freely as you tap. Imagine that you are waking up cells. Explore humming into the bone as you tap.

- Using the soft, inquisitive pads of your fingers, sensitively and patiently explore the sternum, and xiphoid process, if present. Gently press your fingers into the flat hardness of the sternum to determine its size, shape, and topography.

- Palpate to differentiate the edge of the sternum and adjacent end of the ribs at the sternocostal joints.

- Locate the sternal notch at the top and explore the protruding sternoclavicular joints on either side.

- From the sternal notch, slide your fingers slightly below to the prominent horizontal ridge of the joint between the sternal body and manubrium. From there, walk your fingers laterally to feel the second rib articulation.

- Return to the prominent sternoclavicular joint and slowly and gently explore one clavicle at a time with the opposite hand. Feel the top, bottom, front, and back surfaces as you gradually palpate toward the shoulder. Move slowly with focused awareness to register its rounded and spiralic form. Palpate the protrusion of the acromioclavicular joint, the articulation with the scapula at the shoulder.

- Gently massage the soft tissue below and behind the clavicle.

- Take a few moments to attune to any changes in your breath.

### Movement

- Use your finger pads to glide the skin and subcutaneous fascia over underlying bone at different places on the sternum and clavicles.

    - *Does it feel pliable? Glued?*
    - *Does it move more freely in one direction?*
    - *Is it tender?*

- Position the finger pads of one hand on the sternal body and the other on the manubrium. Take several breaths to feel (or imagine) the sternum moving vertically upward on inhalations. Then, use your fingers to emphasize the up and down movement.

    - *Can you do this without your ribs protruding forward?*

    As the sternal body moves upward, visualize the manubrium hinging as it tips backward to wedge and widen the sternal notch.

- Place two fingers in your sternal notch and feel (or imagine) it widen as the clavicles spread on inhalations. Then, move your fingers apart to emphasize the spreading movement.

- Rest the fingertips of each hand on the same side clavicle. Become aware of (or imagine) the clavicles spreading sideways on inhalations, widening the shoulders. Visualize the clavicles spiralling as they spread apart. Use your fingers to emphasize the spread and spiral.

- Place the fingers of one hand on the sternum. Initiate small multiplanar movements from the sternum.

  - *What happens in the rest of your body?*

  Place your fingers on each clavicle and initiate small movements from there.

  - *How does this movement feel different?*

- Redo your baseline reading.

  - *Has your breath changed?*
  - *Are there differences in sternal or clavicular movement?*
  - *Does your head move more easily?*
  - *How does your experience change as you highlight the sternum and clavicles for your nervous system?*
  - *How could you incorporate this new awareness into your daily life?*

## EXPLORATION: DISCOVER YOUR RIBS

### Learning Objectives

- Deepen felt sense of the ribs.

- Understand rib plasticity and elasticity.

### Props

- Two blankets, one folded neatly into quarters and rolled lengthwise to approximately 12 cm (5 in.) in diameter

### Contraindications

- All the explorations in this chapter that include use of a blanket roll are contraindicated for anyone with advanced osteoporosis or existing fractures of the spine or ribs.

- Side-lying positions may be contraindicated for students with painful shoulder or hip conditions.

### Instructions

- Take a baseline in a supine position with straight legs. Notice the sensations of your body resting on the floor. Take a brief baseline of your breathing.

  - *Where do you sense rib movement as you breathe?*

- Place the rolled blanket lengthwise on the mat and arrange your spine, pelvis, and skull on the roll, with knees bent and feet standing. Adjust the roll diameter for comfort if necessary. You may require a second blanket under your head for neck support. Visualize the two halves of the rib basket draping over the roll and sense the widening across your chest.

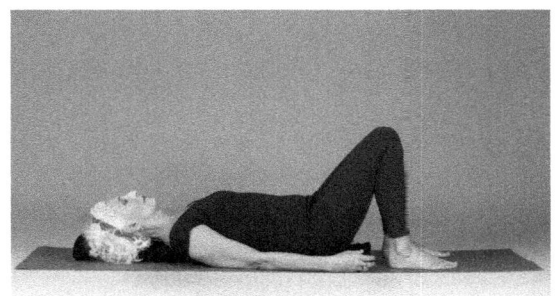

### Palpation

- Gently tap the ribs on one side with the opposite fingertips or cupped hand. Tap the area above and below the breast, the lower rib edge, and as far laterally as you can reach comfortably. Find a speed and intensity that feels good. Sense the vibration and imagine that you are awakening cellular intelligence.

- Use sensitive fingertips to slowly explore anterior and lateral ribs. Find the second rib again at the sternal angle and follow its curved pathway to the clavicle. Then, shift to lower ribs, moving your fingers back and forth across each rib as you trace backward and upward to the lateral rib cage. Avoid tender breast tissue.

- Explore the intercostal spaces on the same side by gently massaging soft tissue *between* ribs with a back and forth movement. Use your finger pads to find a comfortable depth of pressure.

- Continue your exploration on the same side but shift into side-lying position with the blanket supporting your head. With the same side hand, tap and then palpate the lateral and posterior ribs and intercostal spaces as above. Trace the pathway of the ribs from the lateral rib cage toward the spine.

- Palpate the lower two floating ribs carefully as they may be tender.

- After completion, lie on your back and recall your baseline.

  - *How do sensations or breath differ between the two sides?*

- Repeat this exploration on the other side.

- After palpating both sides, move to sitting and notice the effects of this practice.

  - *What do you notice about your ribs? Your breath? Any other effects?*

### Movement

- Still in a seated position, encircle your ribs with your hands. For several breaths, press firmly down and in as you follow the exhale.

  - *Can you sense the plasticity of the ribs?*

- Shift your focus to inhalations. Press into the ribs, then, partly through the inhalation, suddenly release your pressure as the ribs spring back to allow natural inflation of the lungs.

  - *Can you sense the elasticity of the ribs?*

- In your usual physical practice, explore moving with rib awareness and initiating movement from your ribs.

  - *How does rib awareness change your breath? Your movement?*
  - *How does initiating movement from your ribs change the way you move?*

## EXPLORATION: DISCOVER YOUR COSTOVERTEBRAL JOINTS

This practice is adapted from "Mobilizing the Articulations between the Ribs and Vertebrae" in *The Anatomy of Breathing* (Calais-Germain 2006).

The costovertebral joints are often forgotten under layers of tension. This exploration highlights their existence for your nervous system. Tension may ease as the towel cylinder specifically compresses joints and overlying soft tissue. **Dynamic Tension** created between the joints anchored on the towel and moving body parts also induces fascial release.

## Learning Objectives

- Deepen felt sense of costovertebral joints.

- Release excessive tension around costovertebral joints.

## Props

- A thin hand towel approximately 63 cm x 40 cm (25 in. x 16 in.) rolled lengthwise to a 6 cm (2.5 in.) diameter

## Instructions

- Take a baseline in supine.

  - *How are your spine and ribs arranged on the floor?*

- Place the rolled towel lengthwise on the floor. Rest back onto the roll, positioning it immediately to the right of the spine (the location of costovertebral joints) with the bottom end at waist level. Your pelvis, head and arms rest directly on the floor. Bend your knees with the feet a comfortable distance apart. If the roll feels too obtrusive, unroll it to a more comfortable diameter. Tuck any excess towel underneath your neck.

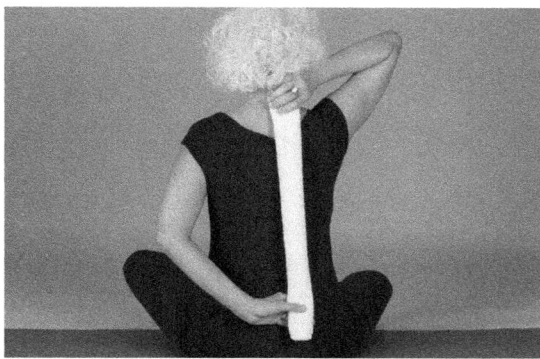

- Take time to adjust to the slight provocation of the rolled towel.

- Direct relaxed inhalations into the line of costovertebral joints pressing into the towel.

Notice the increase in pressure as your ribs expand. With each exhalation imagine your body draping over the towel in a restful way. Continue for several breaths, noticing changes in the sensation of pressure within each breath cycle.

- Continue with this focused inhalation throughout the rest of the exploration, tracking changes in sensations of pressure in the following movements:

  - On inhalations, slowly move your right knee laterally in a comfortable arc of movement, returning to neutral on exhalations. Repeat several times, then remain in the end position for a few breaths, continuing your focus on changing pressure sensations. Then, return your knee upright.
  - Place your arms slightly away from your body, palms facing upward. On each focused inhalation, slowly roll your right palm down and slide it along the floor toward your right foot. On exhalations, return your arm to the starting position. After repeating several times, remain in the end position for a few breaths. Then, return to the starting position.
  - Slowly rotate your head with each focused inhalation, returning to the starting position on exhalations. After repeating several times, remain in the end position for a few breaths, continuing with focused inhalations. Then, return your head to center.
  - Combine all three movements. With each focused inhalation, first move your knee, followed by the arm, then head. Return to neutral position with each exhalation. After repeating several times, remain in the end position for a few breaths. Then, return to neutral position.

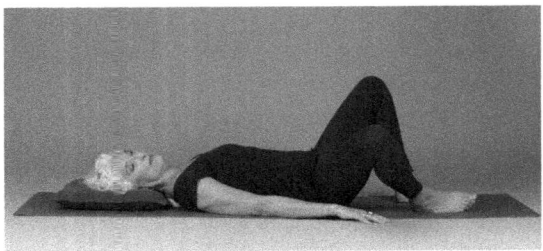

- Straighten your legs and remove the roll to register differences in sensations between sides.

  - *What do you notice?*

- Repeat the exploration on the left side.

- Move into sitting. Visualize the ribs hinging and opening like a book at the costovertebral joints as you inhale. Imagine your spine as the book spine and your ribs fanning open like the book cover.

  - *How does awareness of your costovertebral joints affect your body... breath... state of mind?*
  - *How might this awareness change your movement?*

## EXPLORATION: DISCOVER YOUR DIAPHRAGM

When you develop felt sense of the diaphragm and how it moves, visualizing the movement can initiate inhalation or exhalation. Breathing becomes deeper and effortless.

### Learning Objectives

- Deeper felt sense of the respiratory diaphragm.

- Sense diaphragmatic movement.

### Instructions

- Sit in a comfortable position. Encircle your lower ribs with both hands. Take a few moments to attune to the movement of your breath underneath your hands.

- Visualize the shape, size, and location of the diaphragm as it drapes horizontally over the abdominal organs. The top of the dome aligns with the natural nipple line anteriorly, while the costal attachments extend down to the floating ribs posteriorly.

- Place the soft pads of your right fingers below your sternum and gently palpate the lower border of the right rib basket from

front to back. Pause at several places to explore the topography of the lower ribs and circumference of the rib basket where the diaphragm attaches.

- Curl the fingertips of your right hand under the front ribs with the intention of touching the inner surface. Be gentle! Breathe normally and feel the descent of the diaphragm as it presses into your fingertips on inhalations.

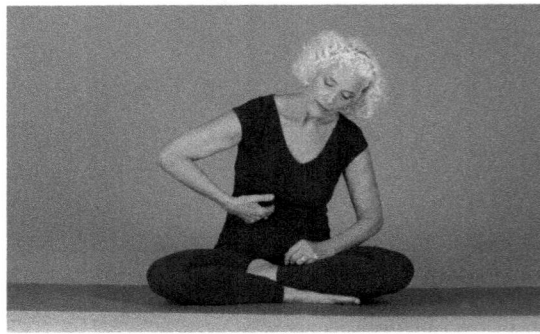

- Make repetitive *K* or *T* sounds to feel the diaphragm pushing into your fingertips.

- Repeat the palpation and sound at several places along the base of the diaphragm.

- Take a few moments to notice sensations on the side you palpated. Then, repeat the exploration on the left side. After completion, encircle your lower ribs with both hands.

  - *Has awareness of your diaphragm changed?*
  - *Has your breath changed?*

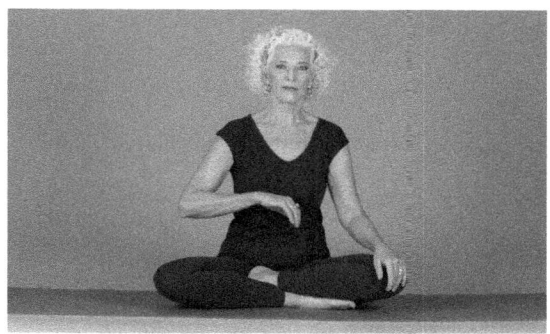

## THE JELLYFISH MUDRA

### Instructions

Watch a mesmerizing YouTube video of jellyfish rhythmically and fluidly contracting and expanding to visualize how the diaphragm moves (see www.youtube.com/watch?v=QzzZ2S5esu8&ab_channel=StephenMorris).

- Hold one hand limply at your solar plexus to mirror the position and shape of the diaphragm. Imagine the diaphragm as a jellyfish and your fingers as dangling crural tentacles.

- Visualize the jellyfish diaphragm flattening and widening as you extend your hand and wrist, widen your fingers, and move your hand slightly inferiorly to mimic the contraction and descent of the diaphragm. As it descends, feel how air can easily flow into the new spaciousness and lower air pressure of the lungs. Visualize the downward movement of the diaphragm initiating inhalations.

- Imagine the jellyfish narrowing and elongating in propulsion as you flex your hand and fingers and draw them superiorly to approximate the doming and rising of the diaphragm toward the chest cavity. Visualize the upward elastic recoil of the diaphragm initiating exhalations. As it ascends, feel how air can easily flow out of the lungs.

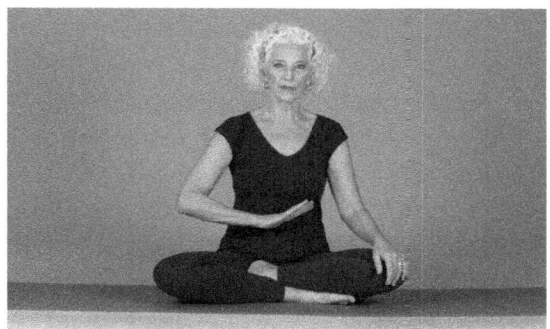

- Repeat these rhythmical movements for several breaths, tracking ascent and descent of the diaphragm. Then, visualize a stronger elastic recoil moving the jellyfish diaphragm higher in the torso as a way of effortlessly extending your exhalations.

- Rest your hand and continue the visualization of your jellyfish diaphragm.

- Sit quietly for a few moments and register any changes in sensation and breath.

  - *Can you sense your diaphragm moving?*
  - *How would your day be different if you recalled the jellyfish image during movement practice and daily activities?*
  - *When would it be most helpful?*
  - *Could it help you self-regulate?*

## EXPLORATION: DISCOVER YOUR INTERCOSTALS

### Learning Objectives

- Develop felt sense of intercostal activation.

- Release intercostal myofascia.

## INTERCOSTAL ACTIVATION

### Instructions

- Sit in a comfortable position and take a brief breathing baseline, noticing rib movement. Using the soft pads of your fingertips, gently palpate along several intercostal spaces to remind your nervous system of the location of the intercostal muscles.

- Encircle your lateral ribs with both hands to provide sensory feedback. As you inhale, visualize the diagonally oriented external intercostals activating in the intercostal spaces to expand and lift the ribs. Repeat several times, relaxing on exhalations.

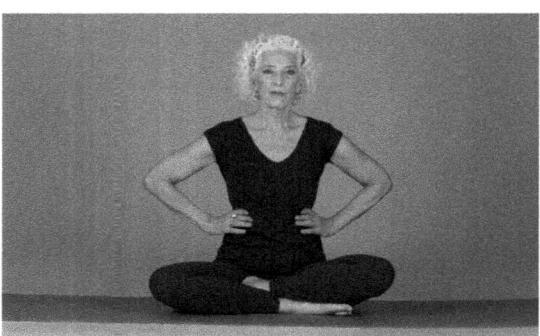

- Now focus on exhalations for several breaths, directing your mind internally to visualize and activate the internal intercostals pulling the ribs closer together and toward the midline, narrowing the thorax.

- Combine conscious activation of internal and external intercostals until you have a clear feeling of their actions.

- To encourage elasticity in respiratory myofascia, create **Dynamic Tension** by visualizing and activating the internal intercostals as you inhale, resisting full rib basket expansion. After several repetitions, do the opposite and visualize and activate the external intercostals as you exhale, resisting narrowing of the rib basket.

- Chant a drawn-out *eeeeee* sound as you exhale to help maintain a wider rib dimension. It's like applying the brakes and accelerator simultaneously.

- Sit quietly to register any changes in sensation, breath, and rib movement.

  – *What are you aware of?*

## INTERCOSTAL RELEASE: THE SKINFOLD PULL

This practice is adapted from "The Skinfold Experiment" in *Ways to Better Breathing* (Speads 1992).

### Instructions

- Begin this exploration either comfortably seated or lying in supine with bent knees.

- With a pincer grip formed by your thumbs and fingers, gently grasp a fold of skin and subcutaneous fascia and lift it away from the underlying tissue and ribs. Begin with the lower right ribs.

- With each inhalation, feel the ribs expanding toward the skinfold. As you exhale, hold the skinfold steady and feel the ribs pulling away, creating **Dynamic Tension**. Continue for three or four breaths or until your inhalation spontaneously deepens.

- Repeat at several places around the circumference of the right rib basket.

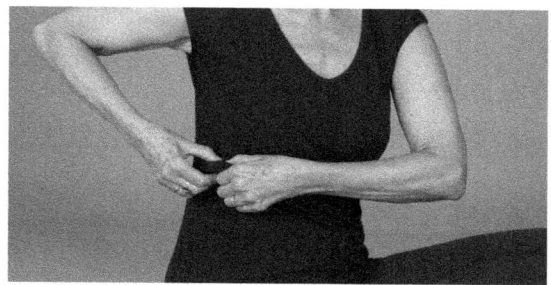

- Pause to register differences in sensations and breath capacity between sides.

- – *What do you notice?*
- Complete the exploration on the left side. If you have an available willing friend, ask them to do this practice on your back ribs.
- Sit quietly and register any changes.
  - – *What are you aware of?*
  - – *Is your breath different?*
  - – *How could daily intercostal awareness change your breath?*

## EXPLORATION: DISCOVER YOUR PELVIC DIAMOND

The Celestial Design Committee fashioned the pelvic diamond to expand and condense with breath. Focusing on this rhythmical movement can help restore both pliability and integrity to pelvic myofascia.

### Learning Objective

- Deepen felt sense of the pelvic floor during breathing.

### Instructions

- Sit comfortably on the floor, a chair, or exercise ball with your pelvis and lumbar spine in neutral position. Use support under your pelvis if necessary. Recall the pelvic diamond image.

- Slowly circle around the pubic bones, right sitting bone, coccyx, and left sitting bone. Circle several times in each direction until you sense the pelvic diamond bones.

- Notice movement in the pelvic floor as you breathe.

  - – *Can you feel it bulging to accommodate organs displaced by the descending diaphragm?*
  - – *What happens as you exhale?*

- Practice each of the following visualizations several times:

  - – As you inhale, visualize the pubic bone and coccyx moving apart. As you exhale, visualize these two points moving closer together.
  - – Imagine widening the distance between the sitting bones as you inhale and moving them closer together as you exhale.
  - – Last, visualize all four points spreading apart on inhalations and condensing toward center on exhalations. Using visual imagery can deepen felt sense of your pelvic floor. As you breathe, you can visualize a flower opening and closing. To reinforce pelvic floor tore, make an "s-s-s-s" sound on exhalations.

- Sit quietly to observe and feel any changes in sensation and breath, then stand and walk a little.

  - – *What's different?*
  - – *Does awareness of your pelvic diamond change how you breathe, sit or walk?*

See Chapter 5 for EA practices for the lungs.

## HEAL IT

Felt sense of structures can be heightened through movement exploration. Liberation of integral breath may be approached from inside out, or outside in; the breath container and contents affect each other. The container can be mobilized externally by either precise or global movement and by applying compression or tensional forces. It can be mobilized internally by directing the breath to specific areas.

## MOBILIZING THE BREATH CONTAINER

### Learning Objectives

- Mobilize components of the breath container to liberate breath movement.

- Isolate movement in specific bones and joints of the breath container.

- Create space for breath expansion.

### EXPLORATION: MOBILIZING RIBS

### Props

- A blanket folded into quarters and rolled from the folded edge into a 12–15 cm (5–6 in.) cylinder. You want comfortable yet firm support so you can release into it and receive sensory feedback. If it's uncomfortable, unroll the blanket to a more acceptable diameter or loosen the roll so it's flatter and wider.

- A pillow for your head

- Pillows or folded blankets for added support, if necessary

### Practice Notes

- Begin by taking a baseline breath reading either sitting or standing.

  - *How do your ribs move as you breathe?*

- Each time you inhale, consciously direct the breath to the area of the ribs pressing into the blanket. Use the feedback of the roll to focus your breath.

### BREATHING INTO THE LATERAL RIBS

In this practice you will consciously direct your breath to specific areas of the ribs. Use feedback from your hand or the blanket roll to focus your breath.

### Instructions

- Arrange the blanket roll horizontally across your mat. Position yourself side lying with the roll placed between armpit and waist. Align your spine and head with the long edge of the mat and support your head on a pillow. The bottom shoulder and hip rest squarely on the floor without your body tipping forward or back.

- Place the palm of your top hand on the lateral ribs. Attune to rib movement as you breathe in a relaxed way. Notice how they spread apart and expand into space and then move together and condense toward your midline. Observe for several breaths, then deliberately direct breath into the ribs underneath your hand and amplify the movement.

- Shift your awareness to feel the pressure on the lower ribs as they expand into the blanket roll on inhalations. Notice the decrease in pressure as you exhale. Continue observing for several breaths, then deliberately direct breath into the lower ribs to amplify the pressure.

- Finally, divide your awareness between top and bottom ribs and direct several breaths equally in both directions. Observe any sensations of inhalations and exhalations.

## RIB ROLLS: RIB INITIATION 📹

### Instructions

- Remain in side-lying position with the palms of your hands together at shoulder height.

- Initiating movement from the ribs, slowly tip forward to roll toward the front ribs. Track sensations point by point as your bottom ribs are compressed by the rolling movement.

- Continue to track sensations as you slowly tip backward, rolling onto your back ribs.

- Repeat several times, initiating forward and back movement from the ribs.

  - *How does your breath want to coordinate with the movement?*

- Contrast the movement by doing a few repetitions initiating the rolling by reaching your arm away from you on the floor.

  - *What's different?*

- Rest for a few breaths.

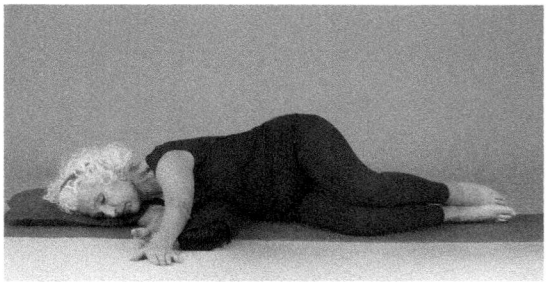

- Add in a twist: Place the palms together with arms resting on the floor at shoulder height. On an inhalation, initiate movement from your ribs to tip backward and roll toward your back ribs. Allow the backward roll to initiate a simultaneous lift of your top arm to 90 degrees.

- On the exhalation, roll further onto your back ribs and continue the arc of arm movement toward the floor behind you. If your arm doesn't reach the floor, stop at your comfortable range or use support, as necessary. Continue to track sensations throughout the movements.

- Rest in the twist for a few breaths, feeling the back ribs expand into the roll on inhalations. On an exhalation, roll toward the front ribs and allow the movement of the rib basket to initiate the return of the arm to the starting position.

- Repeat several times, then rest for a few breaths.

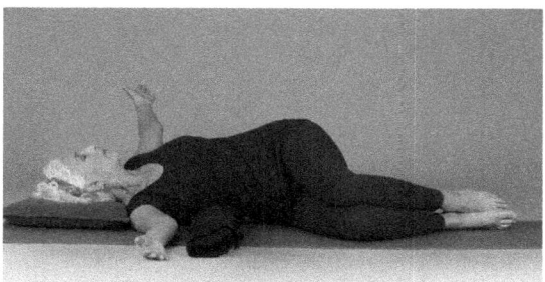

## WINDMILL

### Instructions

- Remain in side-lying position with palms together. Initiating from your ribs, roll backward and drag your fingertips a few inches on the floor in a circular movement toward your head. The elbow, wrist, and fingers remain relaxed and slightly bent. Feel the rib basket compressing on the blanket as you roll incrementally onto the back ribs.

- As your arm circles, pause at random places along the arc of movement and direct several breaths into areas of rib compression. Allow your head to be moved as the torso twists.

- When you reach your comfortable endpoint, start the slow return journey toward the starting position.

- After completing the movements on one side, return to baseline position and notice changes in breath and rib movements.

  - *How does freeing your ribs affect other parts of your body... your breath... the quality of your mind?*

  - *How could flexibility and spaciousness in your ribs change how you move in the world?*

- Repeat the movements on the other side.

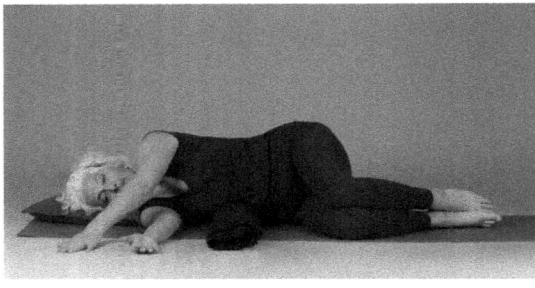

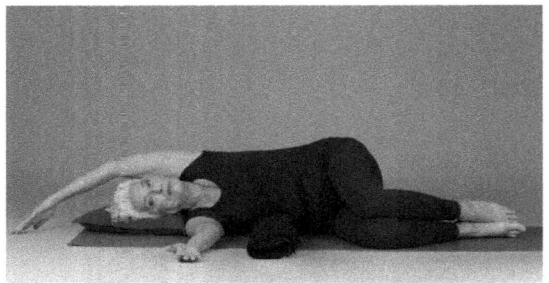

## EXPLORATION: MOBILIZE THE SPINE

### Props

- A yoga belt

### Practice Notes

- Use feedback from the belt to refine precision of breathing into and initiating movement from specific vertebrae.

- Notice areas of restriction and focus on those places.

- You can work with a partner who provides extra feedback with firm finger pressure into the belt on either side of the spine. The partner can also give verbal feedback about extraneous movement or imprecise movement initiation.

### Instructions

- Place the belt across your upper back and under your armpits, holding the ends in each hand. Arrange yourself on all fours with shoulders positioned directly over hands and hips over knees. Adjust the belt to fit snugly across your upper back to provide sensory feedback.

- Direct your inhalations toward vertebrae touching the belt. Initiate movement from those vertebrae, pressing upward into the belt to slightly flex your spine. With each exhalation, release the movement and return to neutral.

  - *Can you refine movement initiation with breath specifically directed to the belt?*

- After several breaths, when your movement initiation becomes more precise, move the belt down the spine and repeat the practice.

- Repeat at several places until you reach the top of the sacrum.

- Sit in a comfortable position to sense any changes in breath and body sensations.

 – *How does your breath change when you have freer movement in your spine?*
 – *What subtle changes do you notice on other levels?*

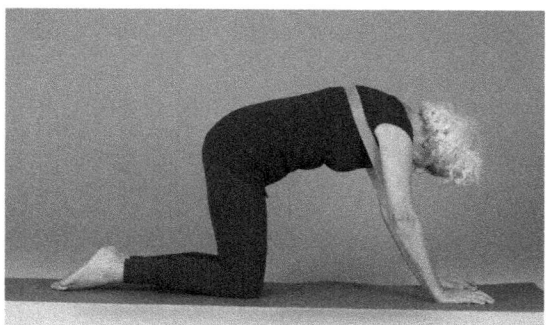
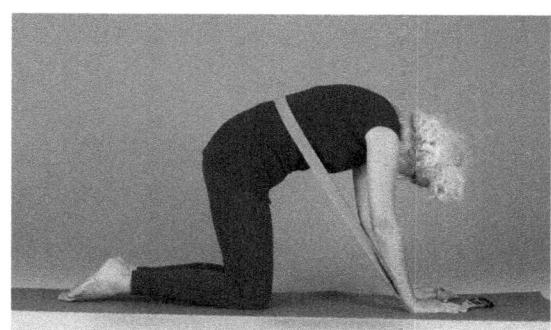

## EXPLORATION: FREE THE CLAVICLES

### Practice Notes

- As you slide your fingertips across your clavicles, use enough pressure to drag the skin and fascia on underlying bone, giving the suggestion of widening and spreading.

- The counterpressure of the bottom arm is equally important as the reach of the top arm in creating **Dynamic Tension** to widen across both clavicles.

### Instructions

- Start on all fours with shoulders positioned directly over hands and hips over knees.

- As you inhale, slide the fingertips of your right hand up the inside of the left arm from wrist to shoulder, then across both clavicles until fingertips rest on the right anterior shoulder, with elbow pointing to the ceiling. Adjust the speed of hand movement to the length of your inhalation or take two breaths, if necessary. Simultaneously, apply equal counterpressure into the floor with the left hand so both arms are activated. Notice the dynamic tension created between the stabilizing bottom arm and the upper reaching arm.

- Remain in the posture for several breaths. Relax slightly with each exhalation and slide your fingers down to the sternum. As you inhale, drag your fingertips across the right clavicle to the lateral end, creating a sense of width through the clavicle. Simultaneously, apply counterpressure into the floor with the left hand establishing a clear line of dynamic tension from the hand pressing into the floor through the torso to the opposite elbow. Allow the breath to move you within the posture.

- Return the right hand to the floor.

- Repeat on the left side.

- Sit in a comfortable seated position, then stand and move your arms randomly.

 – *How have your breath and body sensations changed?*

– *Have your breath and movement habits affected your clavicles?*

– *How does freeing your clavicles affect your arm movements?*

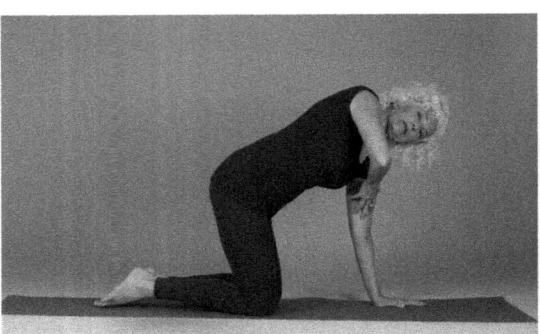

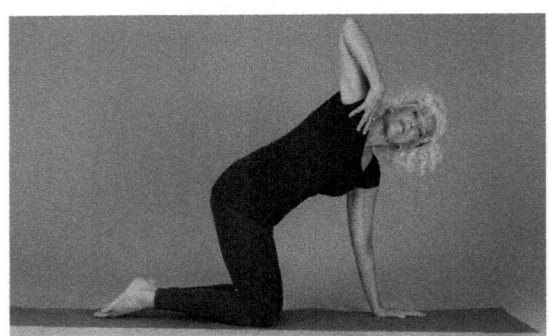

## DOUBLE DUTY FOR THE DIAPHRAGM

### EXPLORATION: THE ELASTIC DIAPHRAGM

The same movement can have different effects when awareness is directed toward specific bony, myofascial, or organ structures. Most movements can refine and release integral breath when done with somatic awareness of the breathing container and contents. For example, the rib basket explorations above would produce different results if done with awareness centered on the diaphragm or lungs (see Chapter 5).

Visualize yourself trying to blow up a new, stiff, and unyielding balloon. Then, visualize softening it and making it more pliable by pulling and massaging in different directions. The diaphragm can be stiff like the balloon and softened in the same way; consciously creating **Dynamic Tension** between anchored and moving structures can increase diaphragmatic elasticity by tensioning its extensive fascial connections with the spine and limbs. Different body positions anchor one or more spinal, rib, or central tendon attachments of the diaphragm, allowing unanchored attachments to move and create **Dynamic Tension**.

Consciously directing descent and ascent of the diaphragm can then amplify tensional forces.

### Learning Objective

- Create pliability and resilience in diaphragmatic myofascia.

### Practice Notes

- As you move, visualize and sense dynamic tension between stabilized and moving parts of the diaphragm.

- You have numerous variables to explore when creating dynamic tension: three diaphragmatic attachments (rib, spine, and central tendon), the spine that moves in multiple planes, and arms and legs that can tension the diaphragm through fascial continuities. Remember how the diaphragm interdigitates with transversus abdominus, quadratus lumborum, and psoas muscles. Activation or elongation of these muscles will affect the diaphragm.

- Any pose, whether done lying down, seated,

or standing, can be used as a vehicle for exploring elasticity of the diaphragm.

- Track sensations as the diaphragm ascends and descends, noticing subtle differences when you move into a posture on inhalations or exhalations.

## Instructions

- Sit on the floor with your left knee crossed over the right with each foot beside the opposite hip. Arms rest at your sides with hands on the floor. Raise your pelvis on a bolster or folded blankets if necessary for comfort.

- Pause to reconnect with felt sense of your jellyfish diaphragm moving with breath. Continue to focus on diaphragm movement as you repeat each of the following movements several times:

### Spinal Flexion and Extension

- As you inhale, raise both arms overhead so your spine extends. As you exhale, lower your arms and round your back in flexion.

- After several repetitions, reverse the breath. Exhale as your arms raise and spine extends and inhale on spinal flexion.

- Remain in the extended position for several breaths. Explore moving your arms separately and together in various ways to subtly increase dynamic tension on the diaphragm through fascial continuities. You can play with internal and external rotation, different angles, levels, intensities, tempos, and combinations of these variables as you track movement of your diaphragm. Moving your spine in different planes and moving on either inhalations or exhalations can also tether diaphragmatic attachments.

- Return to the starting position.

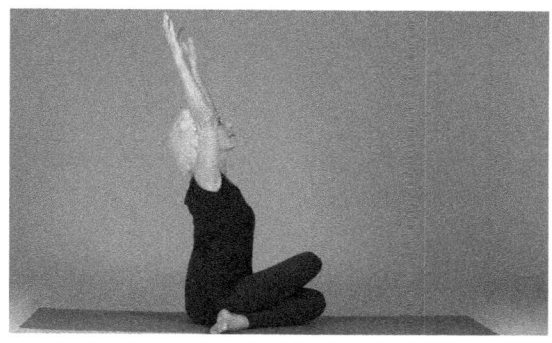

### Side Bend

- As you inhale, sweep your right arm sideways and overhead until your spine side bends to the left. Yield through your left elbow. Return to the starting position as you exhale.

- After several repetitions, reverse the breath, exhaling as you side bend.

- After several repetitions, remain in side bend for several breaths. Track the descent and ascent of your diaphragm and notice how sensations change on inhalations and exhalations. Explore moving your right arm in various ways to subtly increase dynamic tension through the fascial continuities.

- Repeat on the other side.

- Return to the starting position.

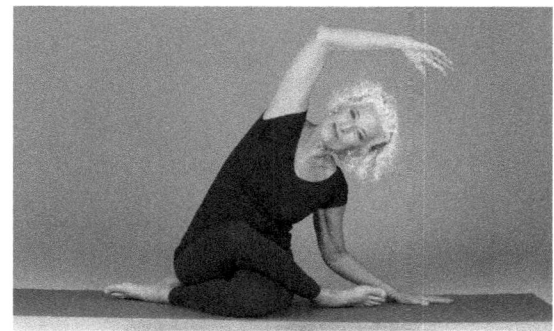

### Twist

- Place your left hand on the right shoulder. As you exhale, move your elbow horizontally to the right so your spine slightly twists. Return to the starting position as you inhale.

- After several repetitions, reverse the breath, inhaling as you move into the twist.

- After several repetitions, remain in the twist for a few breaths. Track the descent and ascent of your diaphragm. Play with moving your arm at different angles to find subtle ways of increasing dynamic tension on the diaphragm through the indirect fascial continuities.

- Repeat on the other side.

- Reverse the position of your legs and repeat the movements.

- Pause to register sensations and changes in breath

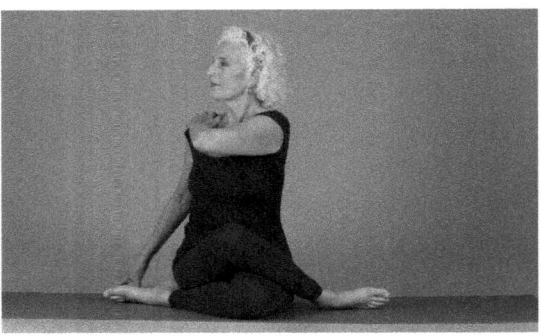

- *How has felt sense of your diaphragm changed?*
- *Which movements give you the most diaphragmatic elasticity?*
- *How does your breath change?*
- *Do you experience any nonphysical effects, like changes in energy or state of mind?*

## EXPLORATION: THE STABILITY DIAPHRAGM

Both breathing and stability functions of the diaphragm can be consciously controlled by isolating and refining awareness and activation of its specific parts. It can be deliberately activated independently of its breathing function to increase intra-abdominal pressure and spinal stability. In asana and other movements, when unimpeded movement of the diaphragm is the primary directive, optimal alignment and motor control often follow naturally. When organized around this intention, the shape or form of a movement decreases in importance. The pose may not be as glorious but will likely express ease, stability, and integral breath.

### Learning Objective

- Access the diaphragm as a source of support.

### Seated Exploration
#### Instructions

- Sit in a comfortable position with your spine effortlessly erect and the diaphragm area open and free.

- Encircle your lower ribs with both hands. Track the ascending and descending movements of your diaphragm.

- On inhalations, visualize the large circumference of the diaphragm activating against the resistance of the weight and volume of abdominal organs, pushing them downward. Feel the lower rib basket widening.

- As you exhale visualize the diaphragm pushing up against the weighted resistance of the heart and lungs. Notice how the diaphragm works harder on both inhalation and exhalation when you visualize it moving against resistance.

- After several repetitions, pause to register sensations and changes in breath.

  - *What do you notice?*

## Triangle Pose (Trikonasana)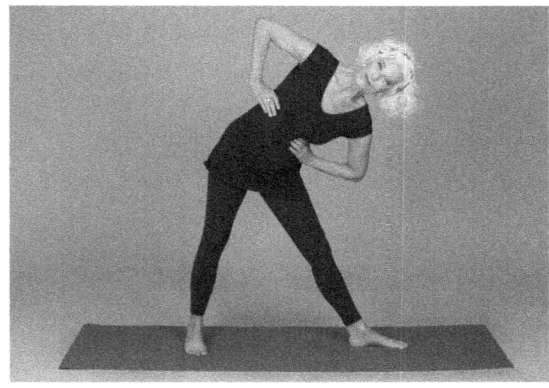
### Practice Notes

- Using the diaphragm as a focus frees you from remembering many alignment details. Whatever details you incorporate are always measured in relation to the freedom of the diaphragm.

- Integrate stability diaphragm awareness into other standing poses, especially balance poses.

### Instructions

- Stand in Mountain pose (Tadasana) and widen your stance comfortably to approximately 60–90 cm (2–3 ft.). Turn your right foot and leg 90 degrees outward and turn your left foot inward slightly. Encircle your lower ribs with both hands and continue to breathe as above, tracking resisted diaphragmatic movement.

- As you inhale, bend sideways from your right **Hip Socket**, tipping your pelvis and spine a few degrees to the right. Pause as you exhale.

- Continue the pelvic side bending incrementally, breath by breath, moving a few degrees at a time. Allow your spine to be carried by the pelvic movement. Stop as soon as you feel challenged to breathe freely into the circumference of the lower ribs.

- Lower your right arm to rest on your leg wherever it reaches comfortably, then raise your left arm toward the ceiling. Continue the resisted breathing for a few more breaths. If it's difficult to maintain a feeling of freedom in your diaphragm, return your hands to your ribs.

- Initiate your exit from the pose with an inhalation.

- Repeat this process, reversing the breathing pattern. Move incrementally into the pose as you exhale and pause as you inhale.

- Repeat the practice on the other side.

- Stand in Mountain pose to register sensations and effects of moving and breathing in this way.

  - *What feels different when you move into the posture on an inhalation or exhalation? Which feels more stable?*
  - *How could the stability diaphragm practice help you to establish mental and emotional steadiness?*

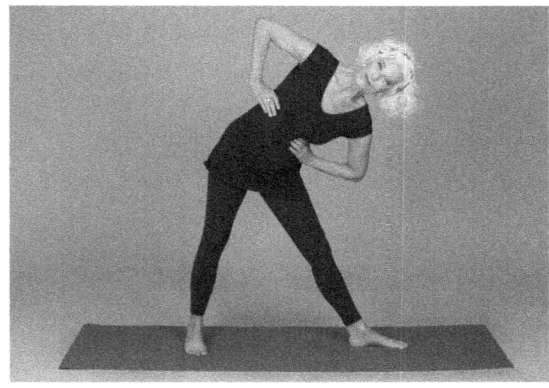

## BREATH PRACTICES

*Where* and *how* we breathe affects our blood chemistry and overall health. By redirecting shallow, upper chest breathing and sinking the breath deeper in the torso, it's easier to access calm and relaxed integral breath. The following practices challenge habitual breathing patterns by deliberately directing breath to the lower ribs or back body. The cumulative effect of consistent practice is efficient effortless, and omnidirectional breath that engages contents and container.

### Learning Objective

- Repattern different modes of breathing to optimize responsive, integral breath and breath chemistry.

### Props

- A yoga belt

### Practice Notes

- Monitor your effort level. Use awareness, ease, and specificity rather than force.

- Have patience with yourself as you refine your ability to direct breath into specific areas.

### FOUNDATIONAL PRACTICE: THORACO-DIAPHRAGMATIC BREATH (SURROUND BREATH)

In this foundational practice, breath is consciously directed to the circumference of the lower ribs. If you are an upper chest breather, then repatterning this mode can radically alter your experience on all koshic levels as blood chemistry levels normalize and the nervous system balances.

Deliberate engagement of abdominal muscles functions as a frontal corset, causing organs to bulge sideways and backward as the diaphragm descends. The abdomen expands minimally, and external intercostal muscles are consciously activated on inhalations. On exhalations, internal intercostals and abdominal muscles are consciously activated.

Engagement of abdominal muscles increases intra-abdominal pressure, which helps to stabilize the spine. The diaphragm strengthens because it must work harder to descend during inhalation. Surround breath can create a mental state of clarity and steadiness, and support movements and tasks that require strength and core stabilization.

### Instructions

- Sit in a comfortable position and wrap the yoga belt around the lower ribs, crossing it below your sternum and holding the ends loosely in both hands.

- On inhalations, visualize the fluidic movement of your jellyfish diaphragm flattening and widening the entire circumference of your lower ribs. Consciously activate your external intercostals.

- Relax your abdomen on exhalations and visualize your diaphragm doming upward. Consciously activate your internal intercostals to condense the ribs toward the midline.

- Tighten the belt snugly and continue surround breathing while maintaining this slight resistance on the ribs. As you inhale, gently activate your abdominal corset and direct breath sideways and backward into the feedback of the belt. Notice areas that are more difficult to access.

- As you exhale, pull the belt a little tighter to emphasize the narrowing of the ribs toward the midline.

- Continue for several breaths.

- When you are finished, sit comfortably to register any physical or energetic effects.

  - *What do you notice?*
  - *In what daily life situations might surround breathing be helpful?*

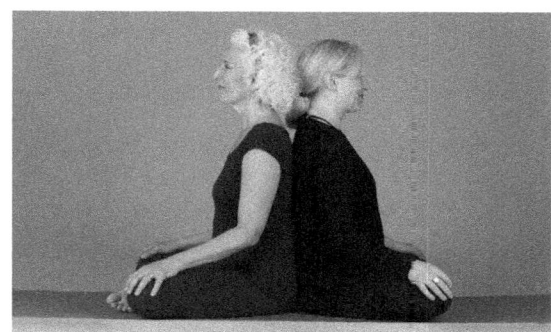

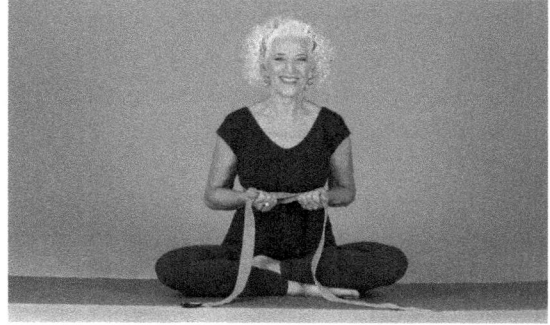

## PARTNER EXPLORATION: BACK BREATHING

This practice is adapted from a practice developed by Sandra Sammartino (1990).

Both breath and movement can transform when awareness is focused on the back body, an often underutilized capacity of the posterior rib basket. Psychologically, it can help you steady yourself and take a step back to observe from a broader, nonintellectual perspective. Many students have reported that back breathing also helps reduce emotional reactivity.

This exploration is best done in partners but may be done alone sitting against a soft surface like an exercise ball.

### Instructions

- Sit comfortably back-to-back with your partner.

- Focus on the contact of your backs. Feel the warmth and pressure of your partner's back. Become aware of breath movement sensations.

- Decide who will "lead," then gradually synchronize your breathing.

- Using the surround breath awareness, direct inhalations into your whole back body, feeling it widen and press into your partner's back. Exhale in a relaxed way.

- After a few minutes, move several inches apart. Focus on sensations of your breath and back body. Notice any feelings that arise.

- Take a few minutes to share your experience with your partner.

  - *What did you notice?*
  - *In what daily life situations could back breathing be helpful?*

## EXPLORATION: I AM BREATHED

After laying the groundwork for integral breath with EA practices, the ultimate practice is to let go of all information and conscious control and allow the wisdom of your body to emerge.

### Learning Objective

- Use breath to connect to subtle realms.

### Instructions

- Sit or lie in a comfortable, supported position.

- Simply witness your breath with open attention. Let go of notions of anatomy or of directing your breath in a certain way.

- Open a place inside yourself for the breath to enter and become receptive to the inward flow of air. Surrender to the outflow. Allow yourself to be moved by the breath.

- Your breath connects your inner and outer worlds. As air flows in, know that you are permitting some of the outer world to enter and permeate your whole being. As air flows out, know that some of your inner Self is moving out to participate in the greater world.

- As air flows in, know that you are filling with life-force energy. As air flows out, know that you are returning life-force energy to the universe. Witness this interchange and sense the oneness of inner and outer worlds.

- Sense your inner aliveness. Silently repeat to yourself *I am being breathed.*

- After 5–10 minutes of practice, sit quietly and allow yourself to receive the fruits of your practice.

  – *What do you notice?*

## THERAPEUTIC APPLICATIONS

> Breathing dysfunction shows more correlation with low back pain than obesity or physical activity levels, and repatterning diaphragm function can reduce both low back pain and urinary incontinence.
>
> *(Smith, Russell, and Hodges 2006)*

Breathing patterns and structure are interdependent. In therapeutic applications of EA, there is wisdom in addressing habitual breathing patterns, respiratory container, and contents. In my clinical practice, I usually start with breath, irrespective of presenting condition. High stress levels have become normalized with the fast pace and demands of daily life and contribute to an epidemic of chronic illnesses like diabetes, heart disease, depression, and immune disorders (Mariotti 2015). Imbalanced blood chemistry caused by chronic hyperventilation constricts smooth muscle in organs and can contribute to dysfunctional physiology in every system. When the sympathetic nervous system works overtime in a sustained state of heightened activity, breathing becomes faster, shallow, and less able to moderate physiological and psychological balance.

In a study examining the relationship between pain and faulty breathing, 87.2 percent of the participants in one community experienced musculoskeletal pain. Almost 60 percent of the study group had disordered breathing patterns in relaxed states and 75 percent showed disordered patterns when taking a deep breath (Perri and Halford 2004). This finding is much higher than the 10 percent of the general population with diagnosed hyperventilation syndrome identified by Thomas *et al.* (2005), and more in line with my anecdotal clinical observations. Perri and Halford highlighted the importance of repatterning dysfunctional breathing for pain relief. Other benefits articulated by research include decreasing both physiological and psychological stress through regulation of respiratory rate, blood pressure, and cortisol levels (Hopper *et al.*, 2019).

Breathing can be compromised by habitual postures like propped military or forward head posture, or by postural responses to anxiety and depression. In the prevalent disordered breathing pattern of upper chest breathing, overuse of secondary breathing muscles causes chronic tension in the neck, jaw, chest, and shoulders, and can cause anxiety. Hyperventilation, commonly associated with upper chest breathing, is an often-undiagnosed pattern that can dysregulate oxygen and carbon dioxide ratios associated with the high incidence of current stress-related pathologies. Reverse breathing is a more severe dysfunction in which the abdomen condenses on inhalations, inhibiting full descent of the diaphragm and lung expansion. Medical conditions like COPD, emphysema, and asthma can cause hyperinflation of the lungs that limits full movement of the diaphragm and leads to deconditioning of the core cylinder of support.

Everyone, but especially people with breathing pattern disorders and respiratory conditions, can benefit from EA breath practices. The explorations are inherently therapeutic by toning the parasympathetic nervous system and creating more physical space for integral breath. Whether the cause of dysregulated breathing is postural, psychological, or physiological, assessment findings often include rigidity of the breath container, underutilization of lung capacity, restricted movement of the diaphragm, and shallow, upper chest breathing.

While discussion of treatment for specific respiratory pathologies is beyond the scope of this book, I will say that my clinical work has shown me how EA practices build self-regulation skills needed to heal dysfunctional breathing and liberate integral breath. Students first use IA to discover habitual breathing, alignment, movement, and mental patterns. As they use EA practices to repattern healthier habits, they connect more deeply to themselves and learn to use breath as both a barometer and modulator of inner experience. This often life-changing process requires time, patience, and education.

The underlying intentions of EA breath practices are to refine breath awareness, awaken somatic intelligence, and optimize alignment and movement of each part of the breathing apparatus to adequately oxygenate every cell. These practices encourage the lungs to maximally inflate, the diaphragm to move freely in its full potential range, rib heads to rotate easily at costovertebral joints, sternum to hinge, clavicles to spiral, and secondary breathing muscles to remain relaxed while primary muscles do their job. With these goals in mind, all parts can work together to liberate the breath. The result is integral breath that is lower in the torso, effortless, more efficient, and adaptable. Rather than something that must be "done" or "performed," we learn to cultivate a sense of allowing themselves to be breathed. As integral breath is revealed, each kosha is affected. As our body finds ease and our mind settles, we can experience and live more from our wholeness.

## KOSHIC CONTEMPLATIONS

### Annamaya Kosha

- *How does your habitual posture affect your breath?*
- *Is your breath container rigid or flexible?*
- *How do you normally breathe during movement and activities?*
- *How have the EA practices affected your movement practice and daily activities?*

### Pranamaya Kosha

- *What is your usual energy level?*
- *What are the energetic effects of your habitual way of breathing?*
- *Do you hold your breath?*
- *When do you breathe freely?*
- *How has your breath changed with EA practices?*

### Manomaya Kosha

- *What have you noticed about the connection between your breath and emotions? Between your breath and stress?*
- *Which anatomical breath structure works best for you as a touchstone for self-regulation?*

### Vijnanamaya Kosha

- *How does your breath reflect your personality and conditioning?*
- *Do you embody any breath metaphors? Are you "waiting with bated breath" or do you "barely have time to breathe"?*
- *How can you use your breath to connect to your deeper Self?*

### Anandamaya Kosha

- *How can you use your breath to feel more connected to the Mystery?*
- *Can you breathe with gratitude into whatever life offers you?*

> As I inspire, with gratitude I breathe in Life.
> As I exhale, I surrender.
> As I inspire, with gratitude I breathe in Light.
> As I exhale, I surrender.
> As I inspire, with gratitude I breathe in Love.
> As I exhale, I surrender.
>
> *Anonymous*

## KEY CONCEPTS

- Breath links mind, body, and spirit and has profound effects on every aspect of life
- Integral breath is relaxed, adaptable, calm, and emanates naturally from a responsive body.
- Interoceptive EA practices can optimize the function of each element of the breath.
- Dysfunctional breathing has a critical impact on emotional states, clarity of thinking, and ability to make good decisions.
- Breathing is the only autonomic function with voluntary control.
- The state of the breath container and contents affect each other.

- The diaphragm has dual functions as the main breathing muscle and trunk stabilizer.
- Health and function of the circulatory and respiratory systems are interdependent.
- The sternum and clavicles are designed to participate in breath.
- Ribs are both plastic and elastic.
- **Thoraco-Diaphragmatic Breath** can balance the nervous system and blood chemistry.
- Breath can be compromised by habitual postures.
- Repatterning dysfunctional breathing patterns can decrease pain and physiological and psychological stress.

## CHAPTER 4

# Fascia: Everything Is Connected

*Unify*      *Separate*
*Sense*      *Support*

From our skin down to the nucleus and cytoskeleton of our 30 trillion cells, we are a continuous body-wide matrix of fascia. This neuromyofascial net is a pervasive metasystem communicating with, connecting, and supporting all other physiological systems to work as a synergistic whole (Langevin 2006). The term *neuromyofascial net* was coined by Robert Schleip to describe the intimacy of the nervous, muscular, and fascial systems (Schleip 2005). The vast fascial network creates unity, continuity, and relationship throughout the body by connecting all structures in one continuous tensional matrix, yet it paradoxically also separates these structures. Without the supportive and coordinating fascial system, life would be challenging for cells, and systems could not function. This body-wide network consists of tensioned tissue that gives us form, keeps us upright and allows us to move.

With an abundance of forms on a continuum from liquid to firm, our fascial system forms a multidimensional, collagenous web surrounding, permeating, and separating structures from top to bottom, inside to outside, and on all levels of scale from cells to gross structures. Compartments and segments within the continuous fascial web create relationships between anatomical parts. Cells, organs, muscles, bones, and neurovascular structures are embedded and integrated within the supportive fascial matrix. The form and qualities of fascia depend on its local function and the biomechanical forces exerted on it both internally and externally. How we move and use our body counts.

> The body-wide continuity of fascia became clear to me when I did a biotensegrity-focused cadaver dissection with John Sharkey and saw how anatomical structures are distinct only when arbitrarily cut away from surrounding tissues.

Fascia has been variously described as the fabric of wholeness, a sensory organ, an organ of form, of innerness, and the medium through which body and spirit communicate (Schleip 2017; van der Wal 2016; Still 1899). All these descriptions attest to its abundant, pervasive nature and multiplicity of function. Contemplating the multidimensionality of fascia can connect us with our own multidimensionality.

The Celestial Design Committee orchestrated a miracle of creation as we unfold embryologically from a single fertilized cell to a full human being with differentiated tissues. We self-organize as internal forces direct the process of differentiation into diverse cells, tissues, organs, and systems, interwoven on all levels by fascia. All collagen-containing structures arise from the middle layer of embryological tissue (the mesoderm). From the one comes the interconnected many (because of fascial continuities, *fascia* also indicates plural). As a result of this continuity, whenever one part of the body is subjected to internal or external forces, the rest of the fascial web is impacted.

From the perspective of the fascial system, body and mind are inseparable, and all movement involves the whole body. As the physical representation of wholeness, fascia can be directly experienced by cultivating felt sense of its presence, structure, and qualities, and by practicing whole-body movements with fascial awareness. As we explore parts of the body, we remember the context of the fascial matrix containing everything, connecting everything, and allowing all parts to communicate. We can embody this awareness of continuity in EA practices to create integrity and flow in movement and life.

As a metasystem, the health of the fascial system affects the health of all other systems. If fascia is pathologically dense, adhered, congested, or inflamed, physiology and movement capacity of surrounding structures suffers. EA practices can support our fascial network to intelligently adapt and support our bodies by consciously balancing compression and tension forces and encouraging resilient elasticity.

## BIOTENSEGRITY

My understanding of biotensegrity owes much to my conversation with Susan Lowell de Solorzano, co-founder of the Stephen M. Levin Biotensegrity Archive, in 2023. Biotensegrity is an emerging wholistic paradigm that challenges the long-established biomechanical model and application of Newtonian physics to biological forms. This evolving paradigm uses the omnidimensional design of the fascial web to describe how living systems work as one integrated whole. The word *biotensegrity* was coined by orthopedic surgeon and biotensegrity authority Dr. Stephen Levin in recognition that biological forms, including humans, reflect the same qualities of tensegrity that govern all scales of existence from cells to organisms.

The word *tensegrity*, coined by Buckminster Fuller, is a combination of the words *tension* and *integrity*. In tensegrity structures, structural integrity is based on balanced relationships between compression elements that do not touch and a continuous tension network containing them. Tension elements pulling in and compression elements pushing out create an efficient architecture characterized by stability, integrity, and the ability to carry and distribute considerable loads. In humans, forces and loads are transferred nonlinearly through this system of tension and compression elements rather than directly passed by compression between bones. In practice, as we move away from biomechanical concepts of "stretching and strengthening" toward establishing "tensional equilibrium" where tension is functionally distributed throughout the body, we are more likely to experience balance, right effort, strength, and integrated movement.

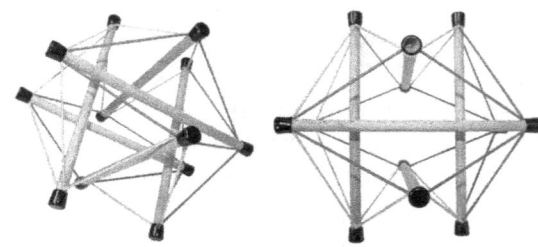

The biotensegrity model unravels movement phenomena that are inadequately explained by the biomechanical model, and firmly places biological movement in the softer, spiralic natural world. We are not machines with straight lines and levers. Like the yogic kosha model, biotensegrity acknowledges our wholeness and continuity, viewing the "parts" as interpenetrating and interdependent facets of the whole. Like the multifaceted jewels in Indra's net, each facet affects, and is affected by, all other facets.

This model offers a sensible explanation for the way humans self-assemble. From embryo to adult, we are in a continuous state of self-creation and self-regulation as we respond to biological forces from within and environmental forces from without. We are endlessly and proficiently reconfiguring tension and compression forces to change shape and move with efficiency and integration. At the macro level, our soft fascia provides the tensional network supporting bony compression elements; however, at the micro level, even the nucleus of cells contains both tension and compression elements (Tadeo *et al.*, 2014). When our tensioned fascial network is balanced and resilient, we can change shape and move efficiently by altering either tension or compression elements. Stresses applied anywhere will be distributed throughout our structure so we can stabilize in any gravitational orientation. At some point, most of us experience a system failure, where our ability to adapt to forces is exceeded and we experience injury, pain, dysfunction, and perhaps psychological distress. The biotensegrity model gives us hope that our ability to adapt and self-create can lead to greater health and function. EA is one pathway of self-creation through remodeling the fascial system.

> We are bees, and our body is a honeycomb. We made the body, cell by cell we made it.
>
> *Rumi (Barks 1995, p. 262)*

## KOSHIC PERSPECTIVES

In annamaya kosha, we explore physical structure, properties, and functions of fascia. A bidirectional relationship exists between structure and movement on one hand, and health and function of the fascial system on the other. Structural misalignment resulting from injury and habitual use can be reinforced by fascial densification and distortion. Alternatively, fascia that undergoes densification and adhesion from injury, unhealthy lifestyle behaviors, and disease processes may eventually cause pain and structural changes. In this physical kosha, we also explore ways to increase fascial health through mindful, multidimensional movement done with variation in range, intensity, tempo, direction, and locus of initiation. As we consciously hydrate fascia and increase glide and elasticity, we can enhance our strength, range, and ease of movement, and encourage cellular health and tissue repair.

In the yogic view, prana circulates through the *nadis* (energy channels), *marma points* (similar to acupuncture points), and *chakras* (energy centers) in pranamaya kosha. Many contemporary yogis and bodyworkers speculate that prana moves through fascia. Corroborating this speculation, research suggests that fascia is the physical medium through which energy flows in line-like structures that correlate with acupuncture meridians (Yu *et al.*, 2011). Energy medicine expert Dr. James Oschman defines fascia as a "semiconducting liquid crystal matrix which stores and processes vast amounts of subliminal or nonneural information. It is the primordial matrix of consciousness" (Oschman 2009). From this perspective, fascia generates piezoelectric currents by transforming mechanical energy produced by tension and compression forces during movement. The resulting electrical fields spread through surrounding tissue, enabling energetic, body-wide communication that supports self-regulation. Oschman hypothesizes that these currents may decrease the viscosity of the gel component of fascia and thereby contribute to fascial health.

Pranamaya kosha governs movement, including transmission of electrical currents and other forms of information like mechanical force, neurotransmitters, nerve impulses, hormones, and immune system components. All of these are transported through fascia. The fascial network transmits and disperses both internal forces generated by muscular effort and external forces such as gravity and ground reaction force (an equal and opposite counterthrust to the force a body exerts on the ground). These forces are diffused throughout the system in an omnidirectional way that minimizes stress on individual structures. *Mechanotransduction* is the conversion of externally or internally generated physical forces into biochemical responses at the cellular level. Through this process, cellular function, even down to the level of gene expression, can be affected (Wagh *et al.*, 2021).

The breath aspect of pranamaya kosha also affects fascial health. Dysfunctional breathing patterns can dysregulate blood chemistry by altering oxygen and carbon dioxide ratios and triggering a cascade of physiological effects, including stimulating the sympathetic nervous system and increasing inflammation. EA breath practices may promote recalibration of oxygen and carbon dioxide ratios and downregulate the sympathetic nervous system to reduce inflammation and myofascial tone.

On the manomaya kosha level, emotions and stress responses may trigger neurochemical responses in the fascial system, provoking tissue stiffening and densification. In fact, fascia has been described as the emotional body, recognizing that physical responses to emotions are experienced first as bodily sensation, then interpreted as specific emotions (Schulz and Feitis 1996). Although controversial and unproven, many bodyworkers and movement therapists

(including me) believe that memories are "stored" in fascia (Tozzi 2014). As evidence, we offer clinical anecdotes describing emotional patterns or unprocessed memories surfacing during bodywork or movement therapy sessions that stimulate significant therapeutic, physiological responses and emotional healing.

> As soon as I placed the foam ball under my painful rib, I started to cry as my suppressed grief was released.
>
> *Judith*

The sensory aspect of manomaya kosha is reflected in the characterization of fascia as the body's largest sensory organ, richly endowed with significantly more sensory receptors than muscle tissue. In this way, fascia may play a role in cultivating body awareness.

Even our experience of Self in vijnanamaya kosha partially arises from interoceptive nerve endings embedded in fascia. These receptors register sensory information that is processed and integrated with other neural inputs in the brain to manufacture a stable sense of self (see Chapter 1). A bidirectional relationship exists between the state of our fascial system and sense of self, including body image. The tone, elasticity and responsiveness of our fascial network can influence the way we feel about ourselves. As an organ of form, fascia will faithfully conform to hold the shape of our embodied metaphors and conditioned responses to life. For example, patterns of overeffort, perfectionism, or resistance can manifest as excessive myofascial tension that restricts movement and force transmission. Our patterns of alignment, breath, personality, and conditioning are in our tissues, just as tree rings record seasons of drought and abundance. As we cultivate felt sense of fascia through interoceptive awareness, we may uncover and compassionately heal these deeper patterns. The good news is that fascia is adaptive, and we can change our fascial "mold" through EA and movement practices. As we learn to embody our fascial self, we may also connect more deeply to our inner spaciousness, resilience, and wisdom.

Fascial awareness can be used as a "touchstone" to wholeness on anandamaya kosha level. Once we sense our inner fascial matrix during movement, that felt sense of wholeness and connection can expand beyond the physical body to our relationship with others, the natural environment, and even the cosmos. In fact, there is an eerie similarity between images from the James Webb space telescope and photos of spiralic fascial structures. When fascia is dense and adhered to underlying tissue, we may experience a sense of operating at less-than-optimal wholeness, a "soul loss." When energy and emotions can't flow through the fascial system, wholeness is more difficult to access; "doing" and fear may replace "being" and love. When we use somatic practices and movement to express and reshape the endless fascial web, all koshic levels of consciousness can work together to create an experience of oneness. We can then move and live more from our wholeness.

> The soul of man, with all the streams of pure living water, seems to dwell in the fascia of the body.
>
> *Dr. Andrew Still, founder of osteopathy (1899)*

## LEARN IT

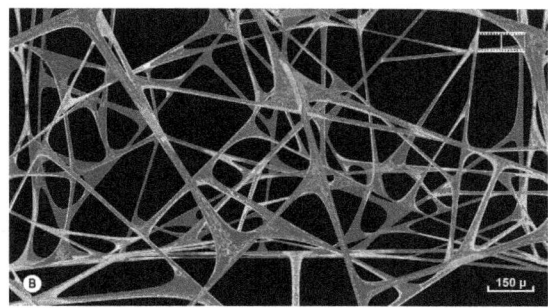

In older definitions, fascia is considered one type of connective tissue; other types include bones, cartilage, and blood. The Fascia Research Society currently defines the fascial system as the three-dimensional continuum of soft, collagen-containing, loose and dense fibrous connective tissues that permeate the body (Adstrum *et al.*, 2017). Fascia is classified according to the composition of its semiviscous matrix, or ground substance, and the different types, quantities, and orientation of non-living fibers and living cells it contains (see Table 4.1). The proportion of these variables determines different types of fascia and their qualities. Ground substance also known as the "vital environment," is a gelatinous, inner ocean facilitating both chemical and molecular exchange of nutrients and waste with cells and between lymph and venous capillaries. We are 70 percent water, on average, and the ground substance can contain up to 90 percent water. Fascial hydration is vital for good health.

On the continuum of fascial densities in the body, fluid fascia like blood and lymph lie at one end and dense, hard bone at the other (Sharkey 2021). In between are:

- abundant, loose, areolar "packing" tissues holding cells and other structures in their rightful place and interweaving with adipose tissue in a subcutaneous "layer" beneath the skin
- dense fibrous tissue surrounding muscle and nerve fibers and bundles of fibers and enveloping organs, forming periosteum, aponeuroses, tendons, ligaments, and deep fascia

- elastic tissue in the dermis and walls of arteries and lungs
- reticular tissue providing scaffolding in glands, organs and bone marrow

- cartilage
- adipose tissue supporting and protecting organs and entwining with superficial fascia.

Table 4.1 Constituents of Fascia

| Constituent | Description | Function |
|---|---|---|
| Fibers | • Collagen fibers—strong, white, spiralic, and inelastic<br>• Elastin fibers<br>• Reticular fibers | • Provide tensile strength<br>• Provide elasticity and resilience<br>• Form inner scaffolding of organs, glands, marrow |
| Cells | • Mainly fibroblasts<br><br>• Fasciacytes<br><br>• Telocytes<br><br>• Immune cells including macrophages and mast cells<br>• Adipose (fat) cells | • Secrete components of fibers and ground substance<br>• Produce hyaluronan, a water-absorbing glycosaminoglycan<br>• Participate in tissue repair, intracellular signaling, and immune function (Stecco *et al.*, 2018)<br>• Immune function<br>• Energy storage |
| Ground substance (mostly water) | • Glycosaminoglycans, predominantly hyaluronan | • Hydration—absorb water<br>• Transport of ions, nutrients, and waste<br>• Provide viscosity and compressive strength<br>• Enable glide between fibers |

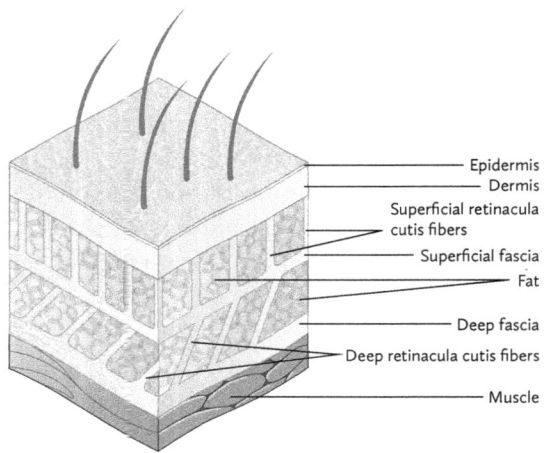

Epidermis
Dermis
Superficial retinacula cutis fibers
Superficial fascia
Fat
Deep fascia
Deep retinacula cutis fibers
Muscle

Although there are no discrete fascial layers, anatomist Gil Headley describes fascia as continuous "textural layers" of varying densities, functions, and properties that are interpenetrated by connecting fascial and neurovascular structures. Fascia can be as tough and strong as leather in tendons and as delicate as cellular cytoskeletons, yielding a unique balance of tensile strength and elasticity, depending on its constituents. It is thickest where stability and stiffness are required and to aid force transmission, as in the iliotibial band.

## Sensory Receptors

The term *neuromyofascial net* acknowledges the rich innervation of fascia. Fascia contains four different types of *mechanoreceptors*, which are sensory receptors activated by mechanical tension and pressure (Schleip 2005). Three types are proprioceptors that respond to specific mechanical forces and qualities of movement and produce distinctive effects, including stimulating vagal tone or altering cardiovascular and respiratory functions. Approximately 80 percent of mechanoreceptors are unmyelinated, free nerve endings; the lack of a fatty sheath slows signal conduction. These receptors transmit interoceptive and nociceptive stimuli, the latter especially when inflammation is present (Langevin 2021). Interoceptive sensitivity can magnify pain perception, yet, paradoxically, may relieve pain through skillful self-regulation (Park *et al.*, 2021).

When interoceptors are stimulated, they activate brain regions mediating emotional states, indicating the strong relationship between myofascia and emotions (Bordoni and Marelli 2017). When we're excited, we feel it in our whole body. The dense concentration of sensory receptors may reflect the evolutionary survival importance of registering our inner experience, emotions, and how we move.

## Properties of fascia

Functional qualities emerge from the nature and structure of fascia.

### THIXOTROPY

*Thixotrophy* is the ability of fascia to transform between viscous and fluid states, partially depending on the degree of thermal or mechanical stimulation. Picture gelatin hardening when chilled and liquefying with stirring. Fascia can hydrate when manipulated through movement or bodywork or thicken when not moved regularly. When fascia densifies, it dehydrates and stiffens, obstructing absorption of nutrients and disposal of cellular wastes. Inflammation may result when cellular access to fluids and nutrients from blood and lymph is impaired. Misalignment, immobility, or overuse of specific movement patterns can cause densification and inflammation leading to adhesion of collagen fibers and hardened lines of tissue tension. This can interfere with organ function and fascial gliding between structures and around joints. Conversely, pliable, hydrated fascia reflects optimal health and function.

### VISCOELASTICITY

Fibers and cells are suspended in ground substance, defining fascia as a *colloid*, a substance characterized by viscoelasticity. This quality combines two properties: the elastic ability to store potential energy during elongation and return to original shape once energy is released (visualize an elastic band), and the viscous ability to resist movement in any direction (visualize pulling bread dough). Viscoelastic properties of myofascia and tendons enable elastic recoil as tissues are loaded and unloaded. Picturing elastic recoil assists us to run gracefully and efficiently like gazelles and walk with a spring in our step. Evoking viscous resistance during movement may contribute to fascial remodeling over time, enabling increased range of motion and more precise motor control. This is helpful when you are a dancer or wish to move with grace and fluidity.

### ADAPTABILITY

Fascia is adaptable. It can remodel according to stresses applied, becoming stiffer and denser along lines of stress. As movement, load, and other mechanical forces are exerted on and within the body, remodeling occurs through collagen fiber breakdown and repair. Habitual alignment and movement (or sedentary) patterns will densify fascia in some planes but simultaneously weaken it in others. This quality of viscoelasticity can be harnessed through EA practices that remodel more elastic, pliable, and resilient fascia. Remodeling is encouraged through movements that vary fascial loading over diverse ranges, angles, and qualities of movement. For example, the quality of elastic recoil can be used to initiate full-body movements that encourage fascial gliding and prevent adhesion. When appropriate levels of force are regularly applied without overloading tissue capacity, fascia will adapt with increased length, strength, and elasticity.

## Movement

Fascia allows us to move our bodies in efficient and coordinated movement patterns. The interwoven fascial compartments surrounding structures at all levels provide a unified, omnidirectional tensional scaffolding of inner support for form, erectness, and movement. When muscle tissues activate, their interpenetrating and enveloping fascia transmits force that moves bones and determines the strength and direction of movement. Fascia can also contract independently of muscular action and may play a role in proprioception, coordination, and joint stability (Schleip and Klingler 2019). All movement is whole-body movement. When one part moves, the fascial network responds and adaptively rearranges tension and compression relationships to support moving parts and maintain uprightness and gravitational balance.

While healthy fascia allows neighboring structures to glide over each other during movement, at a microscopic level mucilaginous filaments and tubules also glide along each other to reconfigure in new relationships and shapes (watch the YouTube video "Strolling under the skin" by Jean-Claude Guimberteau: www.youtube.com/watch?v=DroKc3wo-dA&ab_channel=JeanClaudeGUIMBERTEAU). Spiraled collagen fibers coil and uncoil like springs, allowing fascia to change shape during movement. Without regular uncoiling and gliding, fascia dehydrates, densifies, and forms adhesions. We need to move!

Dynamic tension in myofascia is created when one body part is anchored and another part moves away from it, or when two structures move away from each other. We can embody dynamic tension when we slowly and consciously elongate myofascia while visualizing a simultaneous opposite force, or resistance, to elongation. The quality of viscoelasticity confers this concurrent lengthening and resistance. Whenever we move a body part in one direction, we can visualize fascial resistance at micro and macro levels pulling in the opposite direction and creating dynamic tension. Visualizing these opposing push-pull forces can result in mindful, slow-motion movement. When done with awareness of the continually changing relationships of the parts and of the tissue sensations between the two parts, dynamic tension can educate the nervous system and profoundly improve fluidity, strength, and elasticity of movement (Levin and Martin 2012).

The work of Rolfer and movement educator Hubert Godard establishes that when we visualize two directions of movement our nervous system reorganizes to minimize the number of stabilizing muscles activated, producing stronger coordinated movements more adaptive to specific movement challenges (Newton 1995).

Additionally, when movement is done slowly and consciously with dynamic tension, the nervous system can better register and integrate sensory input, so new information can be used to modulate and refine future movements. Mechanical stresses like dynamic tension also encourage more gel-like extracellular fluid, and cause strengthening collagen fibers to be deposited along lines of tension. This way of moving encourages fascial glide and discourages the dehydration and fiber cross-linking that occurs through inactivity. Awareness of the fascial system and its qualities can invoke felt sense of simultaneous internal spaciousness and support that can lead to more efficient and integrated movement.

## FEEL IT

### EXPLORATION: PLAYING WITH FASCIA

Isaac Newton observed that liquids flow at consistently expected rates. Fluidic fascia defies this prediction by stiffening and holding its shape when sudden pressure is applied, yet softening when patient, light pressure is applied. This non-Newtonian quality explains how heel fascia hardens on impact with the ground to provide thrust during walking and how restrictions in myofascia can release during mindful bodywork or EA practices. If we are unmindful or too forceful, fascia will resist attempts to soften or lengthen. If we establish presence and work patiently, respectfully, and intentionally, fascia will respond by softening. The mixture of water and cornstarch (called Oobleck) used in the first practice demonstrates this phenomenon.

## Learning Objective

- Experience felt sense of fascial qualities of thixotropy and viscoelasticity.

## CORNSTARCH PLAY

### Props

- 500 g (1 lb.) cornstarch, water, a bowl, and strong spoon

### Instructions

- Put the cornstarch in the bowl and gradually add water while stirring with the spoon. When no dry cornstarch remains, cover with an additional 8 cm (3 in.) of water. Leave to stand overnight.

- Place the finger pads of one hand on the surface of the Oobleck. Forcefully try to push your fingers deeper.

  - *What happens?*

- Now center yourself and focus on the sensations of cornstarch beneath your fingers. Set an intention to eventually touch

the bottom of the bowl. With patience and adjustments in your effort level, balance your intention to reach the bottom of the bowl with the resistance of the mixture. Imagine the heat of your fingers melting the Oobleck. This may take some time!

- Once you touch the bottom of the bowl, slowly and mindfully pull your fingers out.

  - *What happens if you try to pull out too quickly?*
  - *Can you imagine the same melting phenomenon occurring in your own body during a slow, compassionate movement practice?*

## PLAY-DOH PLAY

### Props

- Play-Doh, either purchased or homemade

### Instructions

- Manipulate the Play-Doh with your hands by squeezing, pulling, compressing, and twisting it. As you play, notice how it resists manual deformation. As you compress Play-Doh, it pushes back. As you elongate, it pulls back.

- Translate this quality into your own body. In either standing or supine position, explore slow, intuitive, mindful movement as you visualize your fascia responding with the same plastic push and pull qualities.

  - *How does your movement change?*
  - *How does the quality of your mind change? Your breath?*

## EXPLORATION: FASCIAL BREATHING 🔊

### Learning Objectives

- Awareness of how breath affects fascia.

- Access fascial breath as an internal support.

### Instructions

- Start in supine position, supported where necessary for comfort. Observe your natural breath.

  - *Where do you notice breath movement?*
  - *Can you sense any movement in your limbs?*

- Focus on the deep place where breath movement originates: the lumbar attachments of the diaphragm. Notice how your breath emanates from there.

- Visualize your inhalations spreading outward from the diaphragmatic attachments, through the fluidic fascial matrix, to your head... pelvic floor... front... back... sides... and into your limbs. In your mind's eye, picture the ever-widening ripples generated when a stone is thrown into a pond. Let each inhalation initiate breath waves vibrating through your watery fascia.

- As you breathe, visualize the waves of fluidic breath moving omnidirectionally throughout your body. Imagine your whole inner body participating in rhythmic breath pulsations at all levels of scale, from cells, to blood, organs, muscles, and bones. Feel these structures floating and gently rolling in the fluid movement.

  - *What are the sensations of fascial breathing?*

- Refocus your awareness on one leg and track the fluid movement of your breath waves as they radiate from your center, down your leg, through each joint, and into your foot.

  - *Does your leg move subtly as the breath ripples through it?*

- Shift your focus to your remaining limbs, exploring fascial breathing in each individually.

- Finish with full-body fascial breathing, visualizing breath rippling out from your center and reverberating throughout your body.

- Stand up and explore slow, mindful movement.

  - *Can you sense more fluidity in your body?*
  - *How does the quality of your movement change?*
  - *Can you sense internal support?*

## EXPLORATION: FASCIAL PALPATION 🎥

### Learning Objective

- Explore different densities of fascia and the continuities between them.

### Instructions

- In a seated position with the right hand resting on your lap, lightly place your left finger pads on the back of your right hand. Distinguishing the thin layer of skin, use a light touch to move it in random directions over underlying subcutaneous fascia. Carefully glide the skin over the underlying "layer" until you feel a pull or tension between the two densities of tissue. Repeat in different positions on your hand... wrist... forearm... and upper arm.

  – *Can you sense the continuity of the skin with underlying fascia?*

- Use a pincer grip to pick up a tiny fold of skin on the back of your right hand, then let it go. Notice how the elastic skin returns to its original shape (perhaps less so with aging skin). Repeat in different positions on your hand... wrist... forearm... and upper arm.

  – *Where is it easier to differentiate skin from underlying fascia?*
  – *Where is your skin most elastic? Least elastic?*

- Pick up another fold of skin on the back of your hand and tension it in one direction, noticing the lines of pull in the skin and underlying fascia and how far they extend. Repeat in different directions, noticing which have more or less elasticity. Repeat this exploration in different positions on your hand... wrist... forearm... and upper arm.

  – *Does your skin move more easily in one direction in different locations?*

- Place your left finger pads on your forearm, sinking your pressure below the skin into the subcutaneous fascia. Maintaining the deeper pressure, slowly glide the subcutaneous fascia over the underlying myofascia until you feel a pull or tension between the two densities of tissue. Make a fist to activate and differentiate the muscular density. Explore tensioning the tissue in different directions.

- Repeat the tensioning in different positions on your forearm and upper arm.

  – *Where is there more glide? Less glide?*

- Encircle your right forearm with your left hand, sinking your pressure even deeper into the myofascial density. Visualize the myofascia as a soft, malleable tissue "sleeve" surrounding the solid bone "core." Roll the myofascial sleeve laterally around the bone core until you sense tensioning between the two densities of myofascia and periosteum. Repeat the exploration, rolling the sleeve medially... then glide the outer sleeve vertically up... then down... then at different angles... feeling a pull between myofascia and periosteum with each movement.

- Repeat in different positions on your forearm and upper arm.

  – *Can you sense the continuities between fascial densities?*
  – *Where is there more glide? Less glide?*

- Pause to notice sensation differences between right and left arms. Move your arms randomly and notice the contrast between sides.

  – *What do you notice?*

- Repeat the practice on your left arm.

## HEAL IT

## HYDRATION

The volume of fascia is mostly water. Our lifestyle and movement habits, including inactivity, alcohol use, poor diet, and sleep deprivation can dehydrate fascia. "Trying" to stretch dehydrated myofascia is counterproductive: The more you pull, the more it resists. However, we can hydrate and lubricate fascia through specific movements, especially jiggling, oscillating, and bouncing movements that render it more amenable to lengthening. When fascia is adequately hydrated, proprioceptors and interceptors within it function better and motor control is enhanced.

### FOUNDATIONAL PRACTICE: SPINAL WAVE 📹

### Learning Objectives

- Hydrate myofascia and improve lymphatic drainage.

- Consciously transmit force from feet to head.

### Practice Notes

- If lying with legs straight is uncomfortable, bend your knees or use support beneath them.

- Monitor tension levels in your feet, toes, and pelvis to ensure they remain relaxed and passive while the ankles do the work.

- If your legs tire, take a pause.

### Instructions

- Take a baseline reading in supine position.

- With toes pointed toward the ceiling, slowly flex your ankles so your heels push into the floor. Release the ankle flexion, returning your body to its original position.

- Repeat this slow flex and release movement several times. The ankles activate but toes remain passive.

  - *How does the movement impulse sequence through your body to the head? Is it blocked anywhere?*

- Explore effort level, rhythm, and speed to find easy pulsations back and forth from feet to crown. Surrender to the gentle, comforting, pulsing movements for a few minutes.

- Pause to notice the effects of the practice.

  - *How do you feel physically and energetically?*
  - *Is more of your back resting on the floor?*
  - *When you stand up, what feels different?*

### EXPLORATION: GODDESS POSE (UTKATA KONASANA)

When myofascia is elongated or compressed, fluid is squeezed out of microtubules and virtual spaces. When released, new fluid is absorbed. Picture a sponge being squeezed dry and then refilling with water. In this process of fluid exchange, toxins and waste products are removed and nutritional and restorative components are infused.

### Learning Objective

- Refine felt sense of fascial hydration.

### Practice Notes

- Visualize your fascial system as an internal, body-shaped sponge.

- As you enter the pose, visualize the sponge being squeezed and emptied of fluid. As you release the movement, visualize the sponge filling with fluid.

## Instructions

- Take a baseline in standing.

- Move your feet comfortably wide apart and turned out 45 degrees. Place your palms together at your chest.

- On an exhalation, bend your knees and slowly lower your pelvis into a semisquat, ensuring your knees point in the same direction as your toes. Simultaneously, open your arms sideways into a goalpost shape with elbows at shoulder height and fingers spread wide apart.

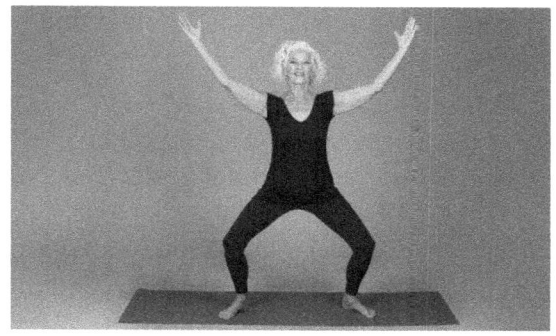

- On an inhalation, press into your feet to return to standing while moving your palms together again.

- Move back and forth several times between these positions, visualizing your fascia being rhythmically emptied and filled with fluid.

- Pause to notice any effects.

  - *How could you take this sponge imagery into other movements?*

## DEEPENING FELT SENSE

### EXPLORATION: CULTIVATING AWARENESS

Intuitive movement arises from inner impulses to move in pleasurable and comfortable ways. Rather than fitting yourself into an externally dictated form that may not consider your individual capabilities and capacities, you are invited to follow inner movement impulses. Exploring intuitive movement bypasses the need to think about what you are doing, so you can experience qualities of movement and sense their effects as you move.

## Learning Objectives

- Refine sensory aspects of fascia through interoceptive awareness.

- Use intuitive movement to deepen felt sense of fascial continuity and qualities.

## Props

- A pillow

## Practice Notes

- Wait until you feel an authentic impulse to move.

- Spend a few minutes exploring each limb.

- As you move, imagine free nerve endings in fascia as sensitive microscopic eyes, ears, and feelers receiving information.

## Instructions

- Position yourself side lying, supporting your head on the pillow. The shoulder and hip rest squarely on the floor without tipping forward or backward. If this is uncomfortable, move into supine position and explore each limb individually. Attune to your inner felt sense.

- Raise your top arm toward to the ceiling.

- Focus on your fingers and the free nerve endings in the skin and fascia. Imagine the receptors as microscopic eyes, ears, and feelers

- Begin to move your fingers intuitively, paying exquisite attention to both internal and external sensations.

- After a while, expand the intuitive movement sequentially to include your wrist... forearm and elbow... upper arm and shoulder... spine... and upper torso.

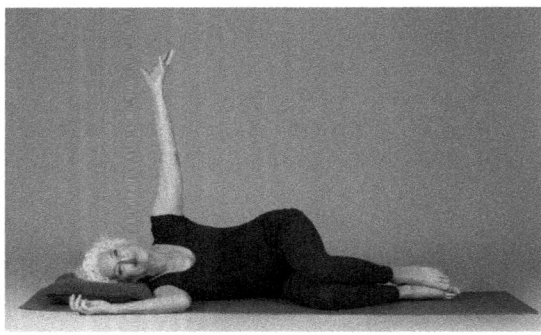

- Rest your arm.

    - *What do you sense?*
    - *Can you sense position of parts... variations in tissue tension... temperature... fluidity?*

- *Can you sense glide... plasticity... elasticity?*
- *Can you sense the fascial continuity from periphery to midline?*
- *What do you sense in the rest of your body?*

- Raise your top leg toward the ceiling without disturbing your pelvic position. Repeat the exploration, beginning with your toes and sequentially including the ankle... calf and knee... thigh and hip... pelvis and spine.

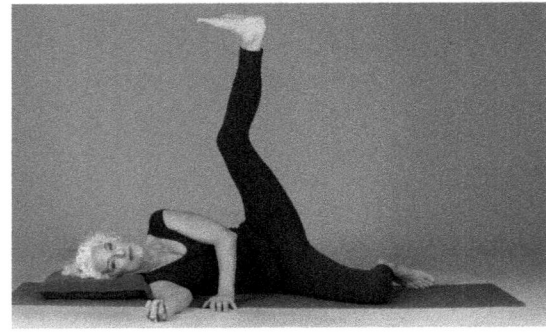

- Lie on your back to sense differences between the two sides.

- Explore movements on the other side.

- Stand to sense any changes in how you stand, then take your increased sensitivity into a familiar standing pose.

    - *What feels different?*

After doing the fascial explorations I had a distinct feeling of my inner fullness, and everything felt connected.

*Jerry*

## MOVING FASCIA

Movement can remodel fascia. In the following explorations you will discover how different modes of mental focus and ways of moving can contribute to fascial health.

### EXPLORATION: DYNAMIC TENSION

Dynamic tension can be deliberately created through practices like "pin and stretch," or by consciously moving two structures apart. Pin and stretch is a myofascial release technique in which one end of a soft tissue structure (a muscle, group of muscles, or myofascial continuity) is "pinned" while the other end is moved. Both practices are done with awareness of shifting sensations and fascial relationships between moving parts. Although usually associated with manual therapy, objects like balls, foam rollers, or even the floor can be used as pins. The parts always stay in relationship; the pinned part stabilizes myofascia so the elongating movement can encourage elasticity and pliability between parts. When done dynamically by rhythmically alternating elongation and release, myofascia is hydrated as fluid is moved in and out of the tissue.

### Learning Objectives

- Experience sensations of fascial spreading during movement.

- Explore ways to hydrate fascia.

- Sense fascial continuities.

### Practice Notes

- Use breath and visualization to amplify effects of dynamic tension and fascial spreading. Useful images that evoke slow spreading movement include **Play-Doh**, flowing molasses, or moving through thick air. Remember your experience playing with **Play-Doh** and **cornstarch**.

- When working with an area of restriction, place attention in that area and visualize the breath softening and hydrating the tissue.

- Track sensations of shifting relationships between anatomical parts. Diffuse your awareness evenly in the volume of tissue between them.

### Exploration: Head to Knee Pose (Janu Sirsasana)
### Props

- A small towel rolled to a 6–9 cm (2.5–3.5 in.) diameter or a 10 cm (4 in.) sensy ball or other pliable facial balls (a pair of 10 cm/4 in. sensy balls can be purchased online)

- Blankets for pelvic or knee support, if required for comfort

### Instructions

- Do a baseline forward bend. Sit comfortably on the floor with legs straight and torso oriented forward.

- Place the sole of your right foot comfortably somewhere on the inner left leg. Use support under your pelvis and knee, if necessary, to position your pelvis in a slight anterior tilt. Bend from the hips to move your spine into a forward bend, maintaining length and natural spinal curves in your spine throughout the movement. Register sensations as you find your comfortable end range of motion.

- Place the towel roll horizontally on the floor under your lower left calf to pin the soft tissue. Join your palms together at the sternum and activate the straight leg by pointing your toes toward the ceiling.

- On an exhalation, bend from your hips to move your spine into a comfortable forward bend.

- On an inhalation, return to the upright starting position and release the foot. Move slowly and dynamically back and forth between the two positions several times. Track the sensation in your posterior body as you move into the posture.

  - *Can you sense dynamic tension between the pinned calf tissue and your back body?*

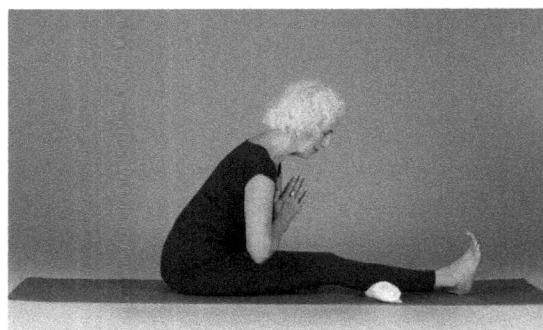

- After several repetitions, remain in the comfortable end range and do several soft, elastic bouncing movements.

- Turn your torso slightly to center it between your legs. Repeat the slow dynamic forward bend and the elastic bounces in end range.

- Move the towel roll higher on the calf and repeat the movements several times.

- Repeat the movements with the towel roll at a few positions on the thigh.

- Remove the roll and do another forward bend.

  - *What's different?*
  - *Has your baseline range of motion increased?*
  - *Have baseline sensations changed?*

- Repeat the baseline and movements on the other side.

## Exploration: Locust Pose Variation (Salabhasana)
### Contraindications

- Pregnancy or recent abdominal surgery.

- Acute shoulder, back or neck conditions sensitive to extension.

### Instructions

- Lie prone with right arm overhead, palm down, and forehead resting on the posterior left hand. The tops of both feet press evenly into the floor. Support the abdomen from groins to sternum with a folded blanket, if necessary for comfort.

- As you inhale, imagine your breath filling the diagonal volume between your right hand and left foot. As you exhale, slide the right arm and left leg further along the floor to create dynamic tension between them.

- On the next inhalation, maintain this dynamic tension as you lift your right arm, head, torso, and left leg off the floor. Align your head with your right arm.

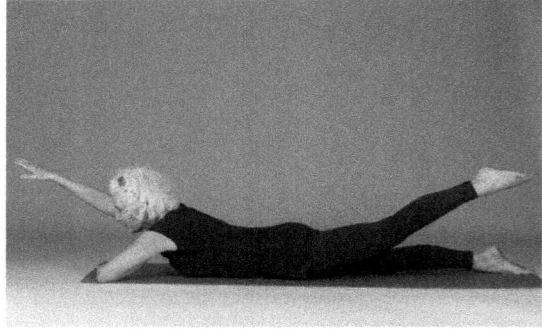

- Slowly release to the floor on an exhalation.

- Repeat several times, then change sides.

- Pause to notice any effects, first lying on your back, then in standing.

  - *What do you notice?*

## EXPLORATION: FORCE TRANSMISSION

As you move, force and momentum sequence through your structure interacting with your body weight, gravity, and the supporting surface. Whether your feet, hands, or other body parts connect with the ground or another surface, Newton's third law applies: For every action there is an equal and opposite reaction. Gravity pulls you down, and the counterthrust of gravity, or ground reaction force, uplifts you to provide support and alignment. Intention, visualization, effort level, and quality of movement can affect how forces sequence through your body. When you vary these elements, you can deliberately and intelligently alter force transmission through bones, organs, fluids, and fascia. Conscious application and direction of mechanical forces can diminish wear and tear by balancing force transmission through joints and soft tissues and relieving individual parts from bearing excessive load.

### Learning Objectives

- Consciously direct force through specific pathways.

- Explore varying qualities of force transmission.

### Foundational Practice: Yield and Push 🎥
Instructions

- Take a baseline in standing with feet shoulder width apart. Register which parts of your feet press more heavily into the ground and how your body weight is distributed between them. Determine your habitual way of transmitting force through your legs and pelvis. Shift your weight side to side, alternately bending each knee, then pushing off the foot to return to full height.

    – *Does force sequence more through one part of your leg or joints?*
    – *Which part of your foot pushes more?*

- Now, actively yield your weight into the right foot, allowing hips, knees, and ankles to bend. As you lower your body into gravity in a slow, controlled way, maintain verticality in your spine.

- Push off equally through your right foot to return to full height and straighten both legs. Now, actively yield into your left foot, then push off equally through the whole foot to return to full height. Imagine your legs as flexible tubes, visualizing a wave of force sequencing through the *volume* of one leg from the ground, up to the hip, across the pelvis, down the opposite leg, to the ground. Yield and push through your legs several times, tracking the pathway of force in your mind.

- Explore different qualities of movement. First, continue yielding and pushing while visualizing the push-off like a rocket ship lifted by ground reaction force on take-off.

- Continue yielding and pushing while imagining your legs as conduits for a bouncing ball that hits the ground with each yield and bounces up with each push-off, travelling up the leg, through the pelvis, and down the other leg to the ground.

    – *Can you harness the buoyancy of ground reaction force?*

- Continue yielding and pushing while playing with the quality of lightness... of heaviness... of speed... of slowness.

- Contrast conscious force transmission with doing the same movement by simply bending and straightening your knees rather than actively yielding and pushing through the feet.

- Repeat these variations in an asymmetrical position, moving one leg forward and turning the back foot out slightly, yielding and pushing back and forth, from front to back leg.

- Stop moving and stand comfortably to notice any effects.

  - *What's different when you consciously transmit force?*
  - *Which qualities help you sense force transmission?*
  - *How does your breath synchronize with the movements?*

## EXPLORATION: WHOLE-BODY MOVEMENT

During movement, the fascial system receives and redistributes forces throughout the whole web, continually making micro-adjustments to fine-tune gravitational forces, strength, and motor control. When you move with awareness of omnidirectional fascial connections in the body, movement is supported from within throughout the whole arc of movement. The part functioning as the supportive foundation is always in shifting relationship with the moving part. As you reach into a cupboard, even your feet are supporting your arm, and, if you pay attention, you may sense your whole body reconfiguring movement and support functions. As you consciously make whole-body movements, you may sense and feel the unity of the body.

### Learning Objectives

- Sense the wholeness of the fascial system.
- Experience how the fascial network responds and reconfigures during movement.

### Practice Notes

- Focus on one body part at a time.
- Occasionally, change levels and positions.
- Integrate the image of fascial receptors having eyes, ears, and feelers.

## Exploration: Intuitive Movement
### Instructions

- Start in either standing or supine position. Recall the abundance of sensory nerve receptors in your fascia, and diffuse your awareness throughout your "innerness," sensing from within.

- Focusing on one arm, begin to move it in simple, easy movements. As you move, imagine your arm as an actor onstage and your fascial network as a connected, supportive, and receptive audience. Picture an audience that listens, sees, and feels the actor, yet maintains awareness of the set and other actors and audience members.

- Explore different shapes, directions, effort levels, tempos, amplitudes, and qualities of movement.

  - *How does the fascial audience support and respond to the actor?*
  - *Can you sense adaptive micro-movements?*
  - *Can you sense how force redistributes through your structure so you remain stable and balanced?*

- Dissolve the image. Now move as though the arm is isolated, like an actor practicing their lines alone.

  - *How are the two modes of moving different?*

- Explore moving from other body parts.

  - *Can you sense the rest of the body supporting the moving part?*

- Pause to register effects of the practice.

  - *What do you notice?*

## Exploration: Archer Pose
## (Akarna Dhanurasana)
### Instructions

- Carry the awareness of "actor and audience" into a yoga posture.

- Stand with your feet wider than your shoulders. Turn your right foot out 90 degrees and adjust the left heel so your body faces right.

- Raise both arms in front to shoulder height, palms facing away from you and fingers pointing up. Form an arrow mudra with the right hand; straighten the wrist and point the thumb to the ceiling, extending the second and third fingers and tucking the fourth and fifth fingers into your palm.

- Move the right elbow straight back as though drawing an arrow on a bow. Simultaneously, press the left palm forward to create dynamic tension between the left hand and right elbow. Sense the foundation of your feet on the floor and the activation of your legs keeping you upright and steady.

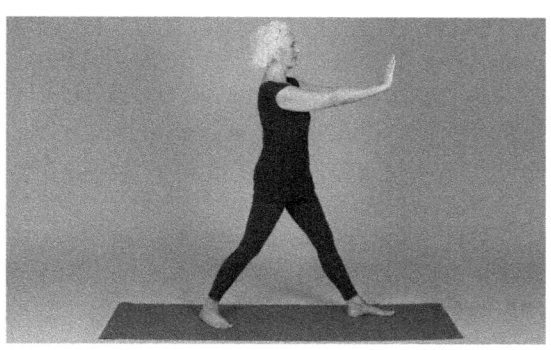

- Work the posture with the breath. On inhalations, "draw the bow." On exhalations,

release the stored kinetic energy and let the arrow "fly," undoing the mudra as you push the right palm forward.

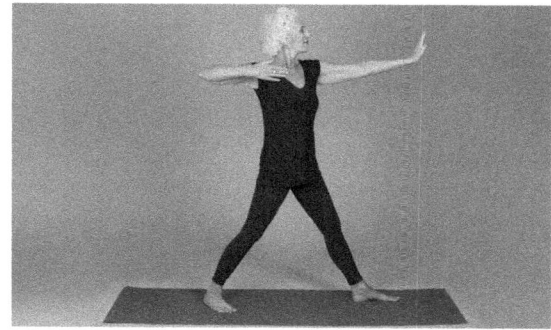

- Move back and forth between the two positions, sensing the alternating elastic recoil and multidimensional dynamic tension throughout your body. Imagine that you create the shape of the posture by reconfiguring tension and compression elements throughout your entire fascial network.

- Move back and forth between the two positions.

- After several repetitions, repeat on the other side.

- Stand with feet together and arms relaxed to register any effects.

  - *What do you notice?*

> After doing the fascial awareness practices, I could sense the "everywhere-ness" of fascia.
>
> *Pauline*

## THERAPEUTIC APPLICATIONS

As the system in which all other systems are embedded, it's unsurprising that fascial health can impact overall health on multidimensional levels. Our understanding of physiology changes when we view fascia as a metasystem connecting and influencing physiological function (Langevin 2006). With this pervasive impact, fascial densification and associated loss of elasticity has been associated with conditions ranging from low back pain to cancer and depression (Bordoni and Zanier 2014). Helene Langevin, a renowned researcher of the role of fascia in pathology, found that most restorative tissue elements occur at the shear zone between different fascial densities. She suggests that increased collagen production (densification) in these areas could decrease shear capacity between zones and thereby harm tissue health, and that healing modalities like manual and movement therapy could improve glide and shear (Langevin 2022).

Fascia has been implicated in diverse musculoskeletal conditions (Ajimsha, Shenoy, and Gampawar 2020). The continuity of the fascial system implies that adverse effects of injury, repetitive movements, or dysfunctional movement patterns in one area will ultimately affect the whole. While healthy fascia with adequate hydration and glide enables efficient, strong, and integrated movement, fascia that is densified, dehydrated, and lacking glide can launch a cascade of effects resulting in pain, inflammation, limited movement, and compromised quality of life (see Flowchart 4.1).

Pathological fascia contains increased densities of free nerve endings that may play a role in both pain generation and perception (Suarez-Rodriguez et al., 2022). With higher fascial sensory innervation than muscle tissue, myofascial pain could be caused by pathological changes in fascial composition and structure rather than in muscles, as was previously believed. Mechanotransduction may therefore be the catalyst for changes in fibroblast activity, density of extracellular matrix, and

inflammation. Additionally, nociceptive signals can be activated by changes in fascial viscoelasticity and result in increased perceived pain (Stecco et al., 2013). A model of chronic back pain developed by Langevin and Sherman hypothesizes that these changes, and the subsequent fear and pain they cause, could initiate a vicious cycle of decreased movement, fascial remodeling, inflammation, and nervous system sensitization leading to further immobility. They suggest that therapeutic fascial remodeling and neuroplastic changes generated through modalities that include manual therapy and movement repatterning could interrupt the cycle, offering a solution to other chronic pain conditions (Langevin and Sherman 2007). More recently Langevin has hypothesized a model linking myofascial pain, proprioception, and fascial mobility, based on observations that both hypermobility and hypomobility of joints and fascia are associated with pain and abnormal proprioception (Langevin 2021). This association may explain how fascial awareness and mindful movement practices can alleviate pain.

The far-reaching influence of fascia also plays a role in numerous (if not all?) chronic diseases (Huston 2022). When the tone of fascial support or the inner scaffolding of any organ is deficient or excessive, organ physiology may suffer from resulting prolapse or restriction. More systemically, research suggests that dysfunction in temperature regulation and lymphatic and superficial vein systems are closely related to excessive stiffening and fibrosis of fascia (Stecco et al., 2015). Even cancer seems to have a fascial component; fascial stiffness and inflammation generated by compromised movement and function may be linked to tumor growth and metastasis (Langevin et al., 2016). Fascia has also been implicated in inflammation associated with autoimmune diseases, including lupus (Noda et al., 2015). Changes in fascial viscoelasticity may even explain morning stiffness and pain in arthritic conditions (Guimberteau et al., 2010).

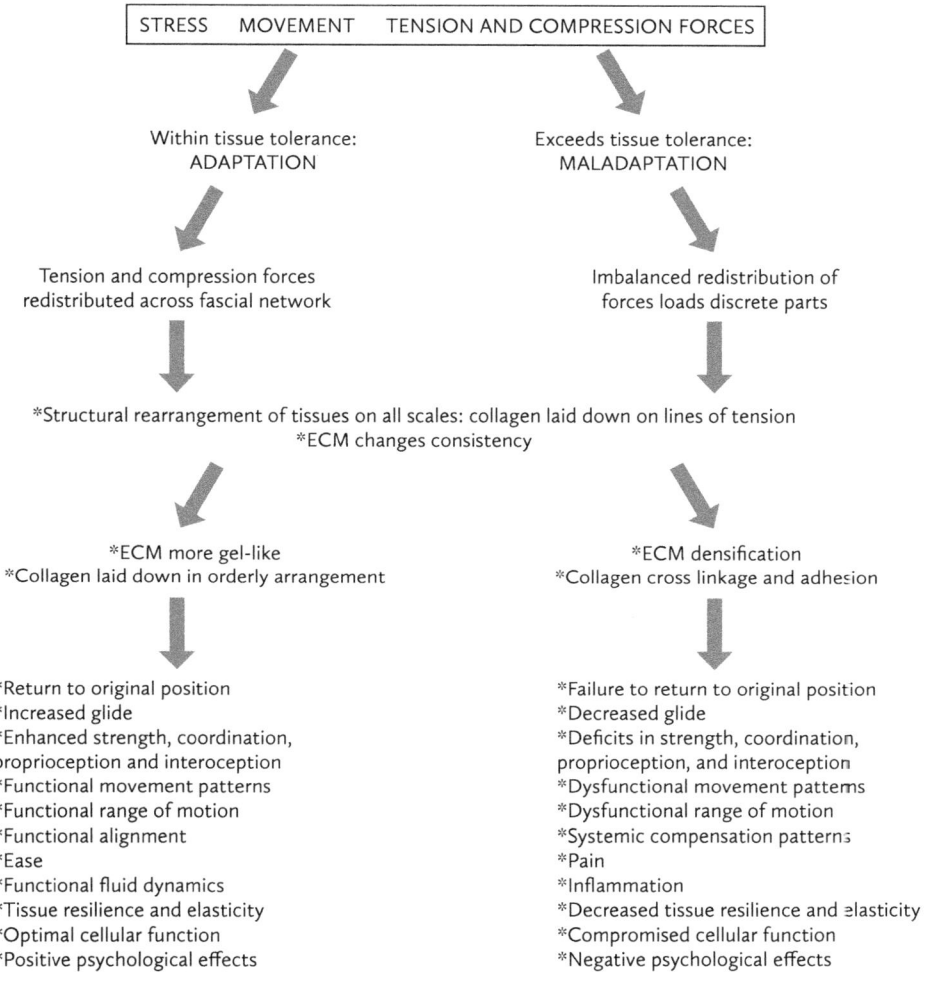

**Flowchart 4.1 Fascial Adaptation**

In the psychological realm, fascial stiffness and inelasticity have been associated with psychological conditions, including depression. Researchers hypothesize that the elevated body tension, posture, and gait patterns associated with chronic depression could increase negative thoughts and emotions (Michalak *et al.*, 2022). Knowing that fascia remodels and conforms according to use, this finding could potentially explain how embodied metaphors and other psychological patterns solidify in the body. It also offers hope that therapeutic practices like EA could play a role in treatment of depression and other psychological conditions.

As practitioners, considering fascia as a contributory cause of structural or organic dysfunction may not be our first thought, but whether clients present with hyperaroused nervous systems, high blood pressure, or irritable bowel syndrome, it behooves us to explore fascial involvement. Fascia asks us to take a global approach to mental and physical health by viewing the human system as an interconnected and interdependent whole rather than separate parts. A whole-person approach is necessitated by the whole-person influence of the fascial system. EA practices reinforce this approach by allowing us to sense fascial continuities and experience the support and fluidity they offer our posture and movement. As we deepen felt sense of the fascial system, we can consciously encourage fascial properties like connection, viscoelasticity, hydration, and capacity to remodel. We can direct appropriate tension or compression forces where required to reconfigure tensional balance. Working with fascia in a gentle and compassionate way can also encourage the nervous system to systemically downregulate fascial tone. We may notice an overflow into our emotional lives as our response-ability becomes more flexible and less reactive.

Awareness of the fascial system may help us feel our way through life as our interoceptive capacity deepens and we learn the lessons of fascia: adaptability, resilience, and flow. When we overlook these lessons, we can get stuck. When we balance push and pull forces in our bodies and lives, the result is effortless effort, gentle strength, and calm action.

## KOSHIC CONTEMPLATIONS

### Annamaya Kosha

- *How does your alignment and movement change with awareness of your fascial system?*
- *How have you modified your movement practice to encourage fascial glide and elasticity?*
- *Have you noticed relief in other parts of your body after working with a specific area?*

### Pranamaya Kosha

- *Has your breath changed after EA explorations?*
- *Have you experienced changes in your nervous system or organic function?*
- *How does your alignment and movement change when you visualize moving force, or prana, through fascial pathways or volumes?*

### Manomaya Kosha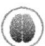

- *Has your felt sense of fascia deepened?*
- *Have you experienced any emotional clearing as you consciously release areas of fascial densification?*
- *Has your level of mindfulness changed?*

### Vijnanamaya Kosha

- *What connections have you made between the condition of your fascial system and your personality and embodied archetypes?*
- *What qualities or visualizations help you access your fascial system?*
- *As you practice these explorations have you experienced more ease or flow in your life?*

### Anandamaya Kosha

- *Are you more aware of relationships and connections within your own body? Of your wholeness?*
- *Are you able to live more in "being" mode rather than "doing" mode?*

## KEY CONCEPTS

- Fascia exists on a continuum of form from liquid to firm, forming a multidimensional, collagenous web surrounding, permeating, and separating structures in the body.
- The fascial system communicates with, connects, and supports all physiological systems to work as a synergistic whole.
- Biotensegrity is an emerging holistic paradigm describing biological structures—from cells to organisms—as systems of tension and compression elements that, when balanced, create stability, integrity, and the ability to distribute load.
- Structural misalignment can be reinforced by fascial densification and distortion, causing pain and further structural changes.

- Fascia has been defined as a semiconducting, liquid crystal matrix storing nonneural information.
- Fascia is the largest sensory organ in the body.
- The state of the fascial network can influence how we feel about ourselves.
- Dehydration can stiffen fascia, obstruct absorption of nutrients, and cause inflammation.
- The property of viscoelasticity enables fascia to remodel according to applied stresses.
- All movement is whole-body movement; when one part moves, the fascial network responds to maintain uprightness and gravitational balance, and support the moving part.

## CHAPTER 5

# Organomics

*I shouted at the top of my lungs.*
*Trust your gut.*
*He has a heart of gold.*
*Her heart is in the right place.*

Organs are not a commonly acknowledged source of support or movement initiation. In fact, we usually ignore them unless they cause distress. However, if we focus our awareness, we can sense the approximately 8 kg (17.5 lb.) of slippery tubes and uniquely shaped organs of varying densities tightly packed inside fascial compartments within our torso. Picture water-filled balloons stuffed into a torso-shaped cloth bag. Like the balloons, the inner volume and compressive force of organs provides shape and support from inside out.

Most fitness and rehab regimes focus on the musculoskeletal system. Yet, when organ awareness is cultivated, and their substance and volume experienced through EA practices, organs can offer an accessible source of support and a fluidic, deep-core locus for movement initiation. They can also play a powerful role in shaping structural alignment. As we develop organ consciousness, our muscles can stop working so hard and we can cultivate **Right Effort**.

## KOSHIC PERSPECTIVES

Annamaya kosha encompasses the three-dimensional presence of organs, their structure, and movement possibilities. Contained within the bony protection of the torso, the state of the container affects organic contents, and vice versa. Healthy organ tone manifests as elasticity, fluidity, and vibrancy, and can influence alignment and tone of overlying structures. When organs are hypotoned, musculoskeletal structures are deprived of inner support and may themselves become slack or compensate with increased rigidity as organs are experienced as "deadweight." Both organic hyper- and hypotonicity add unnecessary stress on ligaments, myofascia, and joints.

Conversely, prolonged external stress from skeletal misalignment or muscular tension can affect tone of underlying organs, compromising cellular function down to the level of DNA expression (Langevin *et al.*, 2005). When cells can't receive nourishment, excrete waste, or produce necessary proteins, physiology suffers. This can explain why significant misalignment and soft tissue damage following musculoskeletal trauma can lead to chronic digestive and other organic issues. This scenario exemplifies a *somatovisceral reflex*, in which somatic stimuli cause a reflexive response in viscera related to the same spinal cord segment (Bath and Owens 2022). Similarly, excessive or deficient tone, or organ pathology, can affect segmentally related myofascia through a visceral-somatic reflex. For example, gallbladder dysfunction can cause reflexive shoulder pain, and menstrual cramps can generate back and leg pain. Accurate diagnosis and treatment may be complicated when these reflexes either mimic or contribute to organ pathologies. As reflexes work bidirectionally, organ function can improve by establishing structural balance to tone and support overlying structures. Visceral manipulation, a manual therapy modality used by specialist practitioners, can also improve organ function.

Organic awareness can discourage excessive, habitual tension and use of overlying muscles. Together with movement initiated from the deep, organic core, this awareness can decrease injury risk. We learn that the outer body will move only as far as internal organ support will sustain and that further movement requires force. When movement unfolds from an internal organic place, energy efficiency increases and strain on joints and soft tissue structures decreases. As we access internal organ support, we can inhibit unnecessary effort required to create a perceived "ideal" posture or movement.

> My arm was partially paralyzed after a stroke. When I access my organs, I feel a sense of aliveness and support that strengthens my movements.
>
> *Paul*

The realm of pranamaya kosha includes the movements of organic processes. From a yogic perspective, prana moves substances in the body; for example, food in the gut, blood in vessels, and sperm through the reproductive tract. Developing felt sense of organs can calm the sympathetic nervous system and activate the parasympathetic system, slowing breath and movement, and encouraging vagal rest and digest functions. When we embody slowness as an organ quality, we might be more willing to support our digestion by changing a habit of eating on the run!

Pranic flow to organs increases when we direct awareness to them. Remember, *where thought goes, prana flows.* As we cultivate organic felt sense, we can tap into the energetic qualities of organs, like grounding and buoyancy.

The emotional aspect of manomaya kosha connects us to our "gut" feelings and raw, unedited emotions often suppressed out of fear or politeness. These habitually suppressed emotions can lead to psychosomatic illness, including cardiovascular and gastrointestinal conditions (Settineri *et al.*, 2019), and may be unearthed during EA explorations of the organs. Chinese medicine associates organs with specific emotions, and uses healing sounds for purification and strengthening. For example, lungs are associated with grief and courage while the heart is associated with love and hate. Jean-Pierre Barral, osteopath and developer of visceral manipulation therapy, describes connections between organs and emotions. Decades of clinical work revealed that organs react to emotions, and those reactions can determine behavioral patterns. He also observed that organ dysfunction can predispose people to particular emotions and that visceral manipulation often resolved both physical and emotional issues (Barral 2007).

EA practices can help us interocept physiological states. When organ messages are consciously received, they may galvanize us to take immediate, self-regulatory action, and even inspire healthier habits. Over time, organ awareness can help us make the long journey from our head into our body. By cultivating IA, internal sensations can be linked with specific emotions, deepening our emotional intelligence. Listening to the language of organs can connect us to our authentic emotional self and encourage compassionate responses. For example, when I feel a distinctive heaviness in my chest, I know I'm feeling grief and need to treat myself with tenderness.

In vijnanamaya kosha, we can deliberately embody specific organ qualities, such as earthiness or slowness, to transform habitual patterns of perception and response. In fact, organ awareness confers a stable sense of self. Our heart, breath, and gastrointestinal rhythms transmit signals to the brain to create a stronger sense of body agency (*this is my body*), location (*this is where my parts are located in space*), and embodied Self (*I am present and authentically responsive*) (Monti *et al.*, 2021).

Developing felt sense of organs and moving from them can awaken us to different levels of consciousness and nourish the deepest layers of Self. As the parasympathetic nervous system is activated, we relax, slow down, and breathe into our bellies. We may sense our inner fullness and be more open to self-compassion and support. With sustained organ awareness, we can feel more seated in ourselves and connected to our inner guidance. As the organs become touchstones for accessing and living from our deeper Self, we can strengthen our *kishkes*, a Yiddish word describing the knowing that comes from gut feelings.

Barral observed that patients often exhibited predictable behaviors or emotional tendencies depending on which organ type they most strongly expressed. In his clinical experience, "heart" people may be excessively attached to a loved one or have a fear of abandonment while "lung" people often have an ambiguous attitude, going from too much to not enough (Barral 2007).

If we listen to our organs, they can teach valuable life lessons:

- Slow down. Pause.
- Nourish yourself first.
- Only work when necessary.
- Work only as much as required.
- Work cooperatively with your neighbors.
- Rest after working.

In anandamaya kosha, working with organs can deepen an experience of oneself as a whole. Connecting with felt sense of inner fullness (and tenderness!) that organs provide can radiate outward into our relationships with others and the greater world.

## LEARN IT

Organs are "the warm, cozy home of our inner sense of fullness, intrinsically expanding in three dimensions regardless of gravity, an expansion that reverberates... to the periphery of the system, sustaining all limbs (head included) to move in an effortlessly, buoyant way" (Miller, Ethridge, and Morgan 2011, p.211).

While all organs can be experienced as movement initiators and support for somatic structures, for the sake of brevity, this chapter focuses on the heart and lungs (see Chapter 3 for lung anatomy). The practices can be modified for other organs.

Organs move in two distinct ways: mobility and motility. *Mobility* refers to movement in relation to other organs and internal structures, like the diaphragm or peritoneal wall. Mobility is supported by lubricating serous fluid that allows organs to slide and fold over or around each other as their functional shape changes. Picture the heart and lungs sliding over each other as they rhythmically expand and condense, or digestive organs sliding over each other in a yoga twist.

Mobility is supported by external movement, and moving our body regularly in ways that encourage organ mobility can improve organic function. Organ mobility and physiology may be impaired by visceral pathology or adhesions, musculoskeletal misalignment, or movement restrictions.

Organs also have inherent *motility*, a slow, low-amplitude, rhythmical movement across all three planes. This oscillating movement is thought to follow the descending spiralic pathway taken by organs during embryological development as they move into their final location in the torso (Barral and Mercier 1988). Each organ has its own rhythm of movement around a unique axis. Motility is palpable by trained practitioners and is a measure of organ health.

### The Heart and Lungs

The spongy, elastic lungs are approximately 24 cm (9.5 in.) in height and weigh on average 840 g (30 oz) in males and 640 g (23 oz) in females. Over half of this weight is blood and blood vessels. Yet the 4–6 l of air that fills their 480 million alveoli doesn't weigh anything! Recall that the lungs fill almost the entire rib basket and encircle the tender heart. The fist-sized heart (average weight of 331 g/12 oz in males and 245 g/8.6 oz in females) is protectively cushioned between the lungs and tirelessly circulating life-giving blood. Further protection is provided by the sternum in front,

the spine in back, and the surrounding ribs. Fascial sacs wrap the heart (pericardium) and lungs (visceral pleura) and are continuous with fascia lining the thoracic cavity (parietal pleura). The heart is tethered in place by ligaments merging into adjacent bone (sternum and spine) and soft tissue structures (diaphragm), while the lungs are stabilized by the upside-down bronchial tree. The heart and lungs slide against each other and the diaphragm, lubricated by serous fluid produced by visceral pleura and pericardium. Developing felt sense of the size, weight, and volume of these organs can affect carriage of the shoulders, neck, and head, the physiology of breath, and the quality and efficiency of movement.

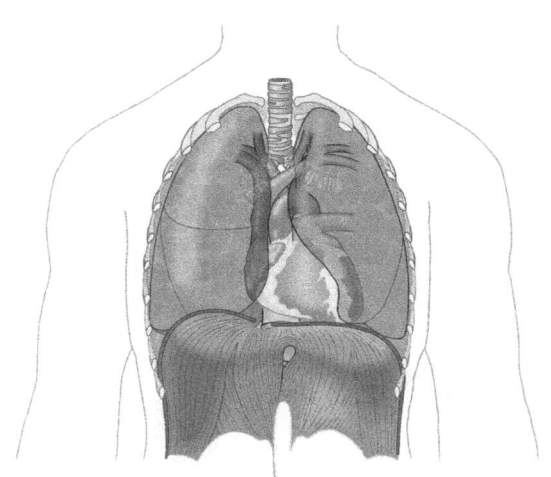

### FEEL IT

*I was hurrying to a meeting and realized how tense I was. As I remembered the support of my heart and lungs, my shoulders immediately dropped, I slowed down and became present.*

DALE

When we picture organs and sense their location, weight, and volume, this awareness can modify movement and alignment. Our movements

unfold from an internal place that bypasses habitual patterns and reduces effort. We may sense that organs are more yielding than bones or muscles, and that they flow and expand in all directions rather than orient in only one (Cranz and Chieii 2014). We can also consciously evoke organ qualities, such as slowness, grounding, earthiness, buoyancy, and support. When awareness expands to include organs, movement conveys a depth, fluidity, and fullness that musculoskeletal focus cannot provide. We can vary quality of movement with interplay between the organic upward moving energy of buoyancy and expression and downward moving energy of weight and earth. With organ awareness we can "organize" ourselves around inner support rather than remembering numerous structural details, like foot position or correct angle of the pelvis.

Bonnie Bainbridge Cohen, in her Body-Mind Centering method, popularized the concept that organs can influence movement, breath, and mind. Some of the following practices are based on her work (Cohen 1993).

## EXPLORATION: ORGAN QUALITIES

### Learning Objective

- Evoke organ qualities of weight, volume, and fluid movement.

### Props

- A latex balloon filled with warm water to a 15 cm (6 in.) diameter

### Instructions

- Sit in a comfortable position and take a baseline.

    – *How do you experience felt sense of your organs?*

- Hold the balloon cupped in your hands. Close your eyes and feel sensations of the balloon pressing into your hands: weight, shape, texture, and temperature.

- Focus on the volume of water as you slowly pour it in different directions. Sense the water rolling and sloshing inside the balloon.

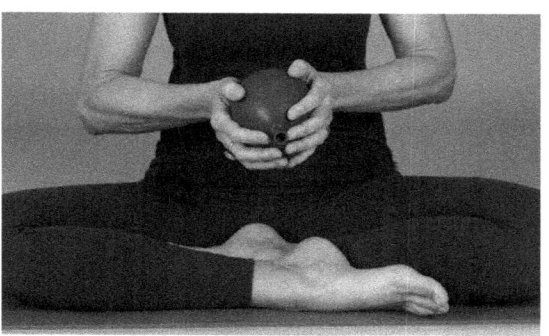

- Vary your movement. Explore pouring slower... faster... jiggling... and moving the balloon through space. Try rolling the balloon between your hands or passing it from hand to hand. Play with it, noticing different qualities and characteristics.

- Place the balloon on the floor and roll it back and forth between your hands or along the floor.

    – *What qualities does handling the water-filled balloon evoke for you?*
    – *What happens to your breath?*
    – *Can you imagine initiating movement by pouring from your organs?*

## EXPLORATION: ORGANIC FELT SENSE

### Learning Objective

- Use visualization, breath, touch, and sound to deepen felt sense of the heart and lungs.

### Practice Note

- Take as much time as necessary with each element of exploration, staying longer with whatever feels interesting.

### Props

- Blanket, cushion, bolster, and water-filled balloon (optional)

### Instructions

- Take a baseline in supine, supporting your head and knees with the cushion and bolster. Cover yourself for warmth, if necessary. Allow enough time to settle and feel your back body on the floor. Let your breath soften and slow.

  – *How do you sense your organs?*

- Connect with your bony skeleton, visualizing its shape and feeling its hardness pressing into the floor. Notice the edges, points, and rounded parts of your skeleton.

- Connect with your myofascia, the weighty soft tissue covering your skeleton. With each exhalation, imagine it draping around your skeleton and settling deeper into gravity.

- Connect with your organ body. Cup your hands on your abdomen as if tenderly holding your organs (or clasp the balloon to your abdomen).

- Imagine your organs as multiple slippery, organ-shaped, water-filled balloons inside your torso. Sense their weight and volume.

- Become aware of your breath and feel the abdominal organs spread and expand into your hands when compressed by the descending diaphragm on inhalations. As you exhale, release their weight into gravity. Imagine them slipping and gliding against each other as you breathe.

### Breath

- Move your hands (or the balloon) to your chest and sense the large lungs expanding and condensing as you breathe. Visualize them pressing multidimensionally into the inner surfaces of the rib basket. Sense how the lungs are held and supported by the rib basket.

- Shift your focus to the 480 million alveoli and imagine each air sac individually expanding and condensing. On inhalations, sense the quality of buoyancy as air inflates the alveoli. On exhalations, sense the quality of earthiness as the weight of the lungs settles into gravity.

- Imagine your lungs as sponges, expanding as they fill with liquid air, then squeezing the air out as you exhale.

- Shift your awareness to the rhythmical contraction of your heart. Imagine you can breathe directly into your heart.

- Sense the considerable combined weight of your heart and lungs yielding into gravity as you exhale.

### Tapping

- Use your finger pads or the palm of your hand to tap your ribs with the intention of creating vibration through heart and lung fluids. Tap systematically over the heart and each lung, covering as much surface area as you can reach. Imagine the fluidic ripples reverberating into areas you can't access.

### Sound

- Place your palms on your chest again. As you exhale, make a hissing sound, *ssss*, and direct the vibration into the depths of each lung for several breaths. In Chinese medicine, this sound is said to transform grief into courage.

- Place both palms over your heart. As you exhale, make a drawn-out *haw* sound, either audibly or whispered. Imagine directing the vibration into the depths of your heart.

Chinese medicine suggests that this sound can transform hate into love and happiness.

- Move onto one side, supporting your head with the cushion. Sense the weight of your organs in this alternate orientation to gravity. Then, roll onto your stomach… then the other side. Spend enough time in each position to sense how organs reorient their weight to gravity. Play with sound and breath in each position.

- Move into a seated position, pausing to register the effects of this practice.

  - *What feels different?*
  - *Which practices did you like best?*
  - *What is the felt sense of your heart and lungs now?*

## EXPLORATION: LOBES OF THE LUNGS

### Learning Objective

- Differentiate different lobes of the lungs.

### Instructions

This practice may be done either seated or supine. Since the left lung has only two lobes and the right has three lobes, we will consider the lower, middle, and upper parts of both lungs.

- Take a breath baseline.

  - *How do you sense your lungs?*

- Place both hands on your lower right rib basket, arranging them to encircle a maximum area front to back. Become aware of the lower lung underneath your hands. Imagine that you are compassionately supporting the lung, welcoming its presence. Sense your hands holding the lung, and the lung rising to meet the invitation of your hands. Imagine the intelligence of your lung cells awakening

with your touch. Direct your inhalations into the volume between your hands.

- After some time, remove your hands and continue to welcome the presence of your lower lung as you breathe. Pause to notice new sensations.

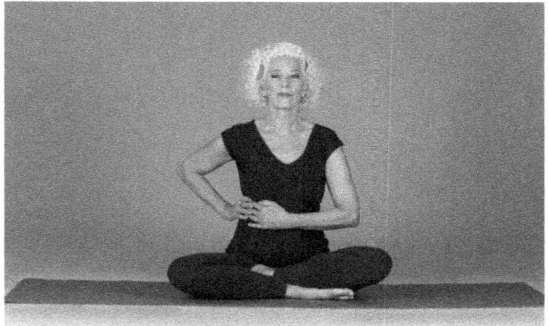

- Place one hand on the ribs underneath your armpit and the other hand on your breast area. Repeat the practice to awaken the intelligence of the middle lung.

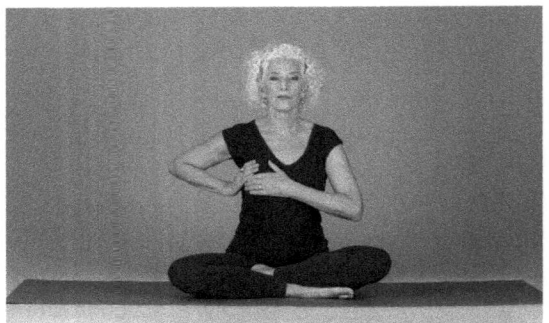
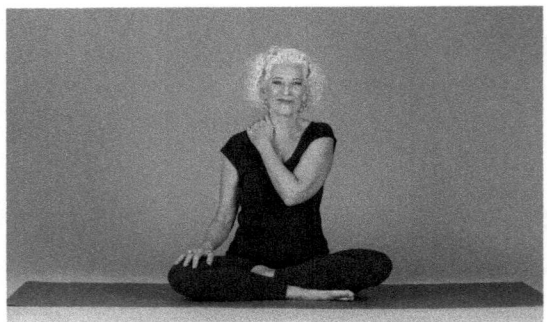

- Place the heel of your left hand below the right clavicle with the fingers draping over the shoulder. Repeat the practice to awaken the intelligence of the upper lung.

- Pause to register effects of the practice and differences between your right and left lungs.

- Move your arms randomly to notice how deeper felt sense of the lungs changes your movement experience.

- Repeat the practice with the left lung.

  - *How does organ awareness change felt sense of your lungs?*
  - *Does your breath change?*
  - *How is your movement different?*

## FOUNDATIONAL PRACTICE: HEART HUG BREATH 🔊

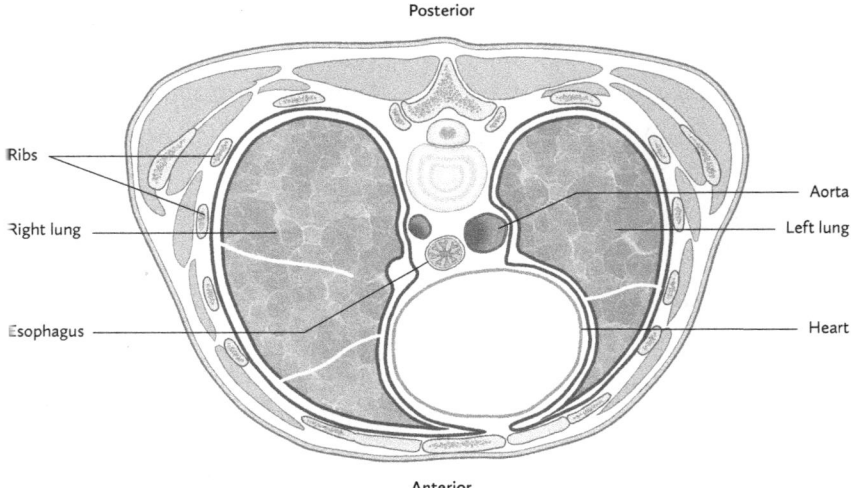

Posterior

Ribs

Right lung

Esophagus

Aorta

Left lung

Heart

Anterior

Self-compassion is an important quality that can be cultivated through EA. Just like muscular strength improves with dedicated and consistent practice, so can the *muscle* of self-compassion. A cross section of the upper torso shows the lungs enveloping the heart in a heart shape. Visualizing this in your body heightens felt sense of your lungs embracing your heart with each breath. It can promote feelings of holding or embracing yourself with compassion, exactly as you are. It's useful any time you need to calm or center yourself, even in the middle of a challenging conversation or situation.

## Learning Objective

- Evoke presence and self-compassion through organ awareness.

## Practice Notes

- If you need strengthening or *tonification*, like when fatigued, focus on imagining the lungs expanding inwardly to embrace the heart.

- If you need *dispersal* of energy, as when feeling overwhelming emotions, focus on imagining the heart expanding outwardly to meet the embrace of the lungs.

## Instructions

- In a comfortable seated position, recall the diagram of the heart and lungs cross section. Translate it into your own body, visualizing your heart-shaped lungs surrounding and holding the heart.

- Place both hands on your chest and imagine tenderly holding your heart and lungs.

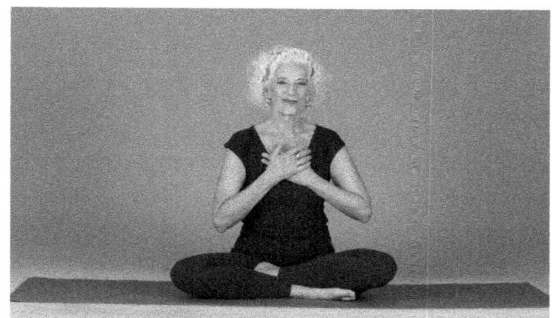

- Attend to the outward expansion of your breath. As you inhale, register your lungs expanding multidimensionally into the front, back and sides of your rib basket. Breathe in a calm and relaxed way, softening on exhalations. Focus on these sensations for several breaths.

- For the next several inhalations, visualize your lungs expanding inwardly to "embrace" or "hug" your heart. Allow this sensation to register in your body. Welcome any feelings, emotions, or images that arise.

- Remove your hands and dissolve the visualization. Pause and register any effects of this practice.

  - *What sensations, emotions, or feelings arose?*
  - *Are there situations in your life where this practice would be useful?*

Doing the heart-hug breath I discovered a place in my heart that felt resistant and emotionally bruised, and was able to soften into it.

*Amy*

## HEAL IT

### EXPLORATION: MOVING FROM THE HEART AND LUNGS

When you consciously initiate movement from an organ, corresponding movement of the musculoskeletal container is supported. Organ-initiated movement has different qualities than muscle-initiated movement and can bypass habitual patterns of muscular activation.

### Learning Objectives

- Explore how organs can support and initiate movement that emanates into musculoskeletal structures.

- Differentiate movement qualities between organ and musculoskeletal initiation.

### Props (optional)

- A water-filled balloon...

- A partner

- A blanket or cushion

### POURING ORGANS

### Instructions

- In a comfortable seated position, spend a few moments sensing the weight of your skeleton and its patterns of pressure on your seated surface. Sense myofascia draping over your bones, settling into gravity. Do a few **Heart Hug Breaths** to center your awareness.

- Become aware of the size, weight, and volume of your heart and lungs. With each exhalation, consciously release their weight into the support of your diaphragm and lower organs.

- Place both hands on your chest as though you are tenderly holding your heart and

lungs. Alternatively, hold the balloon against your chest. Make a connection between the fluid in the balloon and the volume of blood inside your organs.

- Imagine you can initiate *stirring* or *swirling* movements from the blood, remembering the feeling of moving water in your balloon. Use rounded movements that shift your heart through space, carrying the rib basket with it. Lead the movement by directing the volume of organ fluid.

- Play with the qualities of buoyancy and weightiness as your heart moves.

- Stir in both directions.

  - *Do your shoulders or ribs want to take over the movement initiation?*

- Explore slowly pouring the heart and lungs in different directions to initiate spinal movement. On an exhalation, pour forward, receiving the organ weight in your hands. Allow the pouring to carry your spine into gentle flexion.

- Pause as you inhale to sense the weight, then exhale and pour again to move further into flexion. Move incrementally into a comfortable end range.

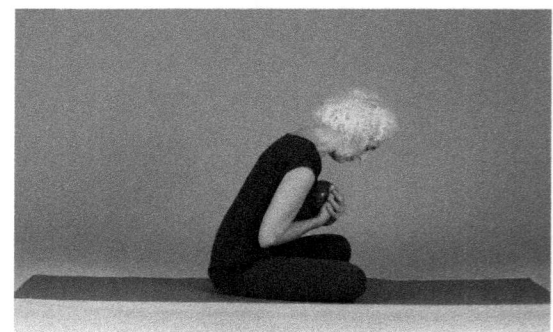

- To return upright, connect with the organic quality of buoyancy. As you inhale, visualize the heart and lungs inflating, or dilating, lifting you with expansive buoyancy.

- Imagine a friend's gentle hands on your back, holding your heart and lungs to receive their weight as you now pour backward. If you have an actual partner, even better. On exhalations, slowly pour the organs into your real or imaginary partner's hands so your spine is carried into slight extension. Move incrementally into a comfortable end zone.

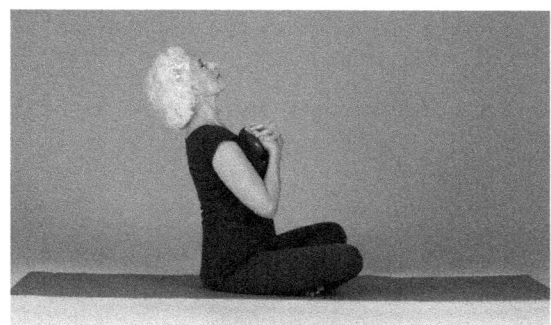

- Visualize the heart and lungs dilating and buoyantly lifting you upright.

- Slowly pour back and forth between flexion and extension and weight and buoyancy. Start with small movements and gradually increase the amplitude to a comfortable end range.

- Initiate the same flexion and extension movements from your spine and register any differences in quality of movement.
  - *How is organ initiation different?*
  - *Which way is easier?*
  - *Do you have felt sense of the difference between qualities of weightiness and buoyancy?*

- Explore pouring your organs in other directions.

- When you are finished with the exploration, pause to register any effects.
  - *What you notice?*

## MOVING THE SHOULDERS

### Instructions

- In either sitting or standing, elevate, depress, and circle your shoulders a few times to establish a musculoskeletal baseline.
  - *What is your effort level, range of motion, and quality of movement?*

- Shift to organ awareness and initiate shoulder elevation and depression from your heart and lungs.

- Still initiating movement from the organs, circle your shoulders several times in each direction.
  - *What's different when you initiate movement from your organs?*

## RIB ROLLS: ORGANIC INITIATION

You have done this practice in Chapter 3, but with a musculoskeletal focus.

### Instructions

- Lie on your right side with hips and knees at 90-degree angles, arms outstretched at shoulder height with palms together. Support your head to comfortably align your spine. Become aware of the weight of your heart and lungs resting into gravity and the compression of the right lung.

- With each exhalation, let the weight of your organs settle into gravity.

- On an exhalation, initiate movement from your heart and lungs to slowly roll forward.

The top arm slides over the bottom arm and your face moves closer to the floor. Visualize the volume of organ fluid pouring forward. Recall the feeling of rolling the water-filled balloon. Track the pouring sensations throughout the rolling movement.

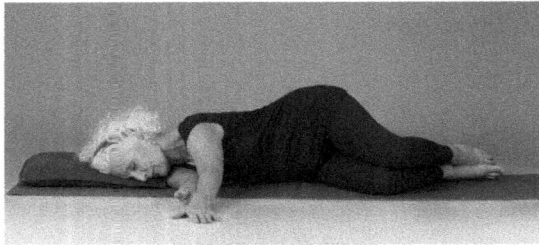

- On an inhalation, continue to track sensations as you slowly pour the organs backward, passing through the starting position and rolling toward your back ribs. Your top arm will slide along the bottom arm.

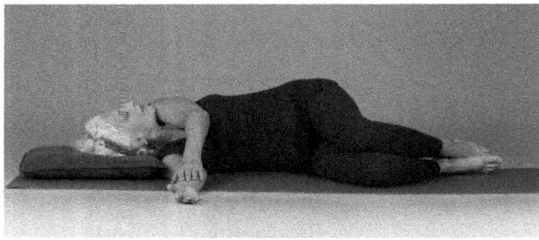

- Repeat several times, slowly pouring your organs forward and backward, then rest for a few breaths.

- Add a twist. On an inhalation, pour your organs backward to roll toward your back ribs. Allow the backward roll to initiate a simultaneous lift of your left arm toward 90 degrees.

- On an exhalation, continue pouring your organs to roll further onto your back ribs and move your arm toward the floor behind you to a comfortable endpoint. Use support if your arm doesn't reach the floor.

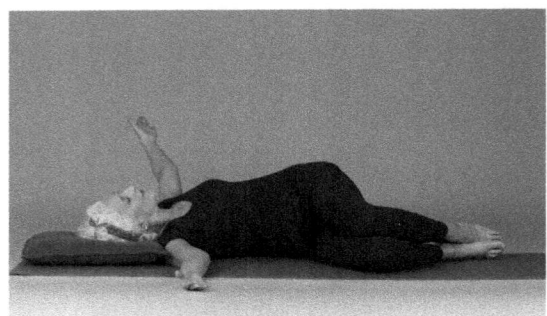

- Remain in the twist for a few breaths, sensing the weight of your organs in this position.

- Exhale as you pour the organs forward to return the arm to starting position.

- Repeat several times, then rest for a few breaths. Move to a seated position and explore a few arm movements to sense differences between the two sides.

- Repeat the movements lying on your left side.

- Move back to a seated position, pausing to sense effects of these movements.

  - *What is felt sense of your organs now?*
  - *How does quality of movement change when you move from your organs?*

## ORGAN SUPPORT 📹

When I sense my heart and lungs supporting my arms, my shoulder doesn't hurt when I reach up.

*Penny*

### Instructions

- Stand in a comfortable position with your arms at your sides, palms facing forward. Set a baseline by alternately rotating your arms internally and externally, initiating movement from the musculoskeletal system.

- Focus on your heart and lungs and sense their energetic connection to your arms. With each breath, imagine heart and lung pranic energy gradually emanating and pulsing down your arms.

- Imagine your anterior heart and lungs dilating and becoming so buoyant that they slightly lift your chest and emanate energy into your arms, causing them to externally rotate.

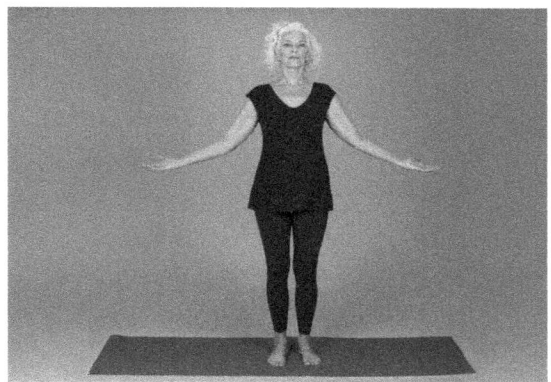

- Now imagine your posterior heart and lungs dilating and becoming so buoyant that your upper back rounds and widens, emanating energy into your arms and causing them to internally rotate.

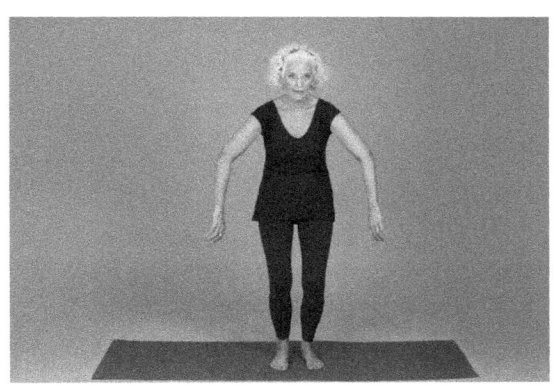

- Alternate dilating anteriorly and posteriorly, imagining heart and lung energy emanating down your arms and initiating the rotation movements.

  - *How does your breath synchronize with the movement?*

- Continue the movements as you visualize your arms as the "wings" of your heart, raising them incrementally to shoulder height.

- Pause with your arms at your sides to register effects of the practice.

  - *How did the quality of your movement change?*
  - *Can you sense the movements unfolding from an inner place?*
  - *Can your heart and lungs emanate vitality?*

- Raise your arms overhead, initiating the movement from your musculoskeletal system. Hold them up for several breaths, then lower them.

- Sense again the connection of your arms to the heart and lungs. Raise them overhead, this time making the movement an expression of the buoyancy and support of the heart and lungs. Lower your arms, still initiating movement from the organs. Repeat the movements several times, imagining your arms as wings of the heart.

- Pause with your arms overhead. Settle them into the organic support of your heart and lungs, allowing your arm muscles to soften. With each exhalation, feel the arms settle deeper into the buoyant support of the organs. After several breaths, lower your arms.

  - *What changes when you rely on organ initiation and support?*
  - *Is it easier to hold the arms up with organ support?*
  - *How could you apply this awareness in your daily activities?*

## EXPLORATION: THE FOUR-CHAMBERED HEART

This practice is adapted from "The Four Chambered Heart" in *The Four-fold Way: Walking the Paths of the Warrior, Teacher, Healer, and Visionary* (Arrien 1993).

In her book *The Four-Fold Way*, cultural anthropologist Dr. Angeles Arrien describes a practice from the native cultures she studied. Daily contemplation of four qualities of the heart was encouraged to maintain emotional and spiritual health. By attuning to the heart daily and nonjudgmentally reflecting on its qualities of fullness, openness, clarity, and strength, we can experience our wholeness.

### Learning Objective

- Contemplate qualities of the heart.

### Instructions

- Sit or lie in a comfortable position with closed eyes. Place your hands on your heart and do several **Heart Hug Breaths**. Rekindle felt sense of your heart and feel it settling into gravity.

- Ask yourself:

  - *How full-hearted am I today?*
  - *Am I feeling generous and motivated to give of myself? Or am I half-hearted about something in my life, feeling like I "should" do something I don't want to do?*
  - *Do I need to change something in my life?*

- Remember a time when you felt full-hearted. Recall the sensations. For several breaths, amplify a feeling of full-heartedness.

- Ask yourself:

  - *How openhearted am I today?*
  - *Can I freely express kindness and warmth? Or is my heart closed, defensive, or self-protective?*

- Remember a time when you felt open-hearted. Recall the sensations. For several breaths, soften your heart and amplify a feeling of openheartedness.

- Ask yourself:

  - *How clear-hearted am I today?*
  - *Do I have clarity about what I am doing? Or do I feel doubt, confusion, or ambivalence?*

- Remember a time when you felt clear-hearted. Recall the sensations. For several breaths, amplify a feeling of clear-heartedness.

- Ask yourself:

  - *How strong-hearted am I today?*
  - *Do I have the courage to be authentic, speak my truth, and hold my ground? Or do I resist expressing my true Self?*

- Remember a time when you felt courageous and strong-hearted. Recall the sensations.

For several breaths, amplify a feeling of strong-heartedness.

- Reflect on which qualities are more accessible to you. Remember these qualities in daily

life and notice what situations and relationships welcome your whole heart.

- – *Which qualities need strengthening?*
- – *Which qualities do you most need now?*

## THERAPEUTIC APPLICATIONS

*With organ awareness, I drop out of monkey mind, ground, and come home to myself.*

SHARON

Awareness of organs gained through EA explorations adds a layer of complexity, depth, and fullness to therapy regardless of which koshic level is being addressed. When organs are directly accessed, adjacent musculoskeletal structures reap the benefits, particularly when underlying organ torsion, adhesions, or hypo- or hypertonicity contribute to structural dysfunction or prevent presenting conditions from resolving as expected. For some people, simply visualizing organ support can radically change movement, alignment, and myofascial tone. Those with rigid posture may learn to soften into the support of their organs, while others with collapsed posture may find spontaneous erectness by embodying organ buoyancy and expression. When a conscious relationship is established with organs, dialogue is possible, and a healing conversation can be initiated between contents and container.

Similarly, working with the musculoskeletal container can enhance organ function. For example, when alignment, mobility, and elasticity of the rib basket, shoulders, and neck are addressed in clients with cardiovascular conditions, imbalanced tension and compression forces affecting cardiac function can recalibrate. Heart mobility and motility may improve, and, in yogic terms, healing prana can circulate freely to and within the heart. Almost a century ago, orthopedic

surgeon Joel Goldthwaite described postural influence on organ function and subsequent failure of tissue adaptation to chronic structural misalignment, observing that when we are out of balance and muscles and ligaments are abnormally tensioned or strained, physiological function suffers (1945).

It's well established that many chronic organic conditions are initiated by sustained overstimulation of the sympathetic nervous system related to high stress levels (Renzaho *et al.*, 2014). Attuning to organs can evoke organic qualities like earthiness, weight, volume, and slowness, which can reduce sympathetic nervous system stimuli and improve parasympathetic vagal tone. Responsive and balanced nervous system adaptation creates an environment that encourages organ repair, health, and resilience.

Interoceptive organ awareness offers benefits beyond the physical body. Cultivating interoception in general has proven helpful in conditions including anxiety, depression, eating disorders, autism, addiction, and trauma (Khalsa *et al.*, 2018). Organ embodiment offers an accessible path of learning to listen and attend to visceral messages signifying emotions, stress, or dysfunction, and to strengthen self-regulation skills. Continued practice refines sensory perception, enhances body awareness, and supports habits of self-nourishment. Connecting to organs with compassionate awareness also improves physiological function, often compromised in psychological conditions.

Learning to access organ support can even

influence personality and behavior. Some students report that connecting with the inner fullness of their organs helped them to meet or push back against external influences and circumstances. Instead of feeling like *the world is against me... I'm powerless*, they found their inner support and resources to face reality. Others discovered that organ awareness provided an inner reference system that helped them establish more integrity between their inner and outer selves.

> With regular organ work I have slowed down. My center seems lower in my body, and somehow more reliable. I'm increasingly in touch with my inner essence and my self-trust has deepened.
>
> *Polly*

## KOSHIC CONTEMPLATIONS

### Annamaya Kosha

- *How does organ awareness affect your alignment and movement?*
- *How does the quality of movement change?*
- *Which organ qualities are most helpful?*
- *How can you incorporate organ awareness into your movement practice and daily activities?*

### Pranamaya Kosha

- *How does your breath change when you focus on organs?*
- *Can you feel your nervous system calming with organ focus?*
- *Have you noticed any physiological changes?*

### Manomaya Kosha

- *Did any emotions arise during the organ explorations?*
- *Are you more aware of emotional or physiological messages from your organs?*

### Vijnanamaya Kosha

- *Do you feel more embodied after doing organ explorations?*
- *Are there specific organ qualities that you could cultivate in your everyday life?*
- *Which lessons from the organs would be useful to incorporate into your life?*

### Anandamaya Kosha

- *Has organ awareness helped you experience your inner fullness and wholeness?*

## KEY CONCEPTS

- Organs can be a source of support and movement initiation.
- The state of the musculoskeletal container affects organic contents, and vice versa.

- Organ awareness can discourage excessive habitual tension and use of overlying muscles.
- Developing felt sense of organs can calm the sympathetic nervous system and

activate the parasympathetic nervous system.

- Organs connect us to our "gut" feelings.
- Organ awareness can confer a stable sense of self.
- Organs have mobility and motility.
- Organ awareness can support and modify movement and alignment.
- Organic support can influence personality and behavior.

# CHAPTER 6

# Standing on Your Own Two Feet

*Keep your feet on the ground.*
*Stand up for yourself.*
*Dig in your heels.*
*Step up to the plate.*
*Take a stand.*
*Walking on eggshells.*

Everything on earth is subject to the force of gravity. Lucky for us humans, there is an equal and opposite uplifting force keeping us upright: ground reaction force, the counterthrust of gravity. Right relationship between gravity and ground reaction force can pattern structural stability and integrity while enabling clear force transmission and resourceful movement. Without right relationship, we must do something to compensate, like holding ourselves up, or distorting other body parts to stay upright. Everyday language reflects this relationship between our legs and the ground. In German, the word for *independent* is *selbstandig*, to stand on one's own (Collinsdictionary.com n.d.). When we feel a sense of safety and belonging, walking in the world with ease and confidence, we can stand on our own two feet. We may be described as grounded.

Lack of right relationship with gravity compromises functional balance between tension and compression forces in the body. As a result, the upward force that anatomist John Sharkey (2015) describes as *lift* fails to provide effortless verticality and buoyancy in standing or provide the ability to self-correct when we lose balance.

Lift helps to create and maintain joint space and expansiveness through soft tissue structures.

Gravity has been humorously described as a negative force, as in the body "losing the battle" with gravity. Although this invisible force is not consciously detected, our nervous system ceaselessly attempts to balance tension, compression, and gravitational forces. As babies learning to stand and walk, our body weight, gravity, and the ground were in constant interplay. As we repeatedly fell, then clumsily and unskillfully found our way to standing, neuromuscular pathways for balance and stability were gradually encoded in our nervous system. As toddlers, we opposed gravity in a beautiful and balanced way, but as we matured, accidents, habitual patterns of use, physical and emotional pain, and life experience disrupted that natural harmonious balance.

Most of us need to relearn what it means to live in an optimally balanced body in which internal forces and gravity interact in ways that produce vitality and economy of energy. When our structure is optimally aligned, it can bear and distribute weight and force in ways that oppose gravity efficiently, and our body can self-correct as appropriate.

> Gravity is the root of lightness.
>
> *Lao Tzu (Cleary 1993, p. 24)*

## KOSHIC PERSPECTIVES

Cultivation of a solid sense of connection to the ground through the lower body has ramifications on all koshic levels. EA awareness and practices for the lower limbs can transform habitual or maladaptive alignment and movement habits that challenge right relationship with the ground, oneself, and the external world.

The lower limbs operate as functional units, extending from hip to foot. Each part influences and is influenced by other parts during force transmission, stability, and locomotion functions. Annamaya kosha exploration of the lower limbs includes learning about anatomy and function and how to cultivate intelligent, optimal alignment and movement. When lower limbs and pelvic bones are in right relationship with gravity, each joint can distribute forces more efficiently to neighboring structures and throughout the body-wide tensional network. When joints of the lower limbs are not balanced, tensional structures often assume the function of stabilizing the skeleton. This gravitational imbalance can initiate a cascade of compensations in the fascial network, causing compromised physiology, pathology, and pain.

Breath and energy levels in pranamaya kosha are affected by the quality of our relationship to the ground. Habits of rigidly holding yourself away from the ground or collapsing into gravity can pattern shallow, upper chest breathing with wide-ranging ramifications on energy levels and physiology. Whenever we lose secure connection with the ground, upper body muscles excessively tense to compensate for lack of support from below and breath is compromised. Finding right relationship encourages free integral breath and energy flow.

We can consciously direct prana and force along defined pathways in the lower limb to establish clear lines of force transmission between the pelvis and ground. Deliberate tracking of force through lower limb joints can balance

distribution of forces through and around joints, increasing movement efficiency and minimizing injury.

Our thinking mind, manomaya kosha, notices alignment and movement habits and their effect on our experience of grounding and stability. We ask, *How do I do that?* Through EA, we learn and embody new information to repattern more helpful ways of relating to the ground. In this process, our interoceptive sense identifies and differentiates sensations signifying optimal functional patterns; we learn sensory signatures of grounding, stability, or clear force transmission.

The sensory aspect of manomaya kosha is represented in extensive innervation of the foot, making it one of our most sensitive parts. Sensory information from feet contributes to our ability to balance and stand upright. Compromised sensory function is associated with poor postural control and fall risk (Viseux 2020). When we consciously sense the ground beneath us, our body awareness increases, our energy settles, and our mind quiets so we can focus more clearly.

We can also notice how our habitual stance affects other koshas, particularly breath and emotions. For example, after working with the **Foot Triangle** practice (provided later in this chapter), one student happily reported her first Christmas holiday gathering without sister fights. Every time she felt her emotions rising, she used her feet as touchstones and was able to stay with herself and respond appropriately rather than react. In this way, establishing structural stability can pattern both mental and emotional stability.

Besides influencing whole-body alignment and movement, the quality of relationship with the ground is echoed in our personality, perceptions, and responses. In vijnanamaya kosha, the shape and way of being in our body may reflect embodied metaphors like "down to earth" or "walking on eggshells." Common compensations for lack of secure foundation are postures of prop and collapse, both of which destabilize our grounding and disrupt tensional harmony (Farhi 1996).

Prop manifests as unconscious pushing away from the ground, with upper body muscles valiantly activating to resist gravity. "Proppers" can be "heady," armoured, and defensive. Collapse can result in slackness, leading to flaccid or droopy posture. This lack of structural integrity and inability to feel support from the ground can contribute to depression or lack of aspiration. In both prop and collapse, the breath is often shallow, adversely affecting multiple physiological systems.

Yield describes a harmonious relationship with gravity, where tension and compression forces are balanced throughout the body, and simultaneous grounding and lift can be experienced. Yield reflects integrity in the fascial network, and balanced effort and ease. Breath is free and unforced, and physiology functions optimally. The experience of physical security provided by right relationship with gravity may generate qualities of presence, trust in life and self, and ability to stay centered amid flux. Embodying yield promotes mental and emotional fluidity, healthy boundaries, and adaptive responsiveness to challenges instead of habitual reflexive reaction.

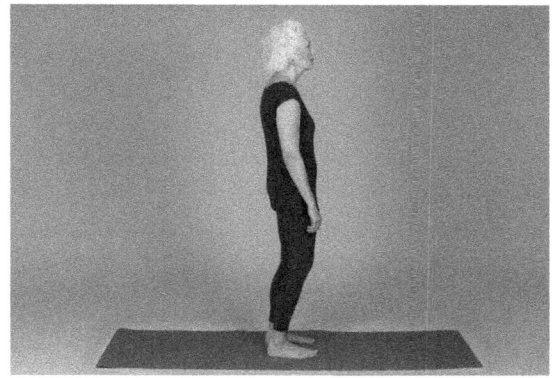

Collapse

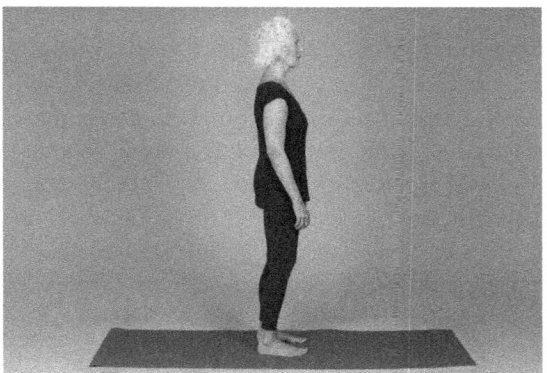

Yield

Cultivating felt sense of support from the earth and right relationship with gravity can result in lift not only through our structure, but also in our heart and mind. This can engender feelings of security, self-reliance, and aspiration. We stand on our own two feet.

> The psychological effect of foot problems of all kinds is remarkably consistent: the deep, unconscious feeling of insecurity.
>
> *Ida Rolf (1989)*

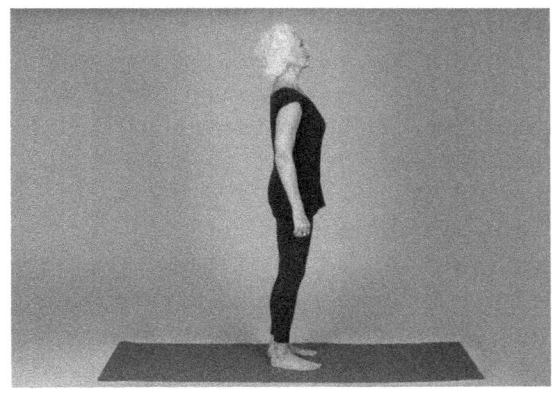

Prop

Exploration of harmonious relationship to the ground helps to integrate lower limbs into the "family" of the body and generate feelings of wholeness and connection in anandamaya kosha. As we establish right relationship with gravity, there may be consequential changes in relationship with self, others, and the cosmos. We may start to treat ourselves with more reverence and gratitude, and other relationships may deepen as we find our ground and stand in our authentic Self.

> If we surrendered to earth's intelligence, we could rise up rooted, like trees.
>
> *Rainer Maria Rilke (Barrows and Macy 1996, p. 116)*

## LEARN IT

It all starts in the feet. The Celestial Design Committee devised these relatively small, delicate, complicated miracles of architecture to efficiently receive and transmit the entire weight of the body into the ground. The complex arrangement of bones and soft tissue creates a stable foundation yet enables spring in our step that provides buoyancy through our structure and propels us through space. As the interface between the body and ground, the ankles and feet can influence tension and compression relationships throughout the body-wide fascial system, resulting in a harmonious (or not so harmonious!) relationship with gravity. The base affects the whole, but the reverse is also true. The feet and legs will shapeshift in response to influences from both the upper body and the ground.

Research has documented structural continuity and force transmission through joints of the lower limbs, pelvis, and lumbar spine in ways that are better explained by an integrated myofascial system than biomechanically (Marinho *et al.*, 2017). Muscles, tendons, ligaments, joint capsules, and associated fascia in this system function synergistically; misalignment or restricted motion in one affects the others. Other research confirms that force is transmitted laterally to synergistic muscles (Huijing 2007) and in multiple planes through some of the myofascial chains proposed by Thomas Myers in his Anatomy Trains Myofascial Meridians model (Krause *et al.*, 2016). We experience this functional integration during lower-limb practices when our upper body releases effort to hold itself up, or during upper-body practices that induce a sense of weightiness and stability in our legs. As we stimulate sensory feedback in our feet, postural regulation and balance can improve (Viseux 2020).

When our legs provide a stable yet flexible foundation, the rest of our body can organize itself around its midline and center of gravity. The nervous system then receives clear input regarding the ground surface and relationship to gravity and can assess, process, and relay motor messages that foster effortless uprightness and balance. Even a small deviation from the central axis can cause imbalances across the fascial matrix, leading to altered movement patterns, increased risk of injury, and challenges to our psychological "footing." When we actively cultivate kinesthetic sense of the relationship between our feet and ground, and consciously stay in relationship with this supportive surface, the resulting fluid stability, strength, and balance affect all koshic levels.

### The Foot and Ankle

Structures in our feet work together to effortlessly transition between functions of stability, shock absorption, mobility, and propulsion. The 26 bones and two tiny sesamoid bones are suspended in a supportive fascial matrix, and 33 joints are stabilized by over 100 ligaments. This arrangement, plus the longitudinal and horizontal arches, permit multiplanar movement enabling us to remain upright on uneven ground. The rich endowment of nerve endings transmits vital information about the ground to the brain to help us navigate different surfaces.

Human feet are pretensioned in a spiral maintained by fascia, primarily the plantar ligament. Our feet can further twist, becoming more rigid to provide support and propel us through space, or untwist to become mobile and adaptable when standing on or traversing uneven surfaces. When feet are pathologically under-or over-twisted, the corresponding slackness or tension can be transmitted upward through fascial continuities, disturbing the balance of tension and compression forces throughout the fascial network. Without this balance, the sensory function of our feet is diminished.

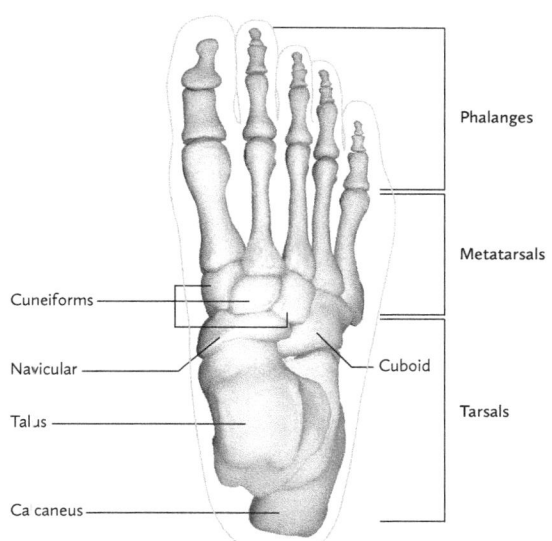

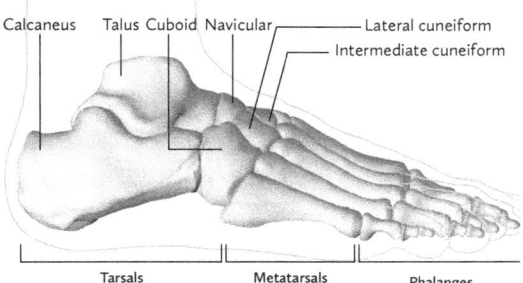

## Bones

Both lower leg bones participate in the ankle joint. The inferior tibia forms most of the joint while the relatively non-weight-bearing fibula fine-tunes movement and provides lateral stability. The malleoli (ankle bones) of the two bones grasp the talus, like ice tongs holding an ice cube, guiding its movement. The seven tarsal bones forming the back half of the foot are irregularly shaped with multiple surfaces fitting together like pieces of a puzzle. Although the gliding movement at individual joints is minimal, collective movement of all the joints is impressive, even allowing circular movement. Strong ligaments stabilize the bones, limit and guide movement, and provide proprioceptive feedback. The talus is extra dense and compact to receive the entire weight of the upper body onto its rounded surface. Weight is transferred posteriorly to the calcaneus and anteriorly to the medial longitudinal arch. Although guided and restrained by ligaments, the talus has no muscular attachments so floats freely in all three planes of movement. The talus is wider in front. When it glides backward on the tibia during dorsiflexion, it wedges firmly between the tibia and fibula to reinforce ankle stability.

The calcaneus (heel bone) receives weight from the talus, then transfers it posteriorly into the ground and anteriorly to the lateral longitudinal arch. In addition to its weight-bearing function, the long calcaneus helps to thrust our body away from the ground during walking. The orientation of the three joint surfaces at the talocalcaneal joint between these two bones allows tiny movements in all three planes for adapting to walking on uneven ground.

The five smaller tarsal bones—the navicular, cuboid, and three cuneiforms—also allow multiplanar movement. Wearing rigid shoes restricts their collective movement, forcing the ankle and knee joints to compensate for foot immobility. When coupled with rigidity or decreased range of motion at the hip joints, this can be a recipe for knee arthritis or other lower limb dysfunction.

The five long bones of the foot, the metatarsals, and their associated phalanges (toe bones) form the front half of the foot. Each toe has three phalanges, except the big toe, which has only two. The first metatarsal is the thickest, reflecting its important role in weight-bearing and thrust. When we sense our toes originating from their articulation with the metatarsal heads our alignment and movement patterns can transform.

## Arches

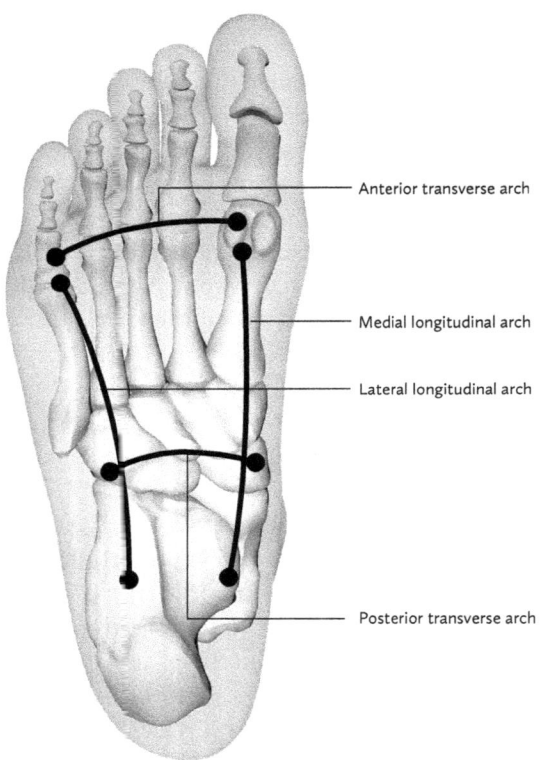

Anterior transverse arch

Medial longitudinal arch

Lateral longitudinal arch

Posterior transverse arch

The medial and lateral longitudinal arches and two transverse arches enable the small surface area of the foot to support our total body weight yet give a spring to each step. The better-known medial arch is formed by the calcaneus, talus, navicular, three cuneiforms, and metatarsals and phalanges of the first three toes. The lateral arch is formed by the calcaneus, cuboid, and metatarsals and phalanges of the lateral two toes. This arch provides stability and supports the more elastic medial arch that enables propulsion by alternately flattening and stiffening during walking. The distal transverse arch is formed by the metatarsal heads while the lesser-known proximal transverse half arch is formed by the navicular, cuboid, cuneiforms, and metatarsal bases, and is completed by the corresponding proximal transverse arch in the other foot. Both distribute weight and play roles in softening and stiffening the foot for propulsion.

## Myofascia

Our foot muscles are part of a myofascial continuity influencing foot, ankle, and knee joints. Twelve extrinsic muscles originate on the lower leg and are responsible for maintaining arches and moving feet and toes. Ten intrinsic muscles within the foot stabilize arches and guide fine motor movements like moving a single toe. Four layers of muscle on the sole of the foot and an associated thick pad of fat absorb shock and provide protection from sharp objects. We can imagine our foot bones suspended in a gel matrix of fascia.

The feet are a feat of economical bioengineering in which minimal materials yield multiple movement and stability possibilities. Foot mobility is maximized by the sheer number of bones and collective movement of many joints. Stability is enhanced partly by the shape of bones and limited movement within individual joints. Strong ligaments further stabilize the foot and ankle as does a retinaculum (fascial band) that "shrink-wraps" ankle and tarsal bones and holds multiple tendons in place. More stability is provided by the extrinsic muscles descending from the leg and wrapping under the foot. Yet, it's still easy to sprain an ankle!

## The Knee

Imagine living life with knees that don't bend. How would we walk? Or sit? Knee joints give us flexibility to move freely and gracefully, and their shock-absorbing function softens the impact of the feet hitting the ground as we locomote. Otherwise, every step would be jarring. The knees transfer ground reaction force upward to enable erectness and lift in our upper body. Healthy and flexible knees allow us to make rapid and adaptable changes in speed or direction of movement.

As the intermediary joint between hips and ankles, our knees are at the mercy of the health and mobility of these neighboring joints. An intrinsically unstable joint, the knee depends on the stabilizing influence of surrounding fascia: the joint capsule and ligaments, overlapping tendons, and cartilaginous menisci. A complex arrangement of ligaments steadies each knee joint from front, back, sides, and within. Range of motion is limited as a trade-off for the increased stability required to absorb and transfer almost all our body weight to the ground. If we carry extra weight, each extra pound (0.45 kg) of weight adds up to six pounds (2.7 kg) of pressure to the knees, increasing the risk of joint wear and tear (Shojania 2010). Both unstable and immobile knees can trigger dysfunction up and down the kinetic chain.

Structurally and functionally, the knee is the largest and most complex joint in our body. It is formed by the two longest bones of the skeleton, the tibia and femur. Although often considered a hinge joint, it's a double condyloid joint; two rounded condyles of the distal femur sit on two shallow convex tibial surfaces separated by an intercondylar ridge. The rounded femoral condyles fit poorly in the flatter tibial plateaus, creating an inherently unstable joint. Two thin C-shaped cartilaginous menisci cushion the joint and create a deeper, more congruent fit. The oval shape of the joint permits only minimal rotation as the articular surfaces are longer front to back.

The fibula is the thinnest bone in the body in proportion to its length. It articulates with the lateral condyle of the femur without participating in the knee joint.

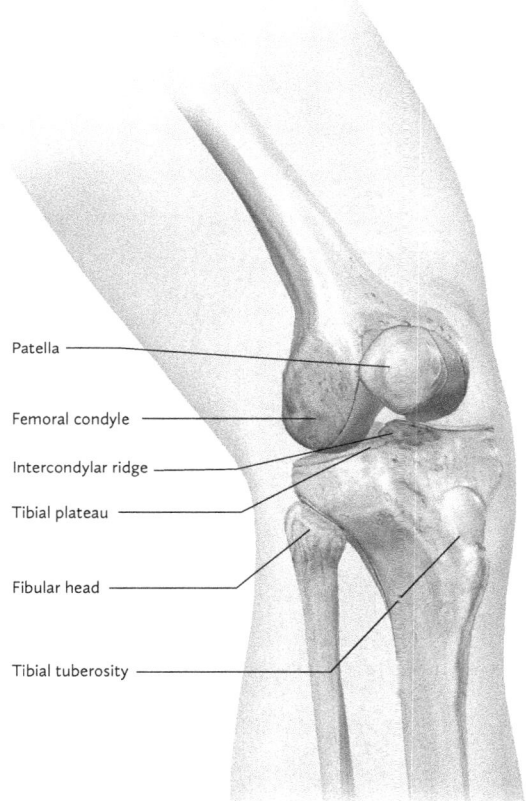

Patella

Femoral condyle

Intercondylar ridge

Tibial plateau

Fibular head

Tibial tuberosity

The patella is a triangular-shaped sesamoid bone embedded within the quadriceps tendon. It covers the knee, protecting it from direct pressure and reducing friction between the quadriceps tendon and femur. It also functions as a pulley, gliding in the groove between the femoral condyles, amplifying mechanical force of the quadriceps muscles.

Multiple myofascial structures cross the knee joint, interweaving and overlapping from multiple directions above and below. Several muscles originate above the hip joint, linking the pelvis and lower leg, further stabilizing the knee from varied angles and inextricably linking knee and hip function.

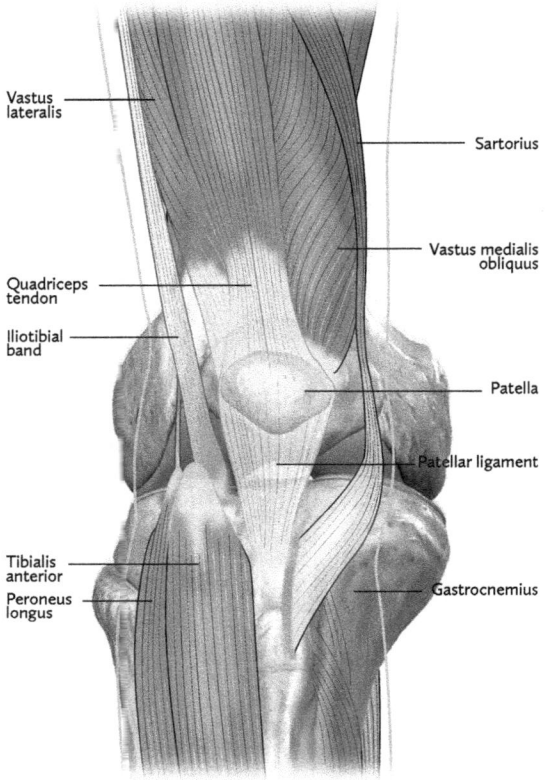

Vastus lateralis
Sartorius
Quadriceps tendon
Vastus medialis obliquus
Iliotibial band
Patella
Patellar ligament
Tibialis anterior
Peroneus longus
Gastrocnemius

## The Hip

The hip joints link the pelvis and legs to determine our direction of movement. The Celestial Design Committee crafted a functional balance between stability and mobility. The magnificent design allows 360 degrees of movement within an intrinsically stable joint requiring great force to dislocate. The deep cup of the hip socket and numerous strong ligaments snugly secure the head of the femur to reinforce and stabilize the joint. Myofascial structures overlap the hip from many different angles to stabilize the pelvis on the femur and support and transfer forces from

above and below. Both stability and mobility are maximized by the design of the ball and socket joints and by the neck of the femur extending the femoral shaft laterally.

The synergy of movement between joints above and below the hip is affected by the condition of the hip joints. Healthy hip joints support both stability *and* efficient movement patterns in the more complicated and less stable joints of the knees or lower back, which often suffer the consequences of tension, misalignment, or injury in the hip. When tension and compression forces throughout the fascial network spread weight transmission through the center of each hip joint, the rest of the body can find optimal alignment and stability.

The hip socket (acetabulum) is a deep concavity formed by fusion of equal parts of the three paired pelvic bones. This design allows force to be transferred and centered in the joint from multiple angles: the pubic bone anteriorly, ischium posteriorly, and ilium laterally. Complete fusion of these bones doesn't occur until 15–20 years of age. The acetabulum articulates with the femur, the longest and strongest bone in the body. The head of the femur is approximately two-thirds of a sphere covered with articular cartilage fitting into the half sphere of the acetabulum, which is deepened and stabilized by the labrum, a cartilaginous ring. Although the elongated femoral neck positions the greater trochanter lateral to the hip joint, the shaft descends diagonally and medially, placing the hip joint directly above the knee joint (helpful in transmission of ground reaction force!). The inner bony architecture of the femoral neck is designed to withstand and accommodate strong bending, shearing, and tensile forces. In excess, these forces contribute to hip pathologies like arthritis and bursitis, while inadequate forces can result in osteoporosis.

Seven strong ligaments stabilize each femur by interweaving with the joint capsule and surrounding myofascia. The ligaments twist around the hip joint to stabilize it in extension, then unwind and loosen in flexion. Structural misalignment can cause ligaments and myofascia surrounding the joint to tighten like a corkscrew, increasing pressure into the socket and eventually damaging the joint capsule and cartilage.

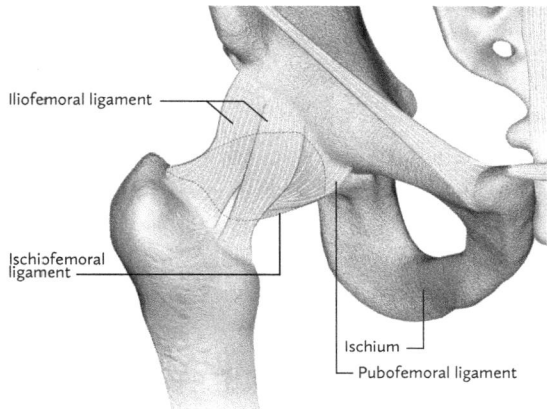

Iliofemoral ligament

Ischiofemoral ligament

Ischium

Pubofemoral ligament

## Component Movement

Joint movement is *helical*, meaning in a spiral like a helix. The round nature of bone with its curved edges and irregular surfaces ensures that movement is never purely in one plane. *Gross* movement occurs when body parts move through space, but the quality and range of gross movement depends on *component*, or intrinsic, movements between articulating surfaces. These internal joint movements ensure long-term integrity of joints:

- *Roll* is a movement in which one joint surface rolls on the other like car tires on a road.
- *Glide* occurs when one joint surface slides across another like a car tire skidding on ice or oil. Roll and glide usually occur together. Without glide, the moving bone would roll off the joint surface.
- *Spin* is a rotational movement in which one bone pivots on another.

Visualizing and encouraging these movements during EA practices can improve joint and myofascial health, decrease pain, and increase comfortable range of motion.

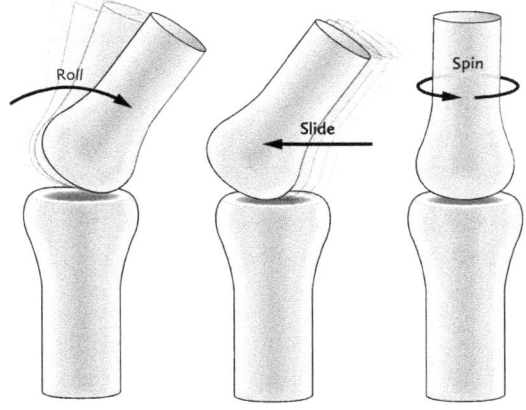

Roll

Slide

Spin

## FEEL IT

Encased in shoes, our feet are deprived of satisfying sensory stimulation, limiting our ability to exploit their rich sensory possibilities and intelligence. We can reawaken "unconscious" feet and amplify our body-mind connection through awareness, imagery, touch, and precise movement that refines the sensorimotor map of our base.

## EXPLORATION: DISCOVER THE LOWER LIMB

### Learning Objectives

- Learn anatomy of the lower limb.

- Deepen felt sense of the lower limb.

### Instructions

- Sit comfortably on a chair or floor and cross your right ankle over your left knee. As you palpate the "geography" and movement possibilities of the bones, imagine them suspended in the gel matrix of fascia.

### *The Foot*

- Start with the phalanges, the toe bones. Take hold of the big toe with the fingers of both hands and sensitively palpate all sides of the two phalanges and their joint. Then, explore the multiplanar movement possibilities by stabilizing the proximal phalange with one hand and moving the distal phalange slowly in all directions with the other hand.

- Repeat this exploration with the other four toes and their three phalanges.

- Locate the long metatarsals. Start with the first metatarsal, palpating its distal rounded ball joint and short, thick shaft. Then, individually palpate the other four long bones.

- With the fingers on top and thumbs on the sole, sink into the space between the first and second metatarsals, compressing the myofascia with your fingers in several places. Then, palpate the spaces between other metatarsals.

- Explore the movement possibilities. Stabilize the lateral four metatarsals with your left hand and move the first metatarsal back and forth, starting at the ball joint and gradually working your way along the shaft to the base. Repeat these explorations with the other metatarsals.

- To locate the tarsals, place two fingers across your instep, then palpate the small bones beneath. Move your foot in all directions to feel movement of the tarsals. Then, immobilize them with your hand and try to move your foot.

   - *Can you sense how the tarsals permit greater foot movement?*

- To locate the talus, plantar flex your foot (point your toes) and place two fingers slightly inferior to an imaginary line drawn between the malleoli (ankle bones). Feel the talus recede as it glides backward when you dorsiflex (move your toes toward your shin).

- Palpate the calcaneus (heel bone) to explore its size, shape, and contours. Press through the fat pad on the heel to access the inferior aspect.

### *The Lower Leg*

- Place your foot flat on the floor. Palpate the contours of the medial malleolus, the distal end of the tibia. From the posterior aspect, find the medial edge of the tibia with your left thumb and use your left fingers to find the sharp anterior edge. Trace both edges of the shaft up to the knee where it flares to form the tibial plateaus at the knee joint.

- Palpate the contours of the lateral malleolus, the distal end of the fibula. Using a back-and-forth movement with your fingertips, follow the shaft upward through overlying myofascia to feel the enlarged fibular head below the knee. Grasp this knob in a pincer grip to move the fibula forward and back in relation to the tibia. Repeat this movement at the distal end. You may feel slight gliding movement in both places.

### The Knee

- Straighten your leg on the floor and palpate the edges and surface of the patella. Press down on it lightly, hold the edges, and move it side to side, then grasp the top and bottom edges and move it up and down.

- Place a finger between the tibial tuberosity and patella, then rhythmically engage and release your quadriceps, feeling the quadriceps tendon stiffen and the patella move.

- Notice that you cannot move the patella when the quadriceps are activated.

- To locate the margins of the knee joint, bend your knee. Place your fingertips on either side of the quadriceps tendon to palpate the horizontal joint margins of the tibial plateaus inferiorly and the femoral condyles superiorly. Flex and extend your knee several times to feel the joint space opening and closing.

### The Thigh and Hip

- To locate the femur, place both hands on either side of the knee joint and palpate the bone of the femoral condyles. The abundance of soft tissue in the thigh makes it difficult to palpate the femur, but you can press firmly through the soft tissue to feel the bony shaft at several places on the anterior and lateral thigh.

- To locate the greater trochanter, straighten your leg, then slide your hand up the lateral femur to reach the protuberance at the top. Explore the topography of the trochanter, then internally and externally rotate your leg to feel it moving.

- Many people mistakenly think the trochanter is the hip joint. To locate the actual hip joint, slide your fingers from the greater trochanter into the hip crease. Flex your thigh several times to feel the thick rectus femoris tendon activating. Sense the hip joint moving deep to the tendon. When you move from felt sense of the hip joint, movement patterns can transform.

- Stand up to sense differences between the two sides.

  – *What do you notice?*

- Walk a little.

  – *How does walking feel different on the awakened side?*

- Repeat the exploration on the other side.

## EXPLORATION: LEG BONE CORE

Although superficial and deep fascia are a continuum linking bones, tendons, and muscles, each has unique tactile qualities that can be palpated. When differentiated through touch, felt sense deepens and neural maps are clarified for each tissue.

### Learning Objective

- Use touch to differentiate bone from surrounding myofascia.

### Instructions

- Take a baseline sitting in a comfortable position on the floor.

  – *What is the felt sense of your legs resting on the floor?*

- Sit with one leg straight and the other bent with the foot on the floor. Encircle the thigh of the bent leg with both hands and visualize the bony "core" of the femur surrounded by a "sleeve" of soft tissue.

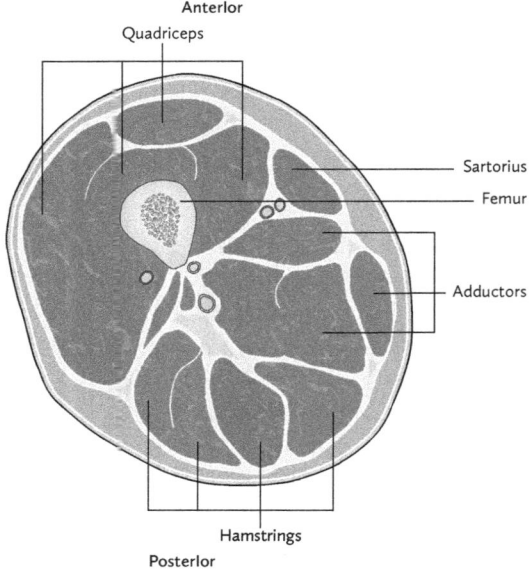

Anterior

Quadriceps

Sartorius

Femur

Adductors

Hamstrings

Posterior

- Using firm pressure, spiral the myofascial sleeve around the bony core of the femur by slowly and mindfully moving it back and forth medially and laterally, without moving the femur itself. Move the flesh enough to sense the tension spiralling through the fascia from skin down to bone.

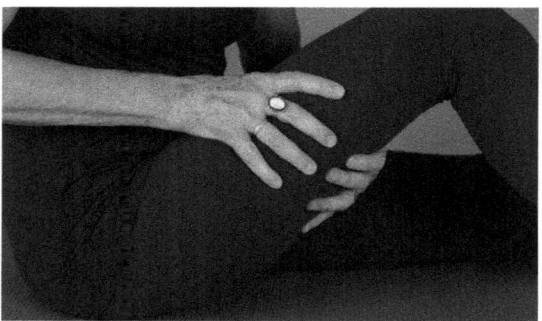

- Move the myofascial sleeve medially, then initiate a subtle, almost imperceptible movement of the bone core, spiralling laterally to create more dynamic tension between the two structures moving in opposite directions. Hold the tension for a few seconds, then stop activating and check if the myofascial sleeve will move a little more medially. From this new place of dynamic tension between the two structures, repeat the process.

  - *Can you sense the continuity between bone and myofascia?*
  - *Can you feel a release in the myofascia?*

- Repeat the process, moving the myofascial sleeve laterally and spinning the bone core medially.

- Repeat the process in additional places on the thighs and calves.

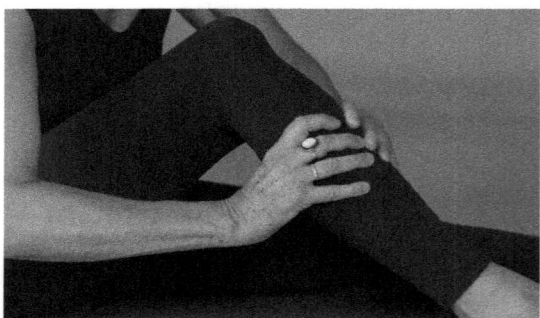

## THE FOOT TRIANGLE

Triangles are the strongest and most materially efficient shapes in nature, stable and able to effectively resist force without deforming. In the foot, tension and compression forces are optimally balanced when standing body weight is transmitted to the ground through triangles formed by three distinct areas of contact on the soles of the feet: the ball joints of the first and fifth metatarsals, and the middle of the anterior calcaneus.

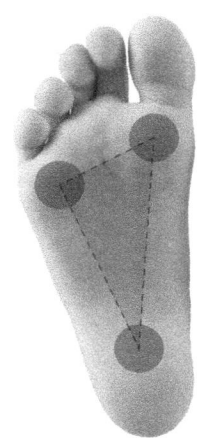

### PALPATING THE FOOT TRIANGLE

#### Learning Objective

- Identify the foot triangle.

#### Instructions

- To find the foot triangle, sit in a comfortable position to easily access one foot with both thumbs on plantar surface and fingers on dorsal surface.

- Use your thumbs to individually explore the first and fifth ball joints, including the size, contours, edges, and movement possibilities. As you palpate the topography of these metatarsal joints for a few minutes each, you're highlighting their existence for your nervous system. Each "point" is more like an area.

- To find the heel point, place the second and third fingers of each hand on the medial and lateral malleoli (ankle bones), then move your fingers down to meet on the sole of the foot, on the border between the tougher, darker heel and the softer, lighter colored arch. Take a few minutes to massage this intersection with your thumbs so it "wakes up."

- Use one finger to trace the outline of the triangle several times in both directions.

### FOUNDATIONAL PRACTICE: THE FOOT TRIANGLE

I developed this foundational practice when my feet were crippled with inflammatory arthritis and "froze" whenever I sat down. I discovered that continual movement prevented the freezing. Students consistently credit foot triangles for transforming the way they stand both physically and psychologically. Even students with balance issues from neurological conditions, including MS and Parkinson's disease, can steady their balance and walk more confidently. Mindfulness of foot triangles provides an effective cue that can undo unnecessary muscular tension, improve physical alignment, establish stability, and refine balance. When you consciously establish a balanced foundation throughout the day, you can repeatedly return to center, connect to the earth, and place yourself squarely in the present moment.

### Learning Objectives

- Deepen felt sense of foot triangles.

- Balance weight distribution in the feet.

- Increase mobility and strengthen feet.

- Pattern stability and balance on all koshic levels.

A 77-year-old student excitedly reported that after diligently incorporating foot triangle awareness into her daily practice and activities, she regained enough balance to stand while pulling on her pants.

Another student exclaimed after her first foot triangle exploration that her back pain was gone.

## Props

- A yoga mat

## Contraindications

- Recent foot or ankle injury, sprain, or fracture.

- Inflamed bunions.

- Fatigue or pain when standing (although this practice can be done seated in a chair or lying on the floor with the feet flat on the wall and hips and knees flexed to 90 degrees).

## Practice Notes

- Do the movements with one foot before repeating with the second foot. For an express version, choose your favorite movements.

- Check in frequently to notice and undo excessive effort or tension. It's easy to overeffort when attempting precision in movement.

## Instructions

- Set a baseline. Stand comfortably in Mountain Pose (Tadasana) on a flat surface, preferably on a yoga mat to utilize the stickiness for fascial release. Use a chair for support, if necessary.

- Breathe easily and settle into open awareness.

- Shift your mind to the interface between your feet and ground surface. Feel the ground with your feet.

- Notice how your weight is sequencing into your feet.

  - *Which parts of your feet touch the floor... press more heavily... don't touch?*
  - *Can you sense differences in your feet when you inhale and exhale?*
  - *Are there areas of clutching or tension?*
  - *Are there any parts that you don't sense clearly?*
  - *Is your weight balanced between the right and left foot?*
  - *Is there more weight in the heels or toes, on the inside or outside of each foot?*
  - *Is weight-bearing the same or different on each foot?*
  - *What does the outline of your foot look like?*
  - *How steady do you feel?*
  - *How much postural sway or subtle movement do you notice?*
  - *Where do you feel tension or ease in your upper body?*

- Slowly and with great awareness, shift your weight incrementally toward your toes and then backward toward your heels. Register each point along the arc of movement as you shift forward and back several times. Notice the response of the rest of your body as you move off the midline. With the same level of awareness, slowly shift your weight back and forth between your right and left foot. Then, shift your weight around the perimeter of your feet, point by point, first in one direction and then the other. Circle twice in each direction.

  - *What happens in the rest of your body as you shift your weight in each direction?*

- *How does your fascial system rebalance tension and compression in response to the shifting foundation?*
- *Notice "any "blind" spots" in your circles and spend a little more time in those places.*

### Wiggle and Spread

- Lift the toes of one foot, then wiggle and spread them for a few moments. Create space between them. Notice which toes move with ease, and which toes "clump" together.

  - *Can you move each toe individually?*

- Choose one toe and try to move it separately. If not, imagine you can.

### Map the Ball Joints

- Lift your heel off the floor. Shift your weight forward onto the first metatarsal (big toe) joint, then shift back to neutral. Repeat a few times, shifting your weight squarely into the joint to precisely differentiate it. Repeat at each joint in the metatarsal arch, noticing the level of sensory awareness at each joint. Spend more time with the joints that seem obscure. Form an intention to consciously establish a body-mind connection at each joint.

- Return the heel to the floor.

### Horizontal Dynamic Tension

- Lift the inner edge of the foot and anchor the little toe ball joint into the stickiness of the mat.

- Reach the big toe ball joint toward the midline, spreading all the metatarsal joints to create dynamic fascial tension between the first and fifth ball joints.

- Maintain dynamic tension as you plant the big toe ball joint into the mat, maximizing the distance from the fifth ball joint. Imagine you are creating space between the joints and spreading the fascial webbing between the long bones of the foot. Allow your body to adjust to this new, wider base.

- Lift the outer edge of the foot and anchor the big toe ball joint into the mat. Reach the little toe ball joint laterally, spreading all the metatarsal joints to create dynamic fascial tension between the first and fifth ball joints.

- Maintain dynamic tension as you plant the little toe ball joint into the stickiness of the mat, maximizing the distance from the first ball joint.

- Repeat the movements a few more times in each direction, monitoring your breath and effort level.

### Wave the Knee

- Lift one heel so your weight is spread over the metatarsal arch.

- Gently anchor the little toe ball joint into the mat, then carefully move your knee a little toward the midline *without* losing the anchor of the ball joint or allowing it to pivot. A gentle fascial tension is usually felt spiralling between the ball of the little toe and the lateral calf.

- Move the knee slowly back to the starting position, then back and forth several times. Notice that you must consciously prevent the little toe ball joint from pivoting.

- Anchor the metatarsal joint of the big toe and carefully move your knee laterally without losing the anchor of the big toe joint or allowing it to pivot. A gentle dynamic fascial tension is usually felt spiralling between the ball joint and inner calf.

- Move the knee slowly back to the starting position, then back and forth several times.

Consciously prevent the ball joints from pivoting by imagining them glued to the mat.

### Circle the Knee

- With the same heel off the floor, slowly massage across the ball joints by moving your knee horizontally in small circles without lifting the metatarsal arch off the floor.

- Circle several times in both directions. Let your mind follow the shifting pressure from ball joint to ball joint as you circle.

### Longitudinal Dynamic Tension

- With the heel still lifted, equally distribute your weight across the metatarsal arch.

- Anchor all five ball joints into the mat as you reach the heel behind you, creating dynamic tension between the metatarsal arch and heel. Maintain this tension while slowly lowering the heel to the floor, maximizing the distance from the metatarsal arch. Visualize spreading foot fascia longitudinally to create more space at the joints.

- Lift the metatarsal arch off the floor. Anchor the heel into the mat as you reach the ball joints forward, creating dynamic tension between the heel and metatarsal arch. Maintain this tension while slowly lowering the metatarsal arch to the floor, maximizing the distance from the heel.

- Repeat the movements a few more times in each direction.

### The Inchworm

- This practice can repattern and strengthen foot arches and tone myofascial structures that provide a spring to your walk. Your newfound awareness of the three foot

triangle points will enable you to actively shorten the middle third of your foot with minimal engagement of the toes.

- Anchor all three foot triangle points into the floor, visualizing the three points as a tripod.

- Create a domed tripod by actively lifting the middle of your foot, condensing the big and little toe ball joints toward the heel point. You can imagine pulling away from a finger emerging from the earth to tickle the middle of your foot.

- Release the effort. Repeat the doming movement several times, inhibiting toe engagement as much as possible.

  - *Are you aware of any activation or lift through your central core as you rhythmically shorten then release the midfoot?*

### Recheck Your Baseline

- Compare the two sides of your body, starting at the ground and slowly scanning to the crown of your head. Walk a little.

  - *How do the two sides differ?*
  - *Are there changes in the way you stand... your balance... amount of postural sway... your walking... your breath... the quality of your mind... energy level?*

Practice some or all these subtle movements several times a day, even when wearing shoes. You can practice in the shower, while brushing your teeth, in line at the bank, during a difficult conversation... in other words, all the time! Whenever you notice yourself in unbalanced weight distribution patterns, you can consciously shift yourself back into balance. As you practice foot triangle awareness in your daily life, notice cumulative physical, energetic, sensory, emotional, and mental effects.

## EXPLORATION: BALANCING THE KNEE 📹

The following two practices are adapted from practices developed by Judith Koltai.

### Learning Objectives

- Build awareness of the interplay between joints in the functional unit of the lower limb.

- Balance tension and compression forces across the knee joints.

### Props

- A sensy ball

- A small towel folded to a 5 cm (2 in.) height

### Practice Notes

- Sustain dynamic engagement of the three foot triangle points throughout the practice so the toes remain pointing upward.

- Do each set of movements 8–10 times, completing all movements on one side at a time.

- Pause after doing each set and allow your nervous system to register sensations.

### Instructions

- Do a baseline forward bend: In a seated position on the floor or firm surface, bend the left knee, externally rotate the leg, and place the sole of the foot in a comfortable position on the right inner leg. Support the left knee if it doesn't reach the floor easily. Activate the right leg by pointing the toes upward. Place the palms together at the chest. On an exhalation, bend forward from the hips without rounding your spine. Notice your comfortable range of motion. Repeat on the other side.

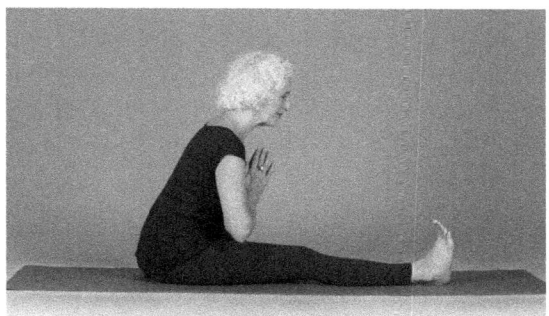

- Place the sensy ball on the towel. With the legs extended, position the ball and towel under your right knee. Bend your left knee with the foot standing on the floor. If necessary, use props to find a comfortable seated posture: Place a cushion or folded blanket under the pelvis, or sit against a wall to support your spine. Balance on your sitting bones to maintain upright posture. Your hands can clasp the bent knee or be placed on the floor behind you.

- For a minute, become aware of sensations in your posterior knee where it rests on the ball. As you inhale, imagine directing your breath there. As you exhale, visualize your knee softening and draping over the ball. Be attentive to subtle shifts and releases. Notice your breath as you rest in listening mode.

### Knee Extension

- On an exhalation, slowly and gently press the back of your knee into the ball, compressing it slightly. On the inhalation, gently release the pressure. Notice sensations of the quadriceps engaging.

- On an exhalation, slowly and gently slide your right heel away from you so the posterior knee passively presses into the ball. Notice sensations of the quadriceps engaging. Gradually relax your leg on inhalations.

### Hip Joint Distraction and Compression

- On an exhalation, slowly plantar flex your ankle, pointing the toes away from you. On the inhalation, dorsiflex your ankle, moving the toes toward your torso. Notice how the sitting bone moves back and forth as your ankle flexes and extends.

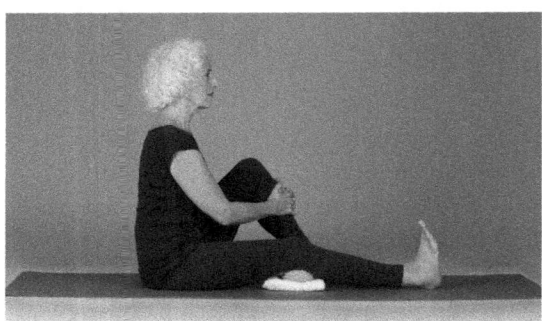

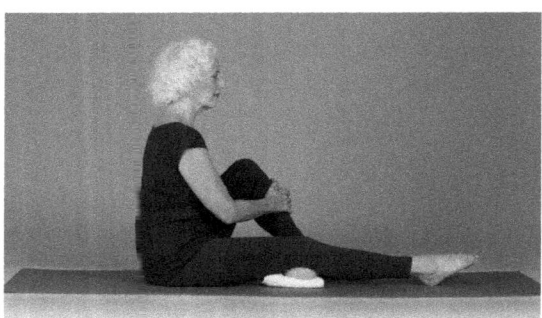

- Imagine a line between your sitting bone and heel that extends beyond your body in both directions. On inhalations, slide your sitting bone forward along the line so the leg moves away from your torso. On exhalations, slide the sitting bone backward along the line. Move the whole leg as a straight unit. Notice how this movement shifts the position of the **Hip Socket** and massages behind the knee.

### Internal and External Rotation

- On exhalations, gently and slowly internally rotate your leg so your toes point toward the midline. On inhalations, externally rotate your leg so your toes move laterally. Notice how the movements roll the ball of the femur in the hip socket and massage the posterior knee.

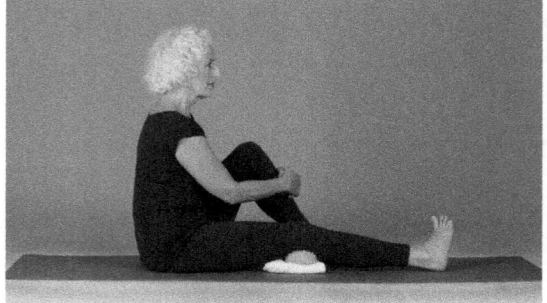

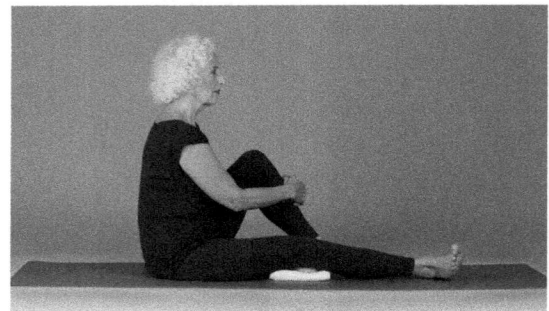

- Circle the foot slowly and gently in both directions, reaching out through the heel and maximizing movement through the ankle. Imagine the gliding movements of the tarsal bones.

- Repeat the baseline forward bend.

  - *How is it different?*

- Straighten both legs.

  - *How does sensation differ between them?*

- Stand and walk around, noticing how felt sense of the right leg has changed.

- Repeat the movements on the other side.

## EXPLORATION: DEFINING THE HIP SOCKET

### Learning Objectives

- Clarify location and felt sense of hip sockets.

- Improve stability and mobility practices.

- Deepen felt sense of component joint movements.

### Practice Note

- Practice all movements on one side at a time.

### Props

- 10 cm (4 in.) sensy ball or other pliable fascial ball

### Instructions

- Lie on your back with the knees bent and feet standing on the floor. Lift your right pelvis and place the ball underneath the soft tissue, slightly medial to the right greater trochanter. Return your pelvis to the floor. Adjust the ball for comfort.

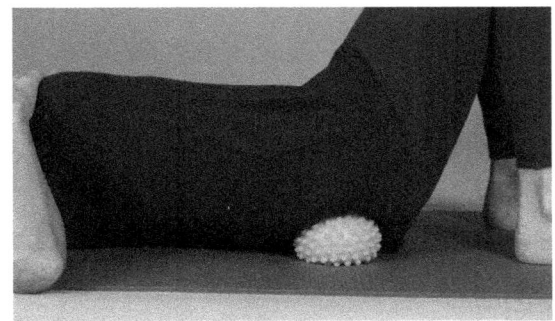

### *External Rotation*

- Initiating movement from deep in the hip socket, slowly move your right knee laterally several inches on an exhalation. Return the knee to neutral position as you inhale.

Repeat several times, visualizing the ball of the femur rolling laterally and gliding medially in the socket.

- After several repetitions, stay in the open position for a few breaths, allowing the knee to sink deeper with each exhalation. Support your knee for comfort, if necessary.

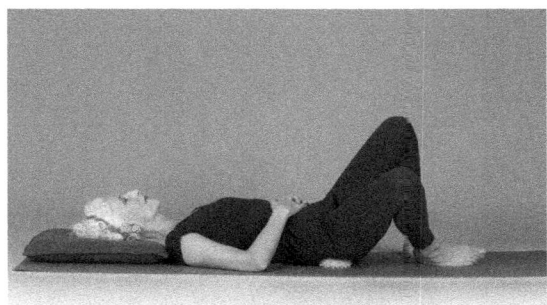

### *Circles*

- Lift your right foot off the floor to position the thigh vertically with the lower leg hanging passively. Trace tiny slow circles in the air with your knee. Imagine the circles as the bottom of a long narrow cone with its tip deep in the hip socket.

- Draw circles in the opposite direction.

  - *Can you visualize the tip of the cone creating spaciousness in the hip socket?*

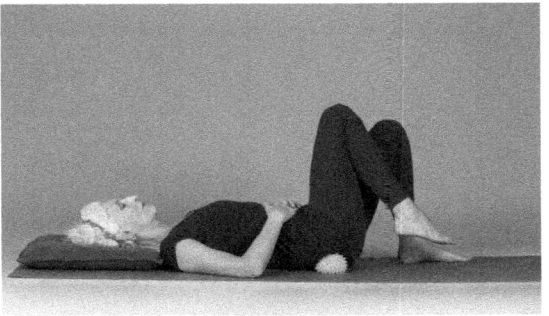

### Internal and External Rotation

- Cross your right ankle above the left knee. If this is challenging, decrease flexion in the left leg until you are comfortable.

- On inhalations, move the right knee toward the left shoulder.

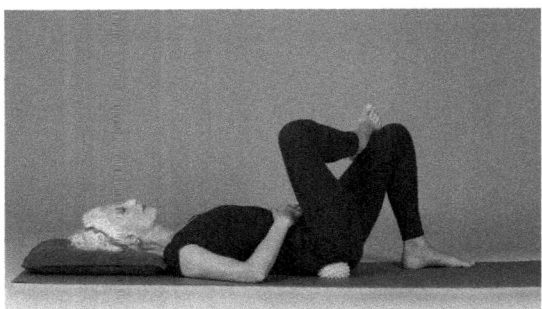

- On exhalations, move the knee away from you, opening the groin area.

- Repeat several times.

  - *Can you visualize the ball of the femur rolling and gliding in the socket?*

### Femoral Spin

- Find the vertical position of the right thigh. Place one finger on top of your knee to help you maintain verticality in the femur as you move. Imagine the line between your finger and the hip socket as an axis.

- On inhalations, internally rotate the femur and visualize the ball of the femur spinning in the socket as the foot moves laterally.

- On exhalations, externally rotate the femur and visualize the ball of the femur spinning in the socket as the foot moves toward the midline. The femur remains vertical during the movements. Repeat several times, initiating movement from the femur, then initiate movement from the foot.

  - *How does initiation locus change the movement? Which direction has more movement?*

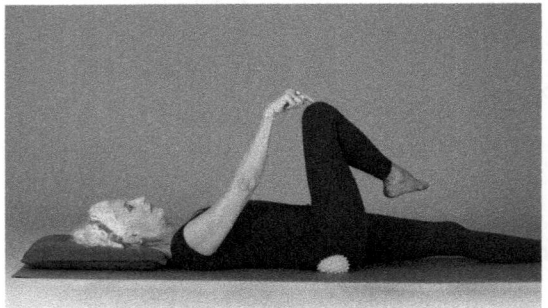

- Straighten both legs and feel the difference between the two sides before doing the movements on the other side.

  - *What do you notice?*

I can't believe how open my hips feel after these practices, even though we didn't do any "hip openers."

*Kathy*

# HEAL IT

## EXPLORATION: ROLL AND GLIDE IN CHAIR POSE (UTKATASANA)

As your knees flex in standing, the femoral condyles roll backward and glide forward on the tibial plateau.

### Learning Objective

- Visualize and explore component movements of roll and glide.

### Practice Note

- As you move, track the experience of shifting weight distribution in your feet.

### Instructions

- Take a baseline reading in standing by bending your knees a few times in your habitual way.

- Bend your knees again, slowly yielding weight into your **Foot Triangles**. Visualize the femoral condyles rolling backward and gliding anteriorly on the tibial plateau. Notice that the bottom of the femur becomes the front of the knee. You can deepen felt sense of roll and glide by forming your hands into fists and mimicking the component movements of each joint as you flex.

- Flex a few times in your habitual way, then return to the roll and glide visualization.

- Pause to notice any effects of the practice.

  - *How do sensations differ between your habitual movements and this exploratory way of moving into flexion?*
  - *How does weight distribution shift in your foot triangles?*
  - *Which way feels more stable? Gives you more range of motion?*
  - *How does the quality of movement change?*

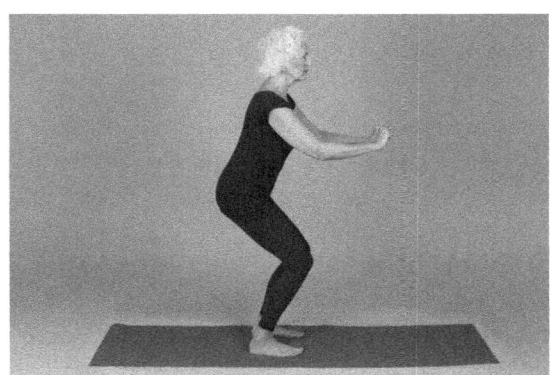

## EXPLORATION: YIELD AND PUSH WITH FOOT TRIANGLES

When you consciously direct force from the foundation of the foot triangles through the middle of each lower limb joint and into the torso, you can experience felt sense of clear, balanced force transmission. Instead of lifting yourself away from the ground with muscular effort in the upper body, you *press* yourself away from the ground, boosted by the counterthrust of ground reaction force and the springiness of fascia.

### Learning Objective

- Explore clear force transmission in the legs through yielding and pushing through the foot triangles.

## Instructions

- Stand with feet shoulder width apart. Distribute your weight equally over both foot triangles.

- Actively yield your weight into the foot triangles, flexing the hips, knees, and ankles. As you slowly lower your body into gravity in a controlled way, maintain verticality in your spine. Notice any habitual tendency you have to over- or under-use specific points and try to yield weight equally into the six points of both foot triangles. Most people tend to unweight the heel points when flexing the legs.

- Push off equally through the six foot triangle points, harnessing the buoyancy of ground reaction force to uplift you to full height as the hips, knees, and ankles extend. As you press into the ground, visualize a flow of energy transmitted upward through the middle of each joint, into the spine, and out through the head, like a rocket ship lifting away from earth.

- Repeat these movements several times, varying your effort level by experimenting with gradations of light-to-strong effort. Then, yield and push with enough force transmission to jump a few times.

- Pause and notice any effects.

  - *What is your optimal effort level?*
  - *Can you yield and push with weight equally distributed within the foot triangles?*
  - *Can you allow your upper body to be uplifted from below?*

## FOUNDATIONAL PRACTICE: GROUNDED MOVEMENT

Foot triangle awareness can help you maintain connection and stability as you move off the vertical axis. Once you have "turned on" this awareness, you can observe your weight-bearing habits and repattern new habits of transferring weight and force through your structure in more balanced ways. All movement can then be experienced in relationship to the ground, and the foundational support of the foot triangles can minimize extraneous muscular effort and encourage optimal alignment. Fascial continuities are more easily experienced when you can sense one part of the body moving away from, yet staying in dynamic tensional relationship to, the foundation of the feet on the ground.

### Learning Objectives

- Explore consciously sustaining connection to the ground through the foot triangles.

- Optimize standing alignment.

### Practice Notes

- To provide clear sensory feedback, you can tape buttons or coins on the foot triangle points. You will sense immediately when your weight distribution is imbalanced.

- As you do the movements, track your sensations.

- Repeat each movement at least three times.

### Instructions

- Stand with your feet parallel and slightly wider than your hips. Establish a baseline in three planes. First, do a forward bend by flexing your hips without rounding your spine. Slide your hands down the front of your legs as you move to a comfortable endpoint without altering your spinal curves, then return to standing. Place your hands on your buttocks and move into a backbend by sliding your hands down the back of your thighs a few inches, then return to standing. Place your hands just above the greater trochanters and do an easy side bend on both sides, moving to a comfortable endpoint. Finally, do a gentle twist with your arms crossed on your chest, twisting a comfortable distance on both sides.

- *What sensations are associated with your habitual way of moving in and out of the position?*
- *How does weight distribution shift in your foot triangles?*

- Repeat these movements in all three planes with the intention of staying firmly grounded in your foot triangles. Stop the movement as soon you feel one or more foot triangle points unweight from the ground.

- *How is the movement qualitatively different?*
- *What changes do you sense in your effort level... range of movement... alignment?*
- *Can you feel dynamic tension between your feet and torso?*
- *When the prime directive is balanced weight distribution in your foot triangles, what adjustments do you make in the rest of your body?*
- *Can you sense fascial continuities between your feet and the rest of your body?*
- Reflect on these questions as you take awareness of grounded movement into standing yoga poses, including balance poses. When you consciously distribute your weight equally between the six points of the two foot triangles, you may discover that you can disregard many common alignment cues regarding positioning of body parts.

## EXPLORATION: FOOT TRIANGLES IN TRIANGLE POSE (TRIKONASANA) 🎥

### Learning Objective

- Integrate foot triangle awareness in a standing yoga pose.

### Instructions

- In standing, move your feet 0.6–0.9 m (2–3 ft.) apart. Turn your left foot 90 degrees to the left and your right foot slightly medially. Balance your weight equally between right and left foot triangles. Place your left hand above the left greater trochanter with fingers in front and thumb behind. Place your right hand on your right hip.

- On an exhalation, initiate movement from the left **Hip Socket** (acetabulum) to roll it around the ball of the femur, tilting the pelvis sideways to move the spine 20 degrees

off vertical. As you move, anchor your right foot triangle into the floor and imagine sending force down the right leg to maintain a strong connection with the ground. Visualize your left hand as a hinge between your pelvis and leg. Pause and inhale.

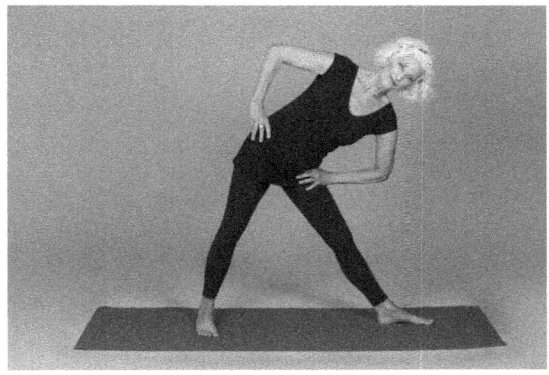

- As you exhale, move another 20 degrees, pausing to check that you are hinging sideways from the pelvis without bending the spine.

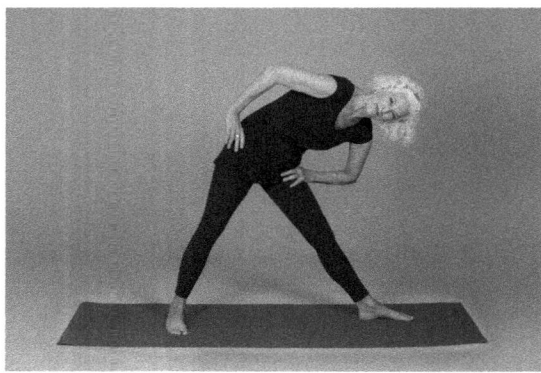

- Continue to move sideways incrementally until you feel the right foot triangle start to unweight from the ground; moving farther will diminish the balanced integrity of the movement.

- Maintain the end position for five breaths, using each exhalation to reestablish a balanced connection between the right foot triangle and the ground.

- To exit the posture, roll the hip socket in the opposite direction to lift the spine upright.

- Repeat the movement without foot triangle awareness and notice how it differs.

- Repeat the movement one more time, anchoring the foot triangle.

- Once you discern felt sense of your foot triangle foundation and of initiating movement from the hip socket, you can add your arms. At the endpoint of side bending, place the back of your left hand on the left leg wherever it reaches comfortably and raise the right arm toward the ceiling. Create dynamic tension between your arms, maintaining the pose for five breaths.

- Pause and reflect on the questions posed in the practice above.

## EXPLORATION: LEGS UP THE WALL POSE (VIPARITA KARANI)

In this restorative pose, the sandbag will help you clearly track force transmission between your feet and lower limb joints.

### Learning Objective

- Track force transmission between the feet and pelvis.

### Props

- A sandbag, 2–3 kg (4.5–6.5 lb.) bag of rice, or a large heavy book

### Instructions

- Lie on your side perpendicular to a wall with your buttocks near the wall and knees tucked into your chest. Place the sandbag beside you.

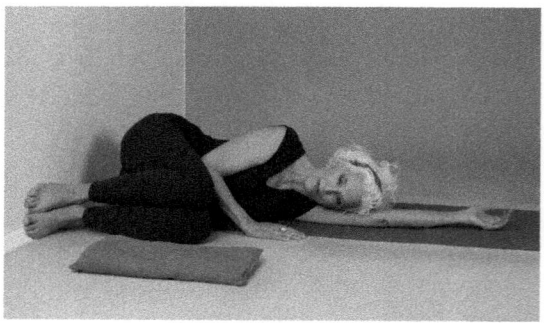

- Roll onto your back and straighten your legs on the wall. Move your pelvis as close to the wall as is comfortable. Bend your knees and balance the sandbag on the soles of your feet, then slide your heels up the wall to straighten your legs.

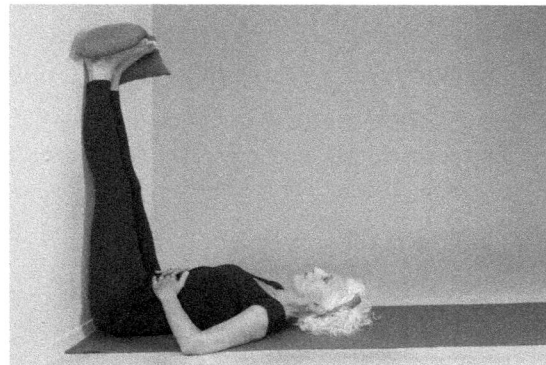

- Feel the weight of the sandbag as it sequences through the bones and soft tissue of your legs and into your pelvis.

  - *Are you resisting the weight, or can you passively allow your legs to receive it?*

- Stay with this awareness for a few minutes, using exhalations to dissolve any resistance.

- Focus on your ankle joints.

  - *Are there any tiny adjustments you can make to spread the pressure of the sandbag equally across the ankle and leg joints?*
  - *As you exhale, can you surrender to the load and allow the bones to receive more weight? Stay with this awareness for a few minutes.*

- Reflect on these questions as you shift your focus to the knee joints for a minute or so.

- Shift your focus to the hip joints.

  - *Can you feel the weight of the sandbag compressing the heads of the femur into the acetabulum?*
  - *Notice which parts of your pelvis receive force as it transfers into the ground.*

- Practice yield and push. Surrender to the weight of the sandbag and actively yield your legs so ankle, knee, and hip joints flex and the sandbag slides down the wall a little. Activate your foot triangle points so the load of the sandbag remains equally distributed. Sustain the activation as you press into the sandbag and slide it up the wall, straightening your legs.

- Yield and push several times as you consciously balance the load of the sandbag equally throughout each leg joint. Visualize force transmission from the feet to the ground on the yield, and from the ground to the feet on the push.

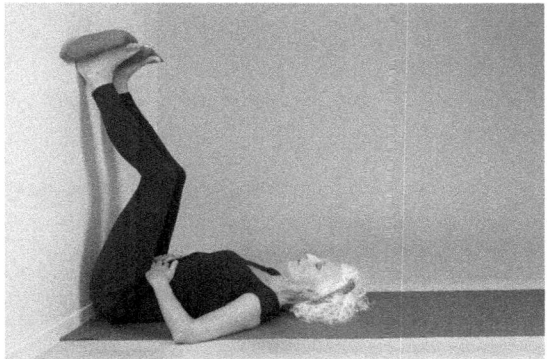

- To exit the posture, bend your knees and remove the sandbag, then roll onto your side and stand up.

  - *Has felt sense of your legs and feet changed?*
  - *How would you describe the sensations?*

- Walk around and notice how this new awareness translates to your walking.

## EXPLORATION: WALKING

> Walk as if you are kissing the earth with your feet.
>
> *Thich Naht Hanh (1992, p. 28)*

When **Foot Triangle** awareness is used as an organizing principle in walking, maladaptive gait patterns can transform as novel sensory inputs are processed in the nervous system. Redistribution of weight in the foot triangles can decrease pain and dysfunction in the lower limb joints and pelvis as force is transmitted more clearly and efficiently. Over time, students find that walking becomes steadier, flowing, and more springy.

### Learning Objective

- Explore the foot triangles in walking.

### Instructions

While walking, spend a few minutes with each of the following steps:

- Focus on each foot triangle point individually for several steps. First, pay attention to the heel point, and as your leg swings forward, reach out through the heel to make ground contact.

- Next, focus on the little toe ball joint, reaching it forward after your heel strikes the ground. Notice how this directs weight to the more stable lateral arch.

- Finally, shift your focus to the big toe ball joint, consciously pushing off the back foot to propel yourself forward in space.

- Track the spiralic movement of your foot as your weight shifts from heel... to lateral arch... to big toe.

- Imagine the three foot triangle points as suction cups gripping the floor as you lift your foot.

- Imagine springs on the bottom of your foot coiling as your foot flattens, then uncoiling to release a wave of elastic rebound through your entire body.

- Imagine that you are walking sole-to-sole with a mirror image of yourself below ground level.

  - *Which images give you the most steadiness, ease, and spring to your step?*

## THERAPEUTIC APPLICATIONS

*I saw an exercise physiologist who asked me to perform some functional movements. He asked how I learned such good alignment and I told him I'm standing in my foot triangles.*

LILY

A balanced relationship with gravity is so consequential that walking patterns can predict future health, sometimes more accurately than traditional diagnostics (Goldberger *et al.*, 2002). When internally and externally generated forces are not transmitted efficiently through the fascial network, our bodies intelligently adapt to the best of their ability by redistributing tension and compression forces. Adaptations may be functional in the short term, but eventually may cause myofascial tension, joint compression, and systemic inefficiency. For example, chronic foot pronation may initially seem benign, but over time could promote neck and shoulder tension that potentially decreases blood flow to the brain, and ultimately affects cognitive function. Lower limb misalignment will likely be overlooked as a contributing cause.

Lack of structural coherence in the functional unit of the lower limb can initiate a cascade of compensations, causing pain, pathology, and compromised physiology. When imbalanced forces compel myofascia to perform structural functions, it may adaptively respond by becoming hard, compact, and rigid like bone. This behavior illustrates Davis's Law, a principle describing how soft tissue remodels according to mechanical demands placed upon it. Form follows function. These changes can compress joint surfaces and decrease range of motion. As excessive myofascial tension constricts neurovascular structures, circulation of blood, lymph, and other fluids is compromised, as is the ability of nerves to register and transmit sensation. Organ physiology may also suffer when the bony container is compromised.

The combination of imbalanced tension and compression forces, compromised mobility, and reduction in sensory function can impair motor control and movement efficiency, and increase chance of injury. Movement may appear uncoordinated and ungraceful. As disequilibrium is perceived by the nervous system, it responds by orchestrating structural compensations in other parts of the body to orient the eyes to the horizon—the prime directive of the righting reflex.

The nervous system may also register a lack of safety, decide the body needs protection, and generate pain. As the body adaptively compensates, a vicious cycle of fear-tension-pain can be perpetuated.

Imbalanced weight-bearing and force transmission between the upper body and ground can cause pain, rigidity, weakness, edema, and restricted movement that contribute to multiple pathologies of hips, knees, and feet. This influence works bidirectionally. Upper body compensations may result from foot pathologies, including over-pronation and supination, plantar fasciitis, and toe deformities like bunions, while these pathologies may have been accelerated by imbalanced force transmission from the upper body. Either way, efficient weight-bearing and force transmission is disrupted throughout the body.

This global perspective of local dysfunction introduces greater healing possibilities. EA practices can redirect compensations by reorganizing the interplay of internal and external forces, awakening connections, and integrating individual structures into the whole. When disorganized tension and compression forces and lack of structural coherence are the lenses through which pathologies are viewed, changing the way we relate to the ground can initiate the healing process. Stimulation of sensory receptors in the feet has been shown clinically to improve balance and postural control in numerous conditions including diabetic neuropathy, aging, and Parkinson's (Viseux *et al.*, 2019). As we develop felt sense of the lower limbs and learn to "stand on our own two feet," the effects reach far beyond the physical. Resilient stability on the physical level can also encourage stability of mind and emotions, and upliftment of spirit.

## KOSHIC CONTEMPLATIONS

### Annamaya Kosha

- *Has deeper felt sense of your feet and legs changed your alignment or movement?*
- *Have chronic pain and tension patterns changed?*
- *How does foot triangle awareness affect the way you stand and move?*

### Pranamaya Kosha

- *As you learn to oppose gravity more efficiently, has your breath changed? Energy level? Physiological functioning?*
- *How does your alignment and movement change when you consciously direct force through defined pathways?*

### Manomaya Kosha

- *Are you aware of habitual ways of distributing weight in your feet?*
- *How are walking and moving different when you attune to the vast sensory capacity of your feet?*

- *Have you experienced greater emotional stability as you integrate foot triangle awareness into your daily life?*

### Vijnanamaya Kosha

- *Do you resonate with any of the metaphors at the beginning of the chapter?*
- *Where do you habitually live on the continuum of collapse, yield, and prop?*
- *Has your position on the continuum changed as you establish structural integrity?*
- *Do you feel like you are standing on your own two feet metaphorically?*

### Anandamaya Kosha

- *Has felt sense of the unity of your body increased with these practices?*
- *As you find more structural integrity through your legs and feet, are you standing more in your authentic Self?*

## KEY CONCEPTS

- Right relationship between gravity and ground reaction force can pattern structural stability and integrity while allowing clear force transmission and resourceful movement.
- The lower limbs operate as functional units, extending from hip to foot, each part influencing and influenced by others.
- The quality of our relationship to the ground can affect all koshic levels.
- Extensive innervation of the feet contributes to the ability to balance and stand upright.
- Prop and collapse are common postural compensations for lack of secure foundation.
- A complex arrangement of bones and soft tissue in the feet creates a stable foundation yet enables spring in our step.
- Structurally and functionally, the knee is the largest and most complex joint in the body.

- The functional design of the hip joint allows 360 degrees of movement within an intrinsically stable joint.
- The foot triangle is a foundational practice that improves alignment, establishes stability, and refines balance on all koshic levels.
- Imbalanced weight-bearing and force transmission can contribute to multiple pathologies of hips, knees, and feet.
- Cultivating felt sense of right relationship and support from the earth can engender feelings of security, self-reliance, and aspiration—standing on our own two feet.

All through life be sure to put your feet in the right place, then stand firm.

*Abraham Lincoln*

# CHAPTER 7

# Supportive Psoas

*Through the psoas practices, I am discovering a strong and resilient resource embedded within, connected to everything. It's like having a new, really good friend.*

JANET

The psoas is arguably one of our most important myofascial structures. Without these paired muscles (plural is also *psoas*), we would have difficulty standing upright or walking. This "buried treasure" has powerful physical effects but also subtly influences our capacity for grounding, wholeness, and authenticity. Although functionally integrated movement can never be reduced to one structure, when the psoas are sensitively accessed and embodied through EA practices, the pelvis, spine, and legs can find right relationship and express graceful, integrated posture and movement.

My clinical practice revealed involvement of the psoas in a majority of presenting conditions. Whether a client presented with back or knee pain, anxiety, or digestive issues, balancing the psoas through awareness and gentle explorations often facilitated profound healing and relief on multidimensional levels. Dr. Janet Travell, coauthor of the classic trigger point manual *Myofascial Pain and Dysfunction*, called the psoas "the hidden prankster" because of its deep location and ability to mimic symptoms commonly attributed to other dysfunctions (Travell and Simons 1992). Students regularly comment that embodying the psoas is the most life-changing EA practice they've learned.

## KOSHIC PERSPECTIVES

A psoas focus in annamaya kosha leads to direct experience of their influence on stability, strength, and coordination. They're not well-known or easily palpated muscles. Hidden deep in the core body, each of their functions can be duplicated by more superficial muscles. When embodied through EA practices, the psoas are experienced as connecting structures, linking upper to lower body, core to periphery, front to back body, and axial to appendicular skeleton. They are also experienced as core structures connecting us to our midline. When movement is consciously initiated from the psoas, we access deep strength, enabling us to move through daily activities with coordinated, integrated movement emanating from our center.

> The psoas is my internal powerhouse. When I initiate movement from it, I feel stronger.
>
> *Laurie*

When the psoas are appropriately toned yet pliable, they contribute to alignment and integrity of the spine, sacroiliac joint, and hip. Grandmother of movement therapy, Mabel Todd, regarded the psoas as the most important muscles in determining upright posture because of their function, relationships, and size (Todd 1937).

In pranamaya kosha, the psoas influence breathing, energy levels, physiology, and transfer of forces. Breath and oxygen availability are affected through extensive psoas fascial continuities and intimate relationship with the respiratory diaphragm. When the psoas are balanced and resilient, the diaphragm is freed to participate in relaxed, full, energy-giving breath. Muscular effort consumes energy; when superficial muscles are doing the job of postural muscles like the psoas, less energy is available for other uses. When the psoas are appropriately engaged, posture and movement are more efficient and consume less energy.

The degree of activation of the psoas can profoundly affect the function of physiological systems, especially nervous, endocrine, and digestive systems. Situated deep in the visceral cavity, excessive or deficient psoas tone will affect nearby organs, glands, and neurovascular structures. Physiological function improves when healthy psoas rhythmically massage visceral structures during breathing, walking, and other movements.

> My long-standing digestive issues resolved after a few months of regularly softening and releasing the psoas.
>
> *Max*

The psoas muscles are the primary physical scaffolding supporting our energetic center. Prana flows more freely throughout the body when healthy psoas support stable and integrated physical structure. Weight and force can also transfer efficiently from the trunk to legs, and vice versa, through the psoas as muscular guides.

Focus on manomaya kosha can reveal emotional dimensions of the psoas and their apparent role as repositories of body memories and instinctual emotion. They are the main muscles activated in the fight, flight, or freeze reflex when the nervous system perceives a threat and triggers survival action. As such, gentle release of psoas tension can sometimes release long-buried emotions, especially fear. Ongoing threat or stress, repressed emotions, and trauma history can chronically activate this reflex and its associated unconscious, persistent psoas tension.

> I unsuccessfully tried to conceive for several years. During a psoas workshop, intense feelings of fear arose. I realized I was unconsciously terrified and resisting motherhood. Two months later I was pregnant!
>
> *Lydia*

The psoas also play a sensory role. Extensive sensory innervation of the fascial component registers and relays information regarding changes in load, position, stress, and ground surface. When received and processed by the central nervous system, the motor response directs psoas myofascial adjustments to maintain upright posture. This sensory role can be impaired when excessive tension compresses fascial nerve endings or the lumbar plexus embedded within the psoas. Perception of physical sensations, feelings, and emotions may be dulled, causing us to lose touch with ourselves. Diminished IA can result, leaving us without an internal guidance system. Conscious connection to, and release of the psoas can refine our perception of body sensation and emotions.

Vijnanamaya kosha is accessed as we discern

more subtle aspects of the psoas. From their deep, central location, the psoas faithfully contort and harden to structurally reinforce our psychological stance and embodied metaphors. With awareness of our patterns and curiosity about their origins, we can explore ways to release the psoas from their role in perpetuating unhelpful patterns. With consistent exploration of the psoas, we may notice gradual changes in our psychological stance, perception, and response.

> Working with the psoas, I realized I was stuck in victim mentality. Accessing spinal support from the psoas helped me to rise to my full height and find inner authority.
>
> *Grace*

As we access the psoas as an inner resource, we generate a sense of being deeply centered in the Self with access to deep inner power and wisdom.

Countless students have experienced spontaneous feelings of self-compassion arise during psoas explorations. Over time, physical posture may change to reflect an attitude of inner poise and dignity.

In its role as the great connector in the physical body, the psoas can lead to felt sense of connection and integration in the larger context of our wholeness in anandamaya kosha. The sense of connection can spill over into our relationships with others, the environment, and the Divine.

> Once I could feel connections between my center and limbs through the psoas, I began to experience a sense of my wholeness. I was able to perceive wholeness as the matrix of my life, and my "problems" were contained within that matrix.
>
> *David*

## LEARN IT

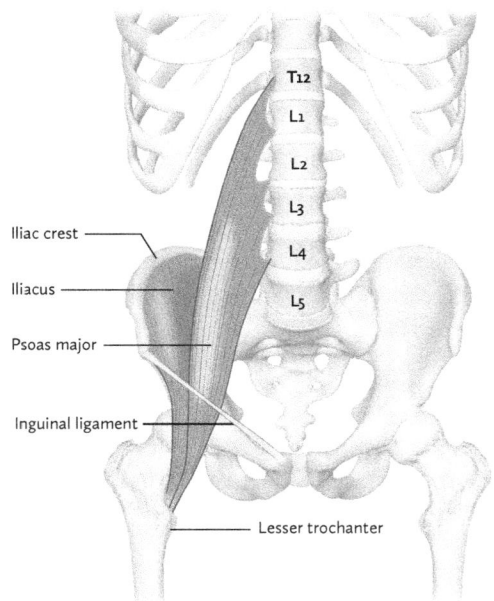

Iliac crest

Iliacus

Psoas major

Inguinal ligament

T12
L1
L2
L3
L4
L5

Lesser trochanter

The psoas major are the largest muscles of the iliopsoas complex that includes the iliacus and psoas minor. They are long (41 cm/16 in.), thick, bulky, triangular-shaped muscles that connect the spine to the legs. They have superficial and deep layers, supplied by two different nerves (Gibbons 2007). The superficial portion arises from the twelfth thoracic and upper four lumbar vertebral bodies and associated intervertebral discs. The deep portion arises from the transverse processes of all five lumbar vertebrae. Both layers pass diagonally forward and slightly laterally over the pubic bone, then dive backward to attach to the lesser trochanter. This reversal of direction creates a pulley-like arrangement that amplifies forces of movement. Numerous muscle bundles formed by these multiple attachments exert varying vectors of force on the spine and pelvis, suggesting that upper and lower psoas may serve different functions. Although historically considered the primary hip flexor, research has challenged this assumption and suggested spinal stability as the primary function (Bogduk, Pearcy and Hadfield 1992). As the deepest core muscles, it's possible that the psoas are meant to initiate movement that other muscles then amplify and direct.

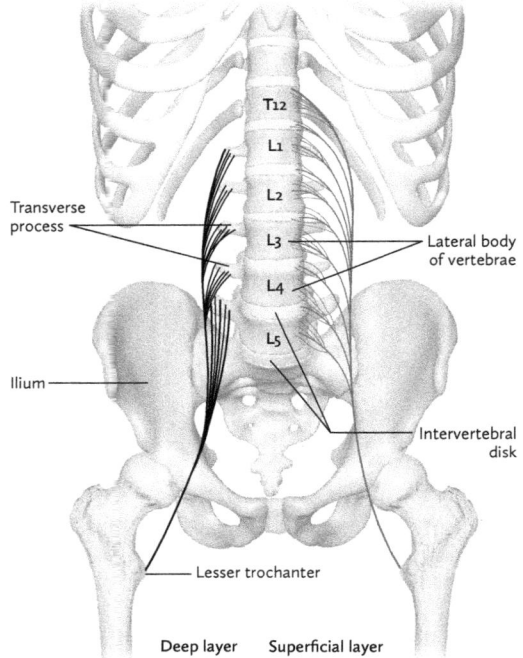

Transverse process

Lateral body of vertebrae

Ilium

T12
L1
L2
L3
L4
L5

Intervertebral disk

Lesser trochanter

Deep layer    Superficial layer

Over- or under-engaged psoas major (hereafter referred to as psoas) can contribute to structural imbalance. The size, strength, and varying vectors of force of the numerous muscle bundles can chronically distort the spine and pelvis. This prevents efficient transfer of force between the pelvis and ground. In their role as lumbopelvic stabilizers, the psoas will lengthen or shorten bilaterally or unilaterally to stabilize the skeleton. Over time, chronically shortened or lengthened psoas will lose pliability and strength, and more superficial muscle groups will compensate for loss of structural and core integrity. This can lead to proprioceptive insufficiency and superficially initiated and less integrated movement. Further structural distortion may result as compensatory misalignments are maintained and reinforced by the psoas, perpetuating a vicious cycle.

The psoas have direct fascial connections to numerous musculoskeletal structures, including respiratory and pelvic diaphragms, quadratus lumborum, multifidus, and anterior spinal ligament. The psoas and respiratory diaphragm interweave at their shared attachments on the lumbar spine, suggesting participation in a continuous interrelated fascial network. Even the arms are fascially continuous with the psoas; we can feel the psoas traction when elevating our arms.

The psoas also have associations with most physiological systems: the lumbar plexus lies between the superficial and deep layers; the urinary system and major arteries follow its muscular pathway; its fibers interdigitate with the respiratory diaphragm; and the muscular shelf formed by the psoas supports pelvic and abdominal organs. While under- or overactive psoas tone can adversely affect physiological function, a healthy, relaxed, yet engaged psoas provides support for organ health. Significant resolution of health issues related to each of these systems has resulted for numerous students after working with the psoas.

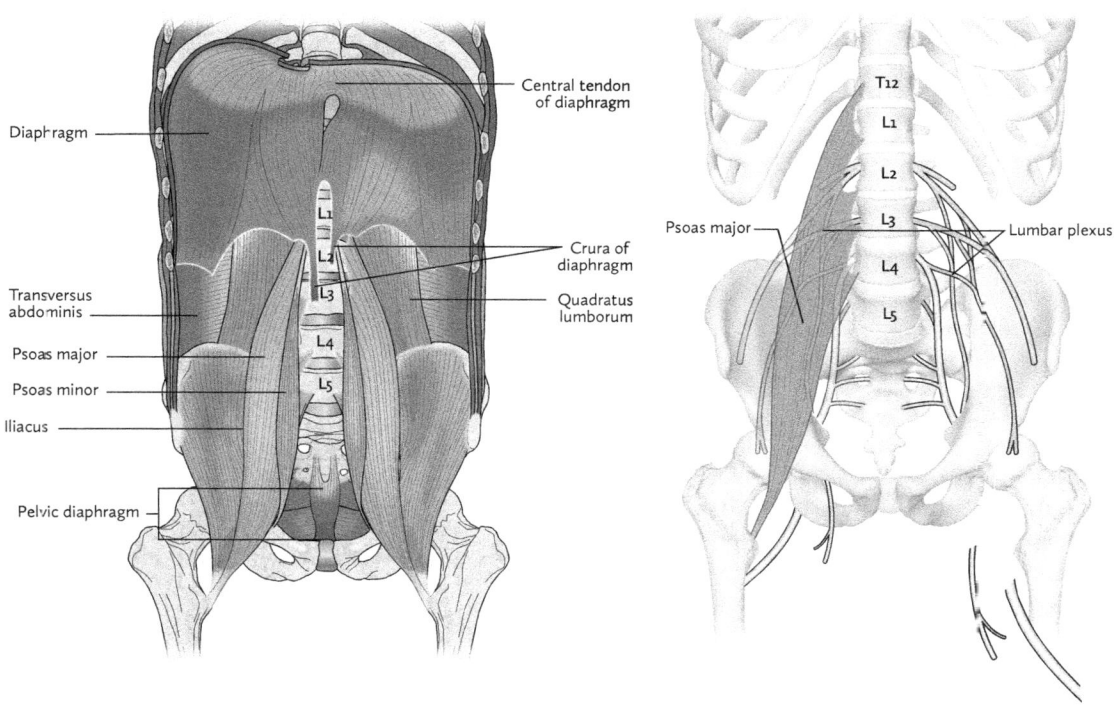

Labels for left illustration:
Diaphragm
Central tendon of diaphragm
Crura of diaphragm
Quadratus lumborum
Transversus abdominis
Psoas major
Psoas minor
Iliacus
Pelvic diaphragm
L1, L2, L3, L4, L5

Labels for right illustration:
T12, L1, L2, L3, L4, L5
Psoas major
Lumbar plexus

## FEEL IT

### The Psoas Protocol

Long periods of sitting or driving, and activities involving hip flexion can leave the psoas either over- or under-activated; the fascial component will remodel to accommodate habitual function. The psoas must first be gently convinced to release unnecessary tension, then find their rightful power. The following psoas protocol progresses from subtle softening and lengthening to conscious activation, and finally to integrating psoas awareness in more complex movements. Following the practices in this step-by-step order builds experiential understanding of the psoas and gradually accesses its pliability, resilience, strength, and spinal support. In the following practices, create "psoas events" by consciously initiating lengthening, condensing, and supporting actions from the deep psoas. You may discover that refining felt sense and moving from the psoas helps to minimize habitual activation of superficial muscles.

I developed this protocol over 15 years of experimentation with accessible therapeutic practices for the psoas that bypassed painful stretching that potentially triggered further contraction. I discovered that coaxing, befriending, and gently persuading the psoas yielded far greater results.

## PSOAS PROTOCOL STAGE I: FIND IT

Understanding placement of insertions and cultivating IA of the central location, size, weight, and volume of the psoas makes conscious connection more accessible. Refining felt sense enables deliberate softening, lengthening, and engaging. Touching the psoas with your own hands clarifies felt sense and increases their presence in the sensory map of the brain.

### Learning Objectives

- Develop felt sense of the psoas, using touch, breath sound, and movement.

- Cultivate a friendly, compassionate relationship with the psoas.

### Practice Notes

- Give yourself at least 10–15 minutes to explore each side in an unhurried, relaxed way.

- Always use the soft pads of your fingers to touch; the psoas are intimate, sensitive muscles and fingertips can be invasive.

### EXPLORATION: LOCATE THE ATTACHMENTS

#### Instructions

The first step is sensing the location of the psoas attachments. Focusing on one side at a time will increase specificity of the sensory experience.

- Start in supine position with the knees bent.

- Find the right upper spinal attachments by first placing the finger pads of your left hand at the midline just below the sternum. Move your fingers down and approximately 4 cm (1.5 in.) to the right so they rest on the upper abdomen just below the ribs. Underneath

your hand, visualize the spinal attachments of the psoas on the transverse processes, bodies, and discs of the upper lumbar vertebrae.

- For several breaths, imagine breathing into these upper fibers as you inhale. As you exhale imagine them softening and falling back into gravity to nestle alongside the spine.

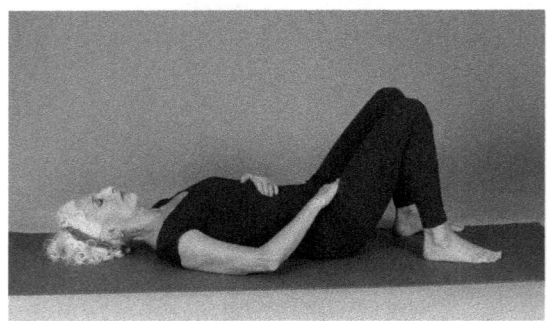

The lower femoral attachments on the lesser trochanter are deeply buried under layers of muscle and you can only infer their location through landmarks.

- Place the palm of your right hand on your inner thigh just below the groin crease. Palpate the landmark of the large adductor longus tendon; it pops up as you move the knee laterally.

- Curl your fingers around the tendon and into the valley between the adductor and hamstring muscle groups. You are now touching the surface directly above the lower psoas attachment on the lesser trochanter of the femur, located near the medial surface of the ischial tuberosity. These adjacent bony features lie in the same plane. When locating the lower attachments in your sensory awareness, or for movement initiation, you can use the medial ischial tuberosity as a landmark.

- Relax your hand and direct several breaths into this area, imagining the lower psoas filling with breath on inhalations and softening on exhalations.

- Pause to register any emerging felt sense of the right psoas before changing sides.

## EXPLORATION: BEFRIEND THE PSOAS

Remember the intimate connections between the psoas and nervous system? If you approach the psoas without gentleness, respect, and compassion, it may contract in defense. It pays to take time to befriend it with visualization, breath, gentle touch, and sound. Chronically contracted psoas muscles are easily agitated, so it's important to know how to soothe them. The hammock position helps psoas muscles relax and soften before palpation.

## Instructions

- Fold a blanket into a long, narrow rectangle approximately 13 cm (5 in.) in height and place it horizontally on the floor. Lie in supine with your pelvis on the blanket and the sacrum fully supported. Slide back on the blanket until your pelvis is tilted slightly posteriorly and your spine sags toward the floor like a hammock.

- Gently place the palms of both hands on the right side of your abdomen atop the pathway of the psoas. Visualize its considerable length as a heavy, thick hammock suspended at one end by the elevated lesser trochanter with the other end resting on the floor. For several inhalations, imagine the entire right psoas filling and expanding with breath. On each exhalation, imagine it softening and surrendering its weight and volume to rest alongside the spine.

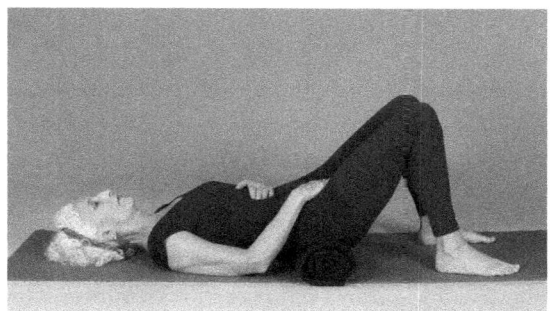

- Using soft hands and light touch, add a tactile cue by stroking your abdomen over the pathway of the psoas muscle from top to bottom. For a few minutes, experiment to discover which type of touch feels most soothing. Light or firm stroking. . patting... jiggling... circling?

- Try humming into your psoas muscle; sound and vibration can be calming. Start by directing your inhalation into the length of the muscle, then exhaling with an *mmm* sound. Direct the vibration into the bulk of the muscle, and visualize it soften and unclench.

- Silently talk to your psoas in a reassuring way, using phrases like *It's okay, I'm here,* or *You're safe now.*

- Pause to register any difference in sensations between the two sides and whether you have a stronger felt sense of the location and presence of the right psoas.

- Repeat these explorations on the left side.

- Remove the bolster and pause to register your experience.

- You can return to these practices any time your psoas feels agitated, or you need to calm yourself. Continue the practice until you sense that the psoas muscle is calm and receptive. Some practices may feel more accessible to you than others.

## EXPLORATION: PALPATE THE PSOAS

Cultivating psoas felt sense creates a clear somatic awareness that enhances the benefits of the practices in this chapter. Although embedded deep in the torso beneath organs and layers of muscle and connective tissue, it's possible to palpate the psoas in a sensitive and nonthreatening way. Avoid invasive palpation; it's counterproductive and can trigger a defensive fight-or-flight response. Approaching the psoas with gentleness, sensitivity, and respect will help you uncover its possibilities.

### Learning Objectives

- Palpate the psoas in a sensitive, nonthreatening way.
- Deepen felt sense of the psoas.

### Practice Notes

- If you have a history of trauma, you may want to discuss with your therapist about palpating the psoas before engaging in this practice. If you become agitated during the practice, do some soothing practices. This palpation practice may not be appropriate for you.

- Give yourself ample time to explore each side. Remember that whenever you work with the psoas you're also working with the nervous system, so establish an unhurried and relaxed atmosphere.

- Your psoas will be more receptive to touch if you do some of the above befriending practices before and after palpation.

- If unsure whether you're feeling the psoas, do not press more deeply into the abdomen. Rather, be more specific and precise with the diaphragmatic breath or the location of your finger pads. If you think that you're feeling the psoas, you probably are.

### Instructions

Recall the intimate relationship of the respiratory diaphragm and psoas muscles. Because they cocontract, the psoas is easily palpable with **Thoraco-Diaphragmatic Breath** (see Chapter 3).

- Lie in supine with knees bent, hip width apart, and feet a comfortable distance from your buttocks. If you feel tension in your legs or abdomen, adjust the distance between your feet and buttocks so the upper and lower legs rest into each other in a relaxed way.

- Place both hands firmly on your lateral ribs with the thumbs wrapping around the back. As you inhale, direct your breath sideways and backward into the pressure of your hands, minimizing breath movement of the abdomen and chest. Continue thoraco-diaphragmatic breathing throughout the practice.

- Recall the location of the right psoas muscle and its diagonal pathway from the solar plexus to groin. Place the finger pads of either hand on your abdomen over the upper attachments.

- With a thoraco-diaphragmatic inhalation, consciously expand your lower ribs. The soft abdomen will expand with the breath, while the muscular psoas will rise from below to meet your finger pads. If unsure whether you are touching the psoas, walk your fingers slightly medially or laterally to differentiate the softness of the abdomen and hardness and vertical orientation of the psoas. You can gently move your finger pads back and forth to feel the underlying ropey texture of the psoas as you inhale. Keep your touch superficial; you want the psoas to rise into your fingers rather than sinking your fingers into it.

- For several breaths, breathe thoraco-diaphragmatically to feel the psoas activate in concert with the diaphragm, rising on inhalations then receding on exhalations.

- To confirm that you're feeling the psoas, lift your right foot from the floor no more than 3 cm (1 in.). The psoas activates in hip flexion and is more palpable. Lower the foot to the floor as you exhale.

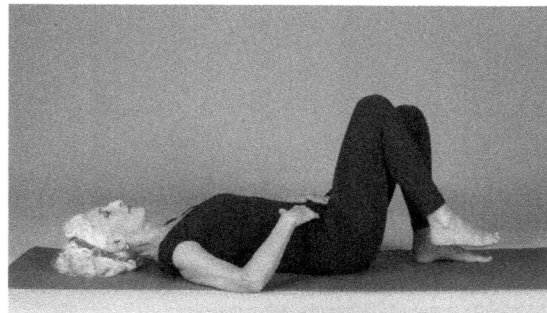

- Repeat a few times to gain confidence that you are feeling the psoas activate.

- Walk your finger pads approximately 3 cm (1 in.) down the pathway of the muscle. Gently palpate activation of the underlying psoas with a few thoraco-diaphragmatic breaths, confirming by lifting the foot. If you experience discomfort, try lightening your touch.

- Repeat this process of superficial palpation at several levels along the course of the psoas, taking three or four thoraco-diaphragmatic breaths at each level. Continue until you reach the groin crease where palpation is more challenging.

- Pause to register differences in sensation between the two sides and whether you have stronger felt sense of the location and presence of the right psoas.

- Repeat the palpation practice on the left side.

## EXPLORATION: CONNECT THE PSOAS AND ARMS

### Learning Objective

- Experience fascial continuity between the psoas and arms.

### Instructions

Recall the abundant fascial continuities between the psoas and arms. You can sense this connection when the upper psoas is tractioned during arm elevation.

- Remain lying supine with knees bent.

- Place your left finger pads on your abdomen overlying the right upper-psoas attachments.

- Slightly lift your right foot to confirm your finger placement over the psoas.

- Slowly raise your right arm overhead toward the floor behind you. Feel the psoas rise into your left fingers.

- Return your arm to the starting position, then repeat the movement a few more times. If your ribs elevate as your arm raises, consciously inhibit their movement.

- Repeat the exploration on the left side.

  - *Is one side more palpable?*

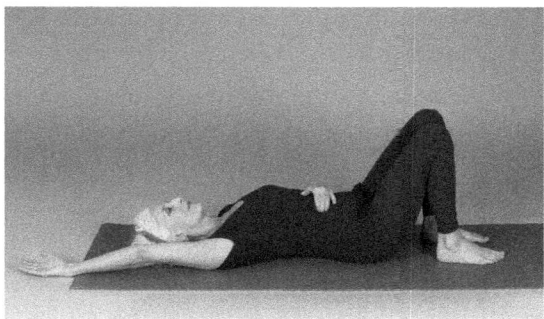

- Pause to register sensations, then stand and walk around moving your arms.

- *Has felt sense of your psoas changed with these practices?*
- *Can you sense a connection between your arms and midline?*
- *How is the rest of your body affected?*

## RESTORATION

Whenever your psoas muscles are agitated, it's important to soothe them by returning to the hammock, breathing, sounding, or stroking practices above.

> All my life I've been very hard on myself. Now when I sense my psoas muscles, I feel a warmth and softening deep inside that reminds me to treat myself more gently.
>
> *Geneva*

## HEAL IT

### PSOAS PROTOCOL STAGE II: SOFTEN IT

### Learning Objectives

- Soften and hydrate psoas myofascia in a gentle, nonthreatening way.
- Release defensive psoas hypertonicity.
- Prepare the psoas to safely participate in movement.

### Practice Note

- Softening, rather than stretching the psoas, is a safe way to encourage psoas pliability and resilience. This helps to restore a neutral position of the pelvis and spine and alleviate compression in the lumbar area and sacroiliac joints.

### EXPLORATION: PRONE HALF BUTTERFLY POSE (ARDHA SUPTA BADDHAKONASANA)

### Props

- A yoga bolster
- A soft, 23 cm (9 in.) inflatable therapy ball

deflated to one-third capacity. Gertie balls are a brand often found in toy shops. Other brands may be found online by searching "23 cm/9 in. inflatable therapy ball." If you don't have a ball, you can substitute a soft, balled-up sweater or shawl.

- Other props as necessary for support

### Contraindication

- If even modified positions don't feel comfortable in your groin, sacroiliac joint, or lower back, this practice may be inappropriate for you.

### Instructions

- Place a bolster lengthwise on a yoga mat or carpet. Add more support if the bolster doesn't underlie your whole torso and head.
- Lie prone with your trunk supported by the bolster and your legs resting on the floor. Bend your left leg to a 30–45 degree angle at the hip, resting the inner knee on the floor in a frog-like position. Raising the trunk reduces potential stress on the lower back

and intensifies sensations of psoas release. Turn your head to the side or support your forehead with a rolled towel. Experiment to find the most comfortable position for your groin and sacroiliac joints.

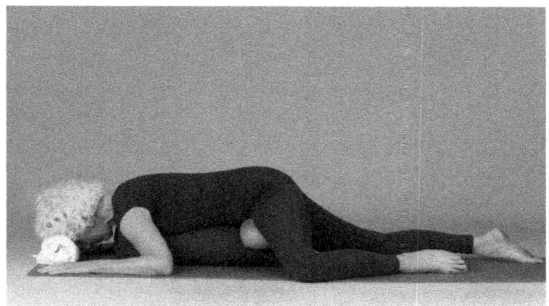

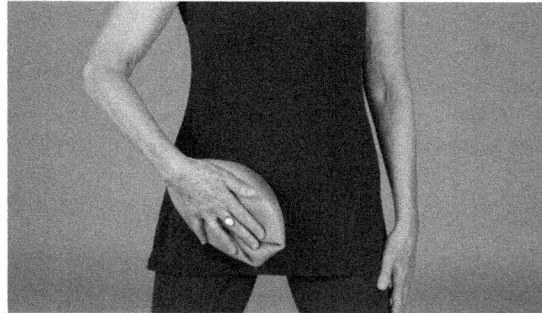

- Place the inside edge of the semi-deflated ball touching the midline of your pubic bone and the bulk of the ball filling the groin space. Rest into the bolster. If the two sides of the pelvis feel radically uneven, deflate the ball more. Find a comfortable arm position.

- On progressive exhalations, consciously soften and release the left groin into the buoyant support of the ball. Visualize your psoas muscle falling forward and draping over the ball.

- Stay in this position for at least five minutes. To intensify the feeling of psoas release, occasionally press your groin gently into the ball as you exhale.

- Remove the ball, then lie in supine and notice any difference between the two sides.

- Repeat the practice on the other side.

- After completion, first lie in supine, then stand to register any effects.

## PSOAS PROTOCOL STAGE III: SUBTLE PSOAS LENGTHENING

Everyday activities and ongoing stress tend to shorten the psoas. An effective countermovement to chronic psoas tension is conscious lengthening, which simultaneously extends the groin and lumbar spine. Although many fitness regimens recommend lunges and backbends that take the psoas into extreme ranges of motion, releasing the psoas gently can inspire graceful posture, greater ease in the spine, and better balance and coordination.

### Practice Note

- You can pin long, thin balloons on your clothes overlying the psoas attachments to add another layer of sensory input during psoas practices. Visual stimuli are very powerful. Even though the balloons are superficial, the visual representation of the psoas helps infer their location deep in the torso.

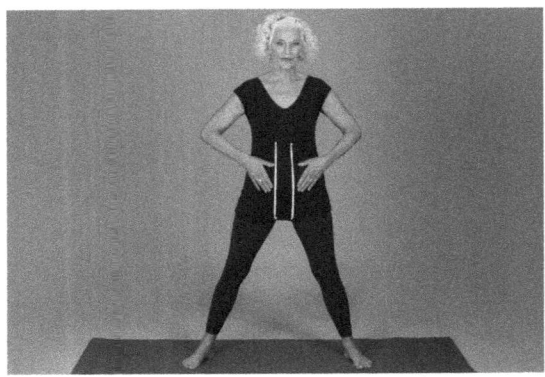

## EXPLORATION: PELVIC MOVEMENT IN THREE PLANES

### Learning Objectives

- Explore pelvic movement in three planes, initiating from the psoas.

- Refine felt sense of the psoas.

- Create psoas events.

### Props

- A thin hand towel approximately 63 cm x 40 cm (25 in. x 16 in.) rolled lengthwise to a 6 cm (2.5 in.) diameter

### Contraindications

- Asymmetrical movements may not be appropriate for those with pelvic or sacroiliac joint instability. If you experience pain during or after this exploration, skip this practice.

### Instructions

- Take a baseline reading in supine. Notice the amount of space between your lumbar spine and the floor.

- Place the rolled towel across T12 (just above the waist) as a sensory reminder of upper-psoas attachments. Adjust the diameter for comfort. Bend both knees with feet flat on the floor.

- Touch your inner ankle bones together to align the feet, then step both heels laterally and move the forefoot to align with them.

- For each of the following movements, place your hands on the upper and lower psoas attachments to help you sense which end is stabilized or moving, and what is happening between them.

## Sacral Rocking
### Instructions

- Move your focus to the triangular sacrum with its tip pointing toward the toes and the base just below the waist.

- Imagine a line down the middle of the triangle. Using this midline as a guide, slowly and gently press down point by point from the base of the triangle to the tip. Notice how the lumbar spine arches.

- Reverse direction and gently press point by point toward the base. Notice how the lumbar spine rounds. This is a rocking movement isolated in the sacrum and pelvis; do not actively press the back of the waist toward the floor or push through the feet.

- Move back and forth from tip to base several times, massaging the midline.

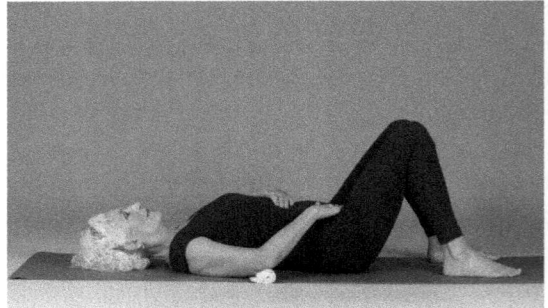

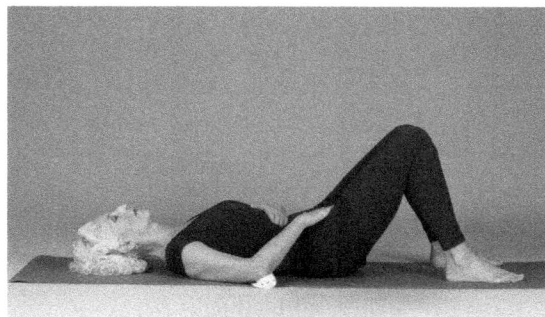

Notice how your breath integrates with these movements.

- *Does it make more sense to inhale or exhale when your spine arches?*

Try both ways to notice differences in sensation, then stay with your preferred way.

- Continue the movement, but now shift your focus to the psoas to create a psoas event. Place your hands over the upper-psoas attachments and gently press into the towel roll to anchor them. Maintain this anchor each time you lengthen the psoas.

- Initiate the movement from both lesser trochanters, tracking the lower attachments as they move toward and away from the anchored upper attachments. Visualize the shape of the psoas changing by alternately lengthening and shortening. Sense the dynamic tension between the two ends.

- Rock back and forth several times, then rest.

- *Is your felt sense of the psoas different side to side?*

## Pelvic Shifting
### Practice Notes

- The pelvis remains flat on the floor throughout the movements.

- Track the lower attachments as the lesser trochanter moves toward and away from the anchored, upper attachments, alternately lengthening and shortening the psoas. Sense the dynamic tension between the two ends.

- Notice which side moves more easily.

### Instructions

- Move your focus to the sitting bones. Recall how their proximity to the lesser trochanter makes them accessible landmarks. Touch your sitting bones to help your nervous system register their location. Imagine a line connecting each sitting bone and same side heel.

- Place both hands gently over the right upper-psoas attachments. Begin by directing several easy inhalations into the upper attachments, softening on exhalations.

- Anchor the upper-psoas attachments by pressing back gently into the towel roll, maintaining this connection throughout the lengthening movement.

- As you exhale, visualize your breath streaming down the length of the right psoas to the lesser trochanter, moving it so the sitting bone slides down the imaginary line toward the right heel. Simultaneously, brush one hand down the pathway of the psoas to provide more sensory input. Use the other hand to help anchor the upper attachments. Sense the psoas muscle lengthening and changing shape and the dynamic tension between the two ends.

- As you inhale, initiate movement from the lesser trochanter to return the pelvis to neutral position. Return your hand to its starting position. Sense the psoas muscle shortening and changing shape.

- Repeat the movement several times on the right side, then rest and notice any differences between the two sides.

- Do a few repetitions the way you would

normally do this movement without psoas awareness.

- Repeat on the left side, then alternate sides several times creating psoas events.

- Pause and register any effects of the movements, then stand and notice further effects.

## Twist

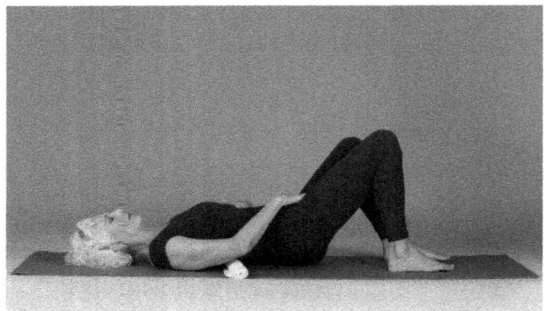

### Practice Notes

- Initiate movement from the lesser trochanter.

- Register shape changes in the psoas as the lesser trochanter moves away from and toward anchored spinal attachments.

- Notice which side moves more easily or has more elasticity.

### Instructions

- Realign your feet to neutral position and place your hands softly over the right psoas attachments.

- As you inhale, direct your awareness to the upper attachments and anchor them by pressing subtly into the towel roll. Maintain this connection as you move.

- As you exhale, visualize your breath streaming down the length of the right psoas to the lesser trochanter and moving it diagonally

away from you, projecting the knee directly over the right foot. Sense the dynamic tension in the body of the psoas as the lesser trochanter moves away from the anchored, upper spinal attachments. Notice how the pelvis twists but keep the movement small to ensure that T12 remains touching the towel as the knee projects.

- Return to neutral as you inhale, releasing pressure on the towel.

- Repeat these psoas events on the right side, then pause, straighten your legs, and register any difference between the two sides.

- Repeat on the left side, then alternate sides several times, creating psoas events.

- Remove the towel roll, then pause to register any effects.

### Variation with a Partner

For many people, this assisted variation clearly "colors" the psoas in their awareness. Before beginning, establish consent to touch.

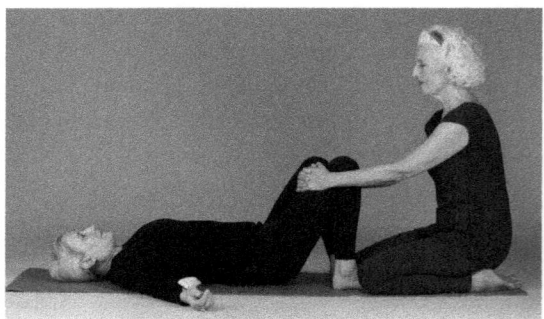

### Instructions

- In the same supine position with bent knees, move your heels closer to your buttocks.

- The partner sits at your feet holding your right anterior thigh with clasped hands. It can be helpful for both partners to coordinate breathing.

- On an extended exhalation, visualize your breath streaming down the length of the right psoas and inner thigh as your partner gently draws your thigh and knee away from the pelvis to encourage passive lengthening of the psoas. The knee projects diagonally directly over the foot and ankle.

- As the partner carefully pulls on your knee, gently anchor T12 into the towel to create dynamic tension between the anchored and moving parts. Repeat the movement three times.

- If you have an area of specific tension or holding in the psoas, you can place your hand there and gently persuade it through touch to participate in the passive lengthening.

- Repeat the practice in a static way. Your partner sustains the mild pull on the thigh for three extended breaths while you continue to visualize streaming each exhalation down the length of the psoas to the knee.

- If your psoas is reluctant to yield, you can encourage lengthening with isometric activation. As you inhale, activate the psoas by trying to gently move your knee toward your chest against the resistance of your partner's hands. On the exhalation, release all effort and allow your partner to carefully lengthen the psoas by pulling on the thigh. Repeat three times.

- Extend your legs and notice how your body is now resting on the floor and any difference in sensation between the two sides.

- Repeat on the left side.

- Pause and notice any effects.

- Stand and notice how you are standing now.
  - *What has changed?*

## EXPLORATION: HALF BOW POSE (ARDHA DHANURASANA) WITH ISOMETRIC RELEASE 📹

### Learning Objectives

- Increase resting length of the psoas.

- Lengthen the lumbar spine and release sacroiliac joint compression.

### Practice Note

- As you found in the previous practice, active engagement of a muscle enhances its ability to release. Attempts to stretch the psoas often result in defensive shortening, but isometric contractions can encourage lengthening. This practice is one of the most effective for releasing unyielding psoas muscles.

### Props

- A soft 23 cm (9 in.) inflatable therapy ball deflated to one-third capacity or substitute a soft balled-up sweater or shawl

### Contraindications

- Those with lumbar spondylolysis, spondylolisthesis, spinal stenosis, or other spinal conditions should use caution. In mild cases, a cushion or folded blanket placed between the groins and ribs will support the spine so this practice can be done safely.

- Pregnancy or recent abdominal surgery.

### Instructions

- Take a baseline reading in supine.
  - *How does your back rest on the floor?*

- Lie prone on a yoga mat with legs hip width apart. Place the partially deflated ball under the right groin with the inside edge touching the midline of the pubic bone and most of the ball filling the groin space. Support your forehead with your hands.

- Flex the right knee and ankle to a 90 degree angle with the sole of the foot facing the ceiling.

- As you inhale, press the right knee into the floor with 20 percent normal effort. As you exhale, visualize your breath streaming down and lengthening the psoas, causing your knee to slide away from your pelvis. Make it a psoas event.

  - *Can you sense how this slight movement also lengthens your low back?*

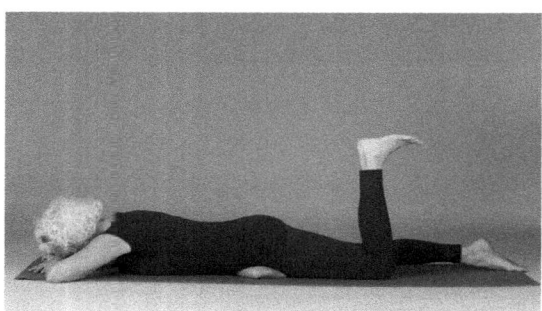

- Inhale a second time and press the right knee into the floor.

- As you exhale, again lengthen the psoas with the breath visualization, then lift your knee

off the floor until you feel a gentle stretch in the anterior thigh and groin. Maintain length as you lift the knee. You can imagine an airplane moving down the runway and gradually lifting off. Face the sole of your foot toward the ceiling to prevent externally rotating the thigh.

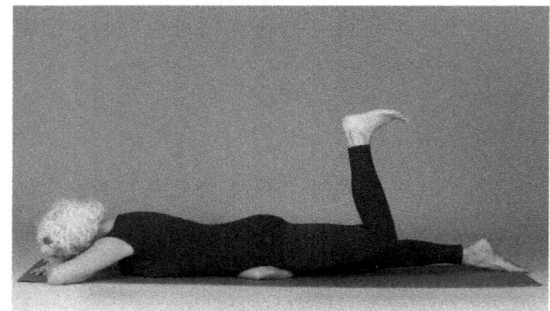

- Repeat several times, then remove the ball and lie prone for a few breaths to notice any changes.

- Roll onto your back and extend your legs, observing any differences between the two sides.

- Repeat on the left side.

- Return to baseline to notice any effects, then stand and walk a little.

  - *What do you notice?*

## PSOAS PROTOCOL STAGE IV: CONSCIOUS ACTIVATION

Once EA practices firmly establish felt sense of the psoas in the neuromuscular landscape of the nervous system, they are more easily deliberately activated. Visualizing the psoas "coiling for power" like a compressed spring creates latent force that, when released, gives momentum and cohesive strength to resulting movement. Viscoelasticity of the extensive psoas fascial matrix supports this dynamic action of coiling and discharge. Although the psoas work synergistically with surrounding muscles, learning to activate and consciously initiate movement from these central, deepest core structures generates maximum power and prevents habitual overuse of superficial muscles. Rectus femoris and rectus abdominis will happily assume psoas functions, but the resulting movement doesn't access core power. Ida Rolf, founder of Rolfing Movement Integration, suggests that during hip flexion the psoas "fall back" toward the spine to support lumbar vertebrae (Rolf 1989). Using this image can help to create psoas events.

## EXPLORATION: ISOLATING PSOAS ACTIVATION

### Learning Objective

- Refine motor control by isolating subtle psoas activation.

### Instructions

- Lie in supine with the left leg straight and right leg bent, foot flat on the floor. Place your finger pads gently in the vicinity of the upper-right psoas attachments. Take a few moments to connect with and soften the psoas with breath, then confirm your location by doing **Thoraco-Diaphragmatic Breath** to feel psoas activation.

- Choose one of the following visualizations to initiate activation of the psoas:
  - The entire muscle condensing, shortening, and widening like a cylinder of **Play-Doh** compressed from both ends.
  - The psoas falling back toward the spine.
  - Upper psoas fibers gliding down and lower fibers gliding up against viscoelastic resistance.
  - The psoas as a water-filled sponge being squeezed dry as the psoas condenses.

- Experiment with each image to see which works best for you.

- As you inhale, imagine filling the length of the psoas with your breath. As you exhale, consciously activate the psoas while visualizing your chosen image.

- Practice this activation for several breaths. You can confirm the psoas is activating by feeling it rise into your hand, although it may be less perceptible than activation with rib breath (see Chapter 3) or lifting the foot. The desired action is a subtle, almost isometric, vertical shortening along the entire length of the psoas muscle, without moving the spine or leg, rotating the pelvis, or hiking the hip. Make it a psoas event. If you don't feel anything, don't worry. Visualizing the image is enough; remember that imagining movement triggers muscular activation.

- Repeat this process with the left psoas. Notice whether one side is more responsive.

- Pause to notice any effects.
  - *What do you notice?*

- Stand, then walk around and notice further effects.

## EXPLORATION: COILING FOR POWER

### Learning Objective

- Harness elastic recoil power in the psoas.

### Instructions

- Lie in supine with knees bent and feet flat on the floor. Loop a yoga belt around the ball of your right foot and extend the leg toward the ceiling.

- On one phase of breath, slightly bend the right hip and knee and visualize the psoas muscle coiling for power. Use your favorite image from the previous exploration to picture the psoas condensing, falling back, and coiling like a spring as the leg attachment moves closer to the anchored spinal attachment.

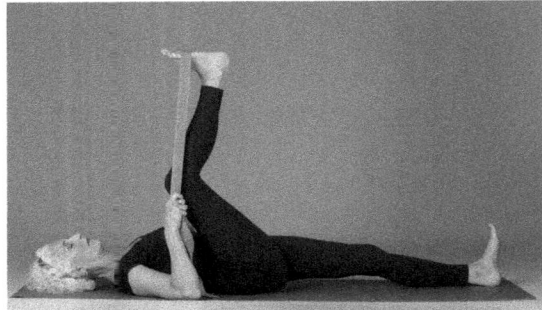

- On the other phase of breath, visualize the coiled power releasing and streaming down the inner leg with enough force to straighten it, pressing the foot into the resistance of the belt.

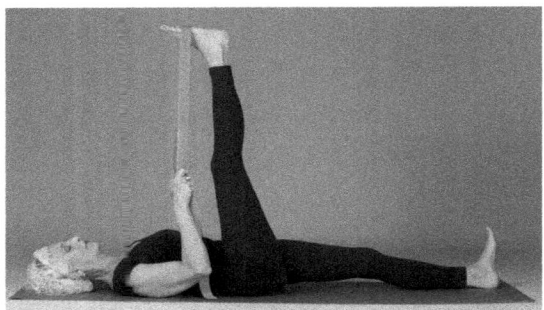

- Repeat these coiling and uncoiling movements several times, tracing the pathway of force from the psoas to the foot on one breath phase, and back to the psoas on the other phase. Make it a psoas event, each time coiling the psoas for power, then unleashing the potential energy like a spring so it does the work of straightening the leg.

- For the sake of contrast, bend and straighten the leg a few times without psoas awareness, the way you would do it habitually before learning about the psoas. Notice how this movement differs.

  – *Where do you initiate movement?*
  – *How does the rest of your body respond?*
  – *How much effort is required?*

- Complete the practice by repeating the movement a few more times as a psoas event.

- Extend both legs to notice any differences between sides.

- Repeat the exploration on the left side.

- Extend both legs and observe sensations in your body. It's common to experience heat sensations in your pelvis after this exploration.

  – *What do you notice?*

Once you've learned to activate your psoas in supine, experiment with more challenging positions, such as side lying, all fours, kneeling, and standing on one or two legs. This will progressively deepen the repatterning of coiling for power and help you integrate your learning into everyday activities like walking and stair climbing.

## EXPLORATION: THE DRAWBRIDGE

When you consciously activate the deep psoas to initiate movement, habitual overuse of superficial muscles is inhibited. The image of a drawbridge is used in both concentric (shortening) and eccentric (lengthening) contractions to bring more precision and refinement to movements of the hip and to create psoas events.

### Learning Objective

- Use imagery to refine psoas-initiated movement.

### Practice Note

- These variations of the drawbridge are progressively more challenging. Start with the first variation and work up to one that, although challenging, can be performed without strain. The first variation helps you learn how to inhibit habitual overuse of superficial hip flexor muscles.

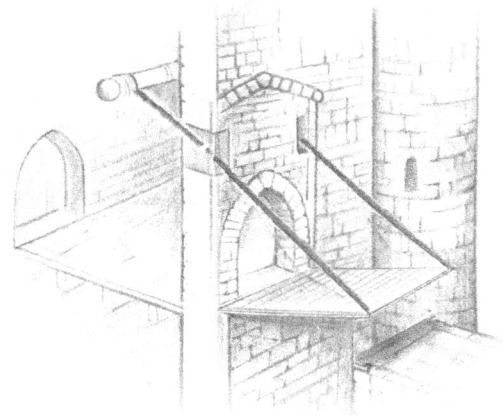

## Contraindications

- Avoid or exercise caution in cases of disc herniation, spondylolisthesis or spinal stenosis, hernia, or acid reflux.

## Props

- A blanket folded into a long, narrow rectangle approximately 13 cm (5 in.) in height or a low bolster
- A yoga belt

## Instructions

- Lie in supine and take a baseline reading.
  - *How does your back body meet the floor?*
- Place the blanket horizontally on the floor and arrange yourself in supine with your pelvis and sacrum fully supported. Bend both knees with feet flat on the floor.

## Passive Variation

In this variation, the leg is lifted passively with the goal of consciously disengaging all hip flexors and uncovering habitual over-engagement of rectus femoris.

## Instructions

- Loop a yoga belt below the right knee, holding the ends loosely with both hands.
- Lift your leg passively by pulling on the belt and using arm strength to raise the right foot 15 cm (6 in.) off the floor.

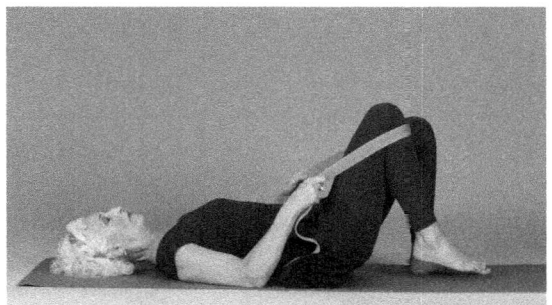

- Imagine the belt as chains raising the "drawbridge" of the thigh. Allow the entire weight of your leg to be supported by the belt. It may be challenging to disengage rectus femoris and allow the leg to be moved passively. You can pull on the belt to bounce or jiggle the leg to dissuade any habitual impulses to "help" hip flexion.
- Slowly lower the foot to the floor passively, visualizing the "drawbridge" lowered by the chains.
  - *Can your hip flexors remain disengaged?*
- Alternate raising and lowering the "drawbridge," gradually increasing the distance between the foot and floor. Pause every now and then to jiggle and bounce the leg to remind it to remain passive.
  - *Is it easier for the leg to remain passive when raising or lowering?*
- Remove the belt and pause for a few moments to notice differences between the two sides.
- Repeat with the other leg.

- Stay with this variation until the hip flexors learn to remain relaxed throughout the passive movement.

## Active Variation

In this variation, you will initially activate the psoas consciously so rectus femoris can activate secondarly in its rightful role as helper, not prime mover. It can be challenging to disengage rectus femoris if it's habitually functioned as prime mover. Maintaining focus on the drawbridge image and creating a psoas event will eventually override unconscious habits of activating superficial muscles in hip flexion. If it's difficult to inhibit rectus femoris, you can do a hybrid assisted version by using the belt to lightly support your leg throughout the movement. It may take some time for rectus femoris to realize it doesn't have to activate so strongly.

### Instructions

- Begin in the same supine starting position as in the passive variation, minus the belt.

- First, sense how you habitually lift your foot off the floor. Forget about psoas awareness for a few moments as you raise and lower your foot several times. Notice how you move.

  – *Where do you initiate movement?*
  – *How does the rest of your body respond?*
  – *How much effort is required?*

- Now monitor rectus femoris activation. Place the finger pads of the right hand in the middle of the upper thigh just below the groin crease.

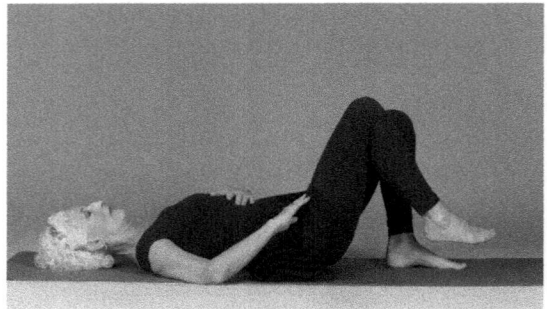

- Feel the rectus femoris tendon pop up as you lift the right foot 3 cm (1 in.) off the floor a few times. Notice the intensity of activation as you raise and lower the foot.

- Recall the location of the trochanteric psoas attachments near the sitting bone.

- To create psoas events, lift and lower your foot again, focusing on movement of these attachments toward and away from the anchored spinal attachments and on the action between them. Visualize your thigh as a drawbridge and the psoas as chains that can be reeled in and out to raise and lower the drawbridge. Monitor and consciously inhibit an over-enthusiastic rectus femoris. You can pat or jiggle its tendon to pacify and dissuade any tendency to lead the movement.

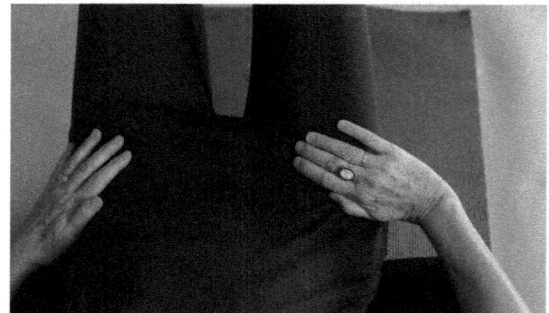

- Each time you lower your leg, visualize the chains reeling out to slowly lower the heavy drawbridge of the thigh and return the foot to the floor. Maintain the mental picture of the psoas "falling back" as it lengthens in eccentric activation.

- Repeat several movements.

- Pause for a few moments to notice differences between sides.

- Repeat on the other leg.

- Remove the blanket and rest in baseline position to sense any changes. Slowly stand up, then walk around and notice any changes.

  - *What do you notice?*

## PSOAS PROTOCOL STAGE V: ENGAGING THE PSOAS

Remember all the psoas muscle bundles with their overlapping attachments and angles of pull? During leg and trunk movement, some muscle bundles work as movers while others are stabilizers. When we consciously activate and visualize these simultaneous functions, it creates cohesion in the psoas and results in stronger, more coordinated movement. The viscoelastic quality of psoas fascia creates a resistance to both shortening and elongation, maintaining a stiffness or pullback in the tissue throughout movement. In the following practices, create psoas events by using appropriate imagery to help you elongate or condense the muscles while simultaneously maintaining spinal support. Once you establish this felt sense, you can integrate it into any movement or daily activity.

### Learning Objectives

- Use the psoas as an organizing principle during movement.

- Experience frontal spinal support from the psoas.

### Practice Note

- When using the psoas as an organizing principle, ask yourself these questions:

  - *Which end of the psoas do I anchor?*
  - *Which end of the psoas do I move? Or do I move both ends simultaneously? Toward or away from each other?*
  - *Where do I sequence force?*
  - *How can the psoas support my spine?*

### EXPLORATION: ASYMMETRICAL FORWARD BEND (PARSVOTTANASANA) 🎥

#### Practice Notes

- Exhale when moving and inhale while pausing.

- Use appropriate imagery to maintain psoas support for the spine.

- Maintain connection between the psoas and the ground throughout the movement. Each time you exhale, imagine sending energy from the psoas down the back leg to anchor into the ground.

#### Instructions

- Stand with your feet hip width apart, then consciously activate your right psoas to step your right foot back approximately 0.5–1 m (1.5–3 ft.). Turn your right foot 45 degrees outward while keeping your hips oriented forward. Place your right palm on your right groin and the left hand at the solar plexus.

- Use imagery to access psoas support for the spine. Imagine that you are sending strong energetic anchors down from each psoas to the ground. Sense right and left psoas muscles like heavy-duty yet pliant pillars supporting your lumbar spine. Or you could visualize your psoas as supportive hands shoring up the front of the spine.

- Initiating movement from the psoas, move your spine forward 20 degrees off the vertical, then pause. Maintain a neutral lumbar curve. As you move forward, simultaneously imagine sending force down the back leg to maintain a strong supportive foundation with the ground while activating the frontal spinal support of the psoas.

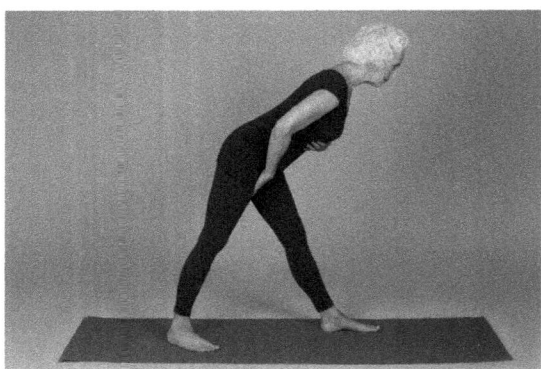

- Move forward another 20 degrees, pausing to check that you're not collapsing at the juncture between the pelvis and lumbar spine or between the lumbar spine and the rib cage. Continue to move forward incrementally until you feel your back heel starting to unweight from the ground. If you go any farther, you'll lose balanced integrity of the movement.

- Maintain the end position for five breaths, using each exhalation to reestablish both frontal spinal support and connection between the right psoas and back foot.

- To exit the posture, bend your left knee and slowly press your foot into the floor to lift your torso back to upright position. Visualize the psoas supporting and lifting your spine.

- Repeat the movement without psoas awareness.

  – *What's different?*

- Do it one more time as a psoas event.

- Once you discern felt sense of the simultaneous actions of the psoas, you can add in the arms. In the starting position, raise your arms overhead and sense the fascial continuity between the psoas, respiratory diaphragm, and arms. Maintain this relationship as you repeat the movement, stabilizing the upper psoas attachments to prevent your lower ribs from jutting forward.

- To exit the posture, move the right foot forward to the starting position by consciously activating your right psoas. Pause in standing to notice differences between the two sides.

- Repeat the practice on the other side.

- Pause in standing and notice any effects.

  – *How does moving as a psoas event change the posture?*

## EXPLORATION: WALKING FROM THE PSOAS

Walking can become a meditation on the psoas by focusing on different psoas events occurring throughout the gait cycle.

### Practice Note

- Break down the gait cycle into individual psoas events and repeat each one several times to firmly establish felt sense of each component. Then, put it all together.

### Instructions

- To establish a baseline, walk on flat ground.

  – *How do you initiate walking?*

- Place your hands over the upper-psoas attachments and visualize your legs starting at the solar plexus. Initiate each step by swinging the leg from there instead of your hip joints.

- *Psoas lengthening and condensing:* As you walk, track the movement of the psoas, alternating between lengthening and condensing as leg attachments move toward and away from spinal attachments on hip flexion and extension. You may be able to palpate their rhythmical, alternating activation.

- *Spinal extension:* As the ball of the back foot pushes off the ground, feel the sequential flow of ground reaction force moving up the leg into the pelvis and spine, creating slight extension through the lower back and lengthening the psoas.

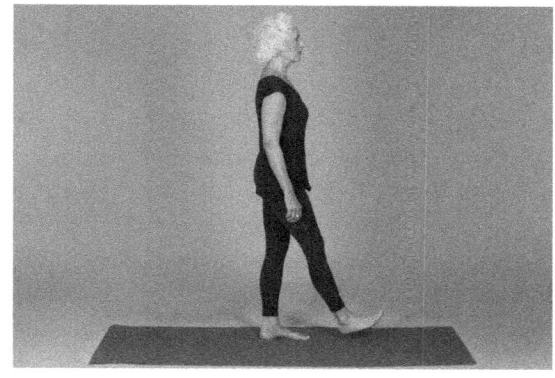

- *Spinal support:* As the back leg draws parallel to and passes the standing leg notice how the spinal support of the psoas helps you balance on one leg.

- *Eccentric activation:* After the heel strikes the ground and the hip moves forward into extension, notice the elongating eccentric activation of the psoas.

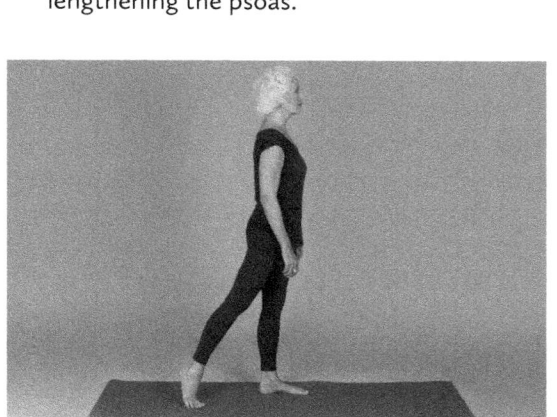

- As the leg swings forward, become aware of the dual function of the psoas: it activates to pull the leg forward and simultaneously offers frontal spinal support to maintain uprightness.

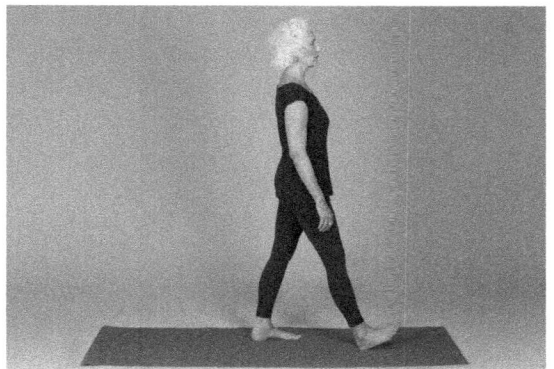

- For a more global experience, imagine the psoas as large industrial-strength springs coiling and uncoiling to give elastic rebound to your steps.

- Continue this walking meditation for at least five minutes.

## THERAPEUTIC APPLICATIONS

As central connecting structures, the psoas have profound multidimensional effects on the koshas. As clinicians, psoas involvement in almost any presenting condition is worth exploring. My own clinical experience and ample research confirm psoas participation in conditions ranging from disc protrusion to PTSD. As deep and hidden structures, they are often-overlooked contributors to pathologies. The extensive fascial connections of the psoas and their contribution to spinal support contribute to these far-ranging effects. In fact, psoas cross-sectional area can predict whole-body sarcopenia (muscle loss), cardiorespiratory fitness, and surgical prognosis in older patients (Chu *et al.*, 2023).

In the musculoskeletal system, bilateral or unilateral psoas imbalance can disrupt equilibrium of tension and compression forces throughout the fascial system, provoking pelvic and spinal misalignments, faulty movement patterns, and imbalanced force transmission. This imbalance can affect even distal structures; shoulder bursitis or knee arthritis may be traced back to structural misalignments initiated by psoas imbalance. Over time, chronically shortened or overstretched psoas eventually lose elasticity, strength, and stabilizing capacity. Other muscle groups compensate for the lack of structural integrity, leading to superficially initiated and less integrated movement.

Chronic shortening of the psoas can contribute to low back pain and sacroiliac joint dysfunction by tilting or twisting the pelvis in any plane, depending on which psoas fibers are involved. Pelvic tilts and twists will compress the femurs in the acetabulum and restrict hip movement, which may transfer rotational torque to either the knees or lumbar spine. In scoliosis, the cross section of the psoas is larger on the concave side of a curvature (Xu *et al.*, 2021) and low back pain associated with scoliosis has been attributed to the psoas (Sanjay *et al.*, 2021). I have

seen many cases of back pain resolve solely with therapeutic psoas work, without treating posterior myofascia. The psoas may also influence pelvic floor functions and balance between pelvic floor movements and the rhythm of the respiratory diaphragm (Siccardi, Tariq, and Valle 2023). Psoas and diaphragm continuity mean that psoas tension prevents full diaphragmatic excursion, potentially giving rise to dysfunctional breathing patterns. Alternatively, shallow or paradoxical breathing can hamper recovery of tight or painful psoas muscles, so breath work may be an important first step in healing psoas dysfunction.

> I had back pain my whole adult life before discovering the secret of the psoas.
>
> *Nina*

Some abdominal and pelvic organs, including the kidneys, rest on and are supported by the muscular shelf of the psoas. This intimate relationship suggests that organs can be affected by psoas tone. Excessive tension in the supportive psoas can be transferred to organs, compromising their movement and function. This connection between the psoas and visceral dysfunction has been recognized for decades; nervous, endocrine, and digestive system imbalance has been attributed to the psoas (Michele 1962). Clinically, I have observed conditions including irritable bowel syndrome and menstrual cramps significantly improve with EA psoas explorations. Relaxed, toned psoas provide support for organs and contribute to healthy function by providing rhythmical organ massage during walking and other movements.

The psoas and nervous system are intimately connected. The lumbar plexus is embedded between the two psoas layers, so whenever we work with the psoas we affect the nervous system, and vice versa. The psoas are the major muscles activated when the nervous system perceives danger; it mobilizes us to escape, fight, or freeze in a protective fetal position. These muscles are recognized as "principal actors in the complex neural network of human psychosomatic experience and the reactive stress system, potentially involved in the incidence, but also the relief, of post-traumatic stress disorder" (Anderson *et al.*, 2017). However, it doesn't take a danger threat to trigger activation; ongoing physical, mental, and emotional stress can chronically contract the psoas and cause persistent overactivation of the sympathetic nervous system. Chronic psoas contraction signals constant danger. Over time, the poor adrenal glands are exhausted from continuously pumping out adrenaline, cortisol,

and other stress hormones, setting the stage for stress-related illnesses.

Balancing the psoas can significantly alter organization of forces throughout the body as the pelvis and spine find their rightful place in gravity and force is transferred efficiently from the torso to the ground. Over time, we learn to access deep power and inner support. We feel more connected to ourselves and others. When interoceptive awareness of the psoas is developed through EA practices, we learn to access inner resources and strength for healing.

> Whenever I feel myself starting to dissociate, I connect with my psoas muscles and come back to myself.
>
> *Anne*

## KOSHIC CONSIDERATIONS

### Annamaya Kosha

- *How have you incorporated psoas awareness into your movement practice and daily activities?*
- *Have you experienced increased stability, strength, or coordination?*
- *Has your upright posture changed?*

### Pranamaya Kosha

- *Have you discovered any relationship between breath and the state of your psoas?*
- *Have your energy levels changed?*
- *Have psoas explorations affected your nervous, endocrine, or digestive system function?*

### Manomaya Kosha

- *Have you had any emotional responses to psoas explorations?*
- *Has your ability to sense emotions changed?*

### Vijnanamaya Kosha

- *Are you aware of a connection between the state of the psoas and your psychological stance?*
- *Do you feel more centered? More connected to your deep inner power?*

### Anandamaya Kosha

- *Do you feel more connected to yourself?*
- *Are you more aware of your wholeness?*

## KEY CONCEPTS

- The psoas muscles are central connecting structures, enabling us to stand and walk, but also subtly influencing our capacity for grounding, wholeness, and authenticity on other koshic levels.
- The psoas has been called the "hidden prankster" because of its deep location and ability to mimic symptoms commonly attributed to other dysfunctions.
- When consciously initiated from the psoas, movement is stronger, integrated, and emanates from the core.
- Breath, energy levels, and force transmission are influenced by the psoas.
- The sensory role of the psoas can be impaired when excessive tension compresses fascial nerve endings or the embedded lumbar plexus.
- Release of psoas tension can release long-buried memories and emotions.

- Psychological stances and embodied metaphors may be structurally reinforced by the psoas.
- The primary function of the psoas is spinal stability, not hip flexion.
- The nervous system is intimately connected to the psoas, particularly in nervous system responses to danger.
- The psoas have direct fascial connections to numerous structures, including the respiratory and pelvic diaphragms.
- Physiological functioning of multiple systems can be affected by excessive psoas tension.
- Refining felt sense and moving from the psoas helps to minimize habitual activation of superficial muscles.
- Interoceptive awareness of the psoas can help us access inner resources and strength for healing.

# CHAPTER 8

# Pelvic Integrity

*He shoots straight from the hip.*
*His tail was between his legs.*
*She's a pain in the butt.*
*They were joined at the hip.*

The pelvis is the center of the body, the hub of the wheel. The center of gravity, usually located at the second sacral segment, is the still point around which our six limbs (arms, legs, head, and tail) move. Along with the development of large brains, upright posture is considered a defining change in human development (Hogervorst, Bouma, and de Vos 2009). Evolution of the pelvis enabled us to leave the sea to walk and eventually stand erect on land. We need our appendicular skeleton, the pelvis, arms, and legs, for locomotion and interacting with the environment.

Structurally, the pelvis is the foundation for the spine and upper body. It is key to upright aligned physical structure, efficient force transfer, and locomotion. Whenever the limbs move off center, the pelvis and associated myofascia adaptively reconfigure to stabilize the body and enable movement. This stabilization function prevents us from toppling over every time we take a step or reach for something! From a biotensegrity perspective, the pelvis adapts to forces by distributing the load through "the tension network of soft tissues that include local pelvic ligaments and extends throughout the entire fascial system and compression network of bones" (Levin 2007).

The pelvis is a movable yet stable structure, constantly shifting and responding to weight and load influences from above and below. When it fails to efficiently adapt to these forces, the body accommodates as best it can, but ongoing compensatory adaptations may eventually result in compromised movement or pain. EA practices endeavor to establish pelvic integrity, that is, an optimal balance of tension and compression forces and of mobility and stability. With integrity, we can experience the pelvis as a center of stability, power, and grounding. Many yoga practitioners emphasize "opening" the hips at the expense of stabilizing the pelvis, and some eventually suffer torn labrums and hip replacements. When we consciously establish a stable yet fluid pelvis through EA practices, we may feel more youthful and vital, or *zaftig*, a Yiddish word meaning lustrous or juicy used to describe sensuous women (Vocabulary.com n.d.). We want to find an optimal place where the pelvis is stable but not rigid and mobile but not unstable.

## KOSHIC PERSPECTIVES

Exploring annamaya kosha in the pelvis includes learning about and developing felt sense of its anatomy, then repatterning optimal alignment and movement to fully experience its capacity for fluid movement, stability, and force transmission. We learn through practice that movement initiated from the pelvis is generally more powerful and integrated, and less effortful.

On the pranamaya kosha level, the pelvis contains our energetic center. Known as *Hara* in Eastern wisdom traditions, it can be a source of great power, equanimity, and creativity. In yogic anatomy, the pelvis contains the first and second *chakras*, spinning energy centers containing elements of earth (stability) and water (fluidity). With pelvic integrity, we can access these elemental qualities more easily.

Pelvic integrity can also optimize physiological functions. The respiratory diaphragm is free to participate in full breathing, and organs and neurovascular structures are adequately supported and have space to move. Even at a cellular level, lack of pelvic integrity can cause compression that disrupts healthy cell physiology.

The pelvis contains the enteric brain, the seat of gut feelings and primal emotions in manomaya kosha. An experience of pelvic integrity can support greater emotional awareness and encourage emotional self-regulation by helping us feel safe and steady. Many students experience a misaligned, rigid, or hypermobile pelvis as a source of pain, compromised movement, and a swamp of stuck emotions. In fact, anxiety, depression, and stress have been strongly associated with chronic pelvic pain (Brooks *et al.*, 2020). Working with the pelvis can sometimes feel like opening Pandora's box! Moshe Feldenkrais, founder of the Feldenkrais method, reportedly said that a decrease in anxiety is experienced as increased freedom of movement in the center of the pelvis.

Pelvic position can reflect patterns of withholding, exaggerating, or authentically expressing emotions. Someone with a tucked pelvis might habitually repress emotions while another who is physically but fluidly centered through the pelvis and legs may appropriately contain or express emotionality. The yoga tradition reminds us that *sthira* (steadiness) contributes to emotional stability and a calm, centered mind.

> When I stabilize my pelvis, it anchors me to myself and gives me emotional clarity.
>
> *Mark*

In vijnanamaya kosha, pelvic position and mobility may mirror our psychology or conditioning and predispose us to distinctive ways of perceiving, feeling, and expressing ourselves in the world. Contrast the pelvis of an anxious perfectionist with that of a confident, easy-going person. Personality traits such as neuroticism have been associated with persistent pelvic pain whereas self-reported extroverted and conscientious women not only experienced less pain but were more likely to resolve pain issues (Xiangsheng *et al.*, 2021). Difficulty in experiencing emotions, creating relationships, and self-management have also been correlated with pelvic pain (Albrecht *et al.*, 2015). Introverts are more likely to exhibit posteriorly rotated pelvic posture while extroverts tend toward the opposite (Guimond & Massrieh 2012). This research leaves us with the chicken and egg question: Is personality a contributing cause or an effect of pelvic alignment, or are they too interconnected to distinguish?

Cultivating felt sense of pelvic structure and function through EA practices can help us feel more seated in our deeper Self and equipped to move in the world with potency and confidence. Many students report feeling more centered, grounded, and balanced after exploring their pelvis with EA and integrating pelvic awareness into their everyday life.

The bony rim of the pelvic bowl forms a circle, the symbol of wholeness; we can view the pelvis as the container of our wholeness. The Zen circle, *ensō*, is a symbol of meditative, dynamic stillness and of *chi*, the universal life-force energy present in all living things. Through the lens of anandamaya kosha, awareness of our habitual orientation of the pelvic bowl can illuminate how our responses, movement, and daily activities may express or deny our inherent wholeness. Through awareness gained in EA practices, this typically subconscious decision can yield to conscious choice. We can choose to be present in our wholeness by shifting conscious awareness to the touchstone of the pelvic circle.

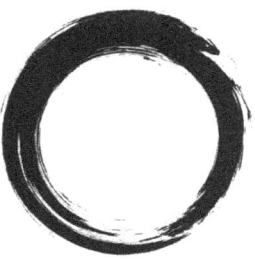

The authentic self is the soul made visible.

*Sarah ban Breathnach (2016)*

## LEARN IT

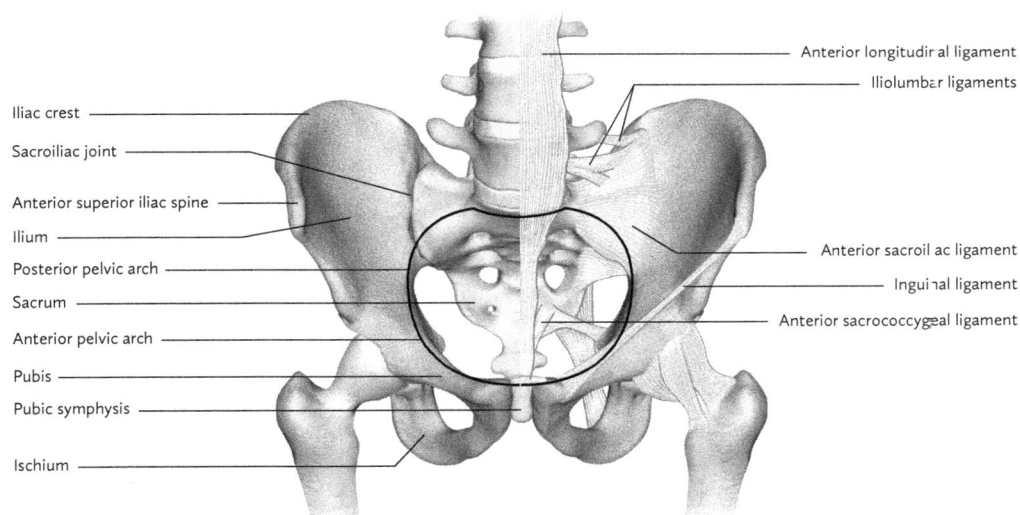

In Latin, *pelvis* means "basin." The shape of the pelvic bones and joints are designed to protect the delicate viscera and spinal cord by absorbing, dissipating, and transferring the impact of heel strike and other movements. The steep sides of the pelvic bowl safeguard digestive, reproductive, and eliminative organs contained within. The inner bowl guides nerves and blood vessels to the legs and provides passage for elimination and birthing. Pelvic nerves transmit motor impulses to organs and muscles so we can move, procreate, and function physiologically. Thirty-six paired muscles radiate from the hub of the pelvis, creating fascial continuities with the arms, legs, spine, and head. The strong diamond-shaped multilayered thoracolumbar fascia merges vertically with myofascia from the sacrum to the neck and horizontally with abdominal, arm, and leg myofascia. No wonder pelvic alignment can have such profound global influence.

## Bones

Three paired bones form the pelvic basin. They are separate cartilaginous structures at birth, partially fuse by age three to provide stability in the hip sockets, and finally fuse in adolescence as cartilage is replaced by bone through progressive weight-bearing and movement. Two independently moving halves of the pelvis join anteriorly at the pubic bones and posteriorly at the sacrum. Each half contains a pubis (pubic bone) anteriorly, an ischium with a tuberosity (sitting bone) posteriorly, and an ilium flaring from the sacrum like a wing. A superior ramus connects the ilia and pubis, while an inferior ramus joins pubis and ischium. The sacrum, suspended between ilia by ligaments, is formed by five vertebrae largely fused by adulthood. Each has rudimentary spinous and transverse processes present in other spinal vertebrae. The sacrum forms the posterior pelvic bowl, with the spine arising from its wide base. The vestigial tail, the coccyx, is formed by three to five fused vertebrae.

The Celestial Design Committee beautifully designed the pelvis to be strong and stable for bearing and transferring the entire weight of the upper body, yet light and flexible enough to permit walking and graceful dancing. Its adaptability is facilitated by the arches, circles, and holes within. Anterior and posterior arches are formed by pubic bones and ilia (anterior arch) and the upper three sacral segments and adjacent thickened ilia (posterior arch). Bone is thickest at the posterior arch for maximum weight-bearing, and thinner elsewhere to provide lightness. The middle of the ilia is so thin that light can shine through! The two arches form a circle that strengthens and stabilizes both arches and transfers weight and force through its curved pathways. Internal hydrostatic pressure from pelvic organs supports and stabilizes both arches. The circle is the boundary between the lower bowl and the upper, incomplete bowl formed by the superior ilia. The "holes" in the pelvic design add more lightness and provide pathways for neurovascular structures: the obturator foramen between the pubic and ischial bones and the greater sciatic foramen created by ligaments closing the notch between the ischial tuberosity and sacrum. The three paired bones meet at the acetabulum of each pelvic half, forming equal thirds of the cup-shaped hip socket. This design makes structural sense when we consider the multiple pathways of forces converging at the hip joints.

## Joints

The pelvis contains five intrinsic joints and three extrinsic joints between the two hip joints and the sacrum and L5 vertebra. While our hip joints allow great movement, the L5–S1 articulation must be stable enough to receive and transmit upper body weight to the legs, favoring stability over range of motion. The paired pubic bones join at the midline through a fibrous cartilaginous disc. This pubic symphysis resists tension, compression, and shearing forces while allowing nominal independent movement of each pelvic half, such as occurs during walking.

When pubic joints move, sacroiliac joints move in tandem. The vertical sacroiliac joints between the upper sacrum and ilia also move minimally. Historically considered immovable, they contain both synovial and fibrous aspects, reflecting both mobility and stability capabilities, although stability prevails. The two large auricular (Latin for *ear*) sacroiliac joint surfaces are irregular and contain "grooves and rails," fitting together to afford greater stability between the vertical surfaces. The joint between the sacrum and coccyx is a cartilaginous articulation that moves very slightly in defecation and childbirth. All these joints absorb the impact of locomotion to protect delicate pelvic organs. Collectively, the limited amount of movement available at each intrinsic joint enables fluid and integrated pelvic movement.

Numerous strong ligaments knit together the internal joints of the pelvis, providing support during weight-bearing and movement, while simultaneously limiting and guiding range of motion. Their subtle elasticity provides springiness for shock absorption and force transfer. The number and strength of ligaments limits pelvic joint movement, favoring stability instead. Asymmetrical ligamentous laxity in pregnancy-related pelvic pain can cause instability, dysfunction, and pain that compromises pelvic structure and support (Damen *et al.*, 2001). The thoracolumbar fascia further assists stabilization of both lumbosacral junction and sacroiliac joints (Willard *et al.*, 2012).

> Apparently rock and roll liberated the pelvis and it hasn't been the same since.
>
> *Emma Thompson (1995)*

## Myofascia

Of the 36 (!) paired muscles connecting the pelvis to other body parts, several radiate from the pelvis to the ribs, spine, head, and arms while the majority connect the pelvis to the legs. The latter include the abdominals, posterior trunk muscles, iliopsoas complex, hip adductors and abductors, quadriceps, hip extensors, external rotators, pelvic floor muscles, and latissimus dorsi. The numerous muscles and associated fascia form "spokes" radiating from the hub of the pelvic wheel, providing considerable mobility and postural support.

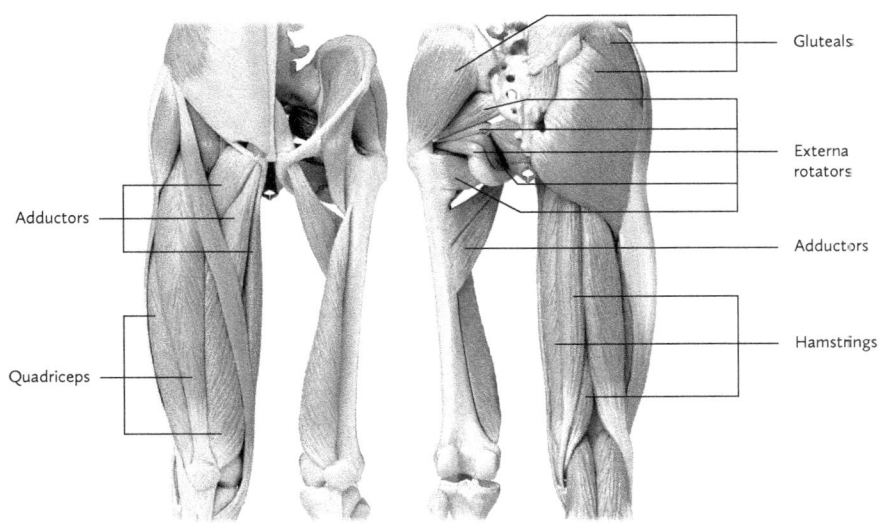

Adductors

Quadriceps

Gluteals

External rotators

Adductors

Hamstrings

Several pelvic muscles have triangular shapes that contribute precision and motor control across multiple vectors of movement. Force and energy sequence from the pelvis to limbs and vice versa through these myofascial structures. Each structure exerts a distinct angle of tensional pull. When structures have too much or too little tone, the pelvis is subjected to multidirectional vectors of force that imbalance tension and compression forces. This can negatively affect range of motion, strength, and force transfer. The health and longevity of pelvic joints depends on balanced tone of these numerous myofascial structures.

When elastic and resilient, the horizontal fascial planes of the pelvic floor and respiratory diaphragm also assist in stabilizing the pelvis (see Chapter 3). Like the feet, both diaphragms function as resilient foundations supporting structures higher up and contributing to upright stability.

## FEEL IT

Mapping the pelvis through touch, breath, and movement builds three-dimensional felt sense that clarifies its structure, size, and location for the nervous system. When you consciously situate your awareness within the pelvis, it can be experienced as a source of support, power, and (paradoxically) stillness.

## EXPLORATION: DISCOVER THE PELVIS

### Learning Objective

• Map the pelvis through touch.

### Props

• Support for the head.

### Practice Notes

• An anatomical model or anatomy book can be helpful for reference.

• The pelvis is a sensitive area, so give yourself ample time in a quiet environment for this exploration.

• Use gentle, slow, and respectful touch to palpate the topography of bones and differentiate soft tissue textures.

• Experiment using your fingers, thumbs, and palms to palpate.

• Be curious about the location, size, roundness, and orientation of bony structures and their relationships to other structures.

• Explore the dimensionality of bones—top, bottom, inside, and outside. Use a

back-and-forth movement of your fingertips to palpate bony edges.

• Palpate attentively to register and anchor awareness of each structure in your nervous system.

### Instructions

• Lie in supine with your hands resting on your abdomen. Take a baseline reading of current felt sense of your pelvis as you lie on the floor.

• Explore the most prominent points of the pelvis on either side of your abdomen, the anterior superior iliac spine (ASIS).

• From the ASIS, follow the pelvic crests posteriorly, palpating the thickness of their edges. Slide your fingers medially to feel the inner surface of the ilia in a few places, then slide your fingers laterally to feel the outer surface through overlying myofascia.

• Returning to the ASIS, slide your fingers inferiorly to the groin crease. Trace it medially until you feel the lateral edges of the pubis. Define the different dimensions of the pubic bones—anterior, superior, and inferior surfaces. Trace medially to the pubic symphysis—a small depression between the two pubic bones—and explore its contours.

- Roll onto one side with your knees and hips at 90 degree angles, with ample support under your head. Find the top of the pelvic crest at your lateral waist and slowly explore it back to the sacrum. Use your flat finger pads to find the slight depression or dimple indicating the sacroiliac joint. Find and palpate the posterior superior iliac crest (PSIS), the small protrusion located lateral to the dimple.

- Use the palm of your hand to palpate the curved bony surface of the sacrum, outlining its triangular shape and locating the vertical bumps of vestigial spinous processes in the midline. Curl one finger around the coccyx as it curves into the body and explore its dimensions.

- Use the heel of your hand to massage through the gluteal muscles to feel the flared surface of the ilia. The large amount of soft tissue makes the bone challenging to palpate, but you can infer its shape. Work your way laterally to the hip joint and palpate the size and contours of the greater trochanter.

- Slide your hand down to the sitting bone and outline its size, shape, and dimensions. Follow it anteriorly, lifting your leg to follow the ramus to the pubic bone. Trace the shape of the **Pelvic Diamond** (see Chapter 3), connecting the four points of the coccyx, pubic and sitting bones.

- Lie on your back and register any difference in sensations between sides, then complete the exploration on the other side.

- When finished, register any changes in felt sense of your pelvis in sitting, standing, and walking.

  - *Are you more aware of your pelvic diamond in sitting?*
  - *How has felt sense of your pelvis changed?*
  - *Has your standing or walking changed?*

## FOUNDATIONAL PRACTICE: THE HARASPHERE

We can be reminded of our wholeness through anatomical awareness of the pelvic circle, where the Hara, or energetic center, is located. Remember that the circle is a symbol of wholeness. In Oriental medicine, a person's health is measured by the strength of the Hara. When you consciously breathe into or initiate movement from your Hara, core muscles engage automatically, and movement is stronger and more integrated. The *Harasphere*, an imagined yellow sphere centered in the pelvis, is used in this practice to help you focus your awareness and give you a physical location to access your wholeness.

### Learning Objective

- Explore the pelvic circle through breath and movement.

### THE HARA BREATH

### Learning Objectives

- Use breath to deepen awareness of the pelvic circle and Hara.

- Calm the mind and settle the body.

## Instructions

- Sit in a comfortable seated position. Imagine a bright yellow sphere wedged in the pelvic circle formed by the anterior and posterior arches.

- With your hands resting in your lap, form the Mandala Mudra, a hand gesture associated with wholeness (Le Page and Aboim 2013). Place your right hand in the left palm and join thumb tips together to form a circle mirroring the pelvic circle. Close your eyes or gaze downward.

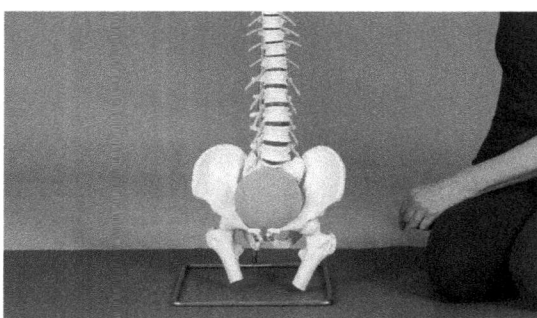

- With each inhalation, visualize the sphere expanding and pressing into the bones of the pelvis. Breathe calmly and with ease.

- First, focus on the sphere pressing simultaneously forward and back against the inner surfaces of the pubic bone and sacrum. With each exhalation, visualize the sphere condensing into its center.

- After several breaths, focus on the sphere pressing sideways against the inner surface of the lower bowl of the ilia.

- Visualize the sphere pressing simultaneously up toward the diaphragm, and down to the pelvic floor. Feel the pelvic diamond expanding and condensing with each breath.

- Finally, visualize the sphere expanding omnidirectionally as you inhale, condensing into its center as you exhale.

- Sit quietly to register the effects of this practice.

> The Hara Breath helps me define my boundaries. When I sense the bony pelvic container, I feel centered and contained enough to set boundaries with others.
>
> *Patricia*

## EXPLORATION: THE PELVIC DANCE

### Learning Objective

- Explore pelvic anatomy by initiating movement from different structures.

### Instructions

- Start on all fours with the knees and hands a comfortable distance apart.

- Initiating movement from your sacrum, move your pelvis in gentle anterior and posterior tilt, side bend, circles, and other spontaneous movements. Allow your knees and elbows to respond to or follow the pelvic movement.

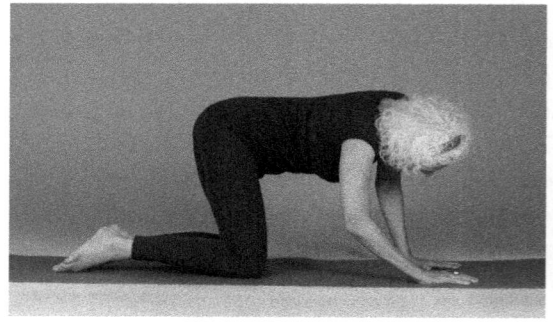

- Explore moving from different structures: Shift your awareness to one of the three pelvic bones and initiate moving from there.

- Explore moving from the other two bones, the pelvic floor, pelvic organs, and the Harasphere.

- Stand and continue your pelvic dance, focusing on each structure individually.

- Pause and notice any sensations.

  - *Which structures are most accessible to you? Inaccessible?*
  - *How does pelvic initiation change your movement?*
  - *Has felt sense of your pelvis changed?*

## HEAL IT

Sometimes, practicing mobility, flexibility, or strengthening movements without pelvic awareness can reinforce existing imbalances in pelvic tension and compression forces. When preliminary practices are done to repattern the pelvis closer to its anatomically balanced position, the benefits of subsequent movement are maximized.

## FOUNDATIONAL PRACTICE: THE PELVIC RESET

The pelvic reset is an osteopathic, self-help technique using subtle rhythmical isometric activation. When the femoral heads are centered in the **Hip Sockets**, forces are transferred more efficiently between the upper body and ground, and we feel more balanced and centered. The resulting redistribution of tension and compression forces throughout the pelvis can sometimes immediately ease pain. From a koshic perspective, this self-adjustment can contribute to physical, mental, and emotional stability and inspire a sense of safety. Commonly, students stand up after doing this technique exclaiming, *Oh, there I am. I'm back.*

### Learning Objective

- Reposition and stabilize the pelvic bones closer to neutral position.

I originally learned this technique as "The Shotgun," so named because it can alleviate pelvic, low back, hip, and lower limb pain and dysfunction generated by a variety of causes.

### Precautions

If you have sacroiliac joint issues, try this technique with legs hip width apart only. To find this neutral alignment in supine, touch your inner ankle bones together to align your feet, then step your heels laterally and move your forefeet to align with them. As with all EA practices, if this sequence causes discomfort, pause, and explore whether modifying your breath or effort level is helpful. If not, discontinue the practice and consult with your health professional.

### Props

- Yoga mat and belt

- Hard foam yoga block (8 x 15 x 23 cm/ 3 x 6 x 9 in.). If you don't have a block, you can improvise with lightweight objects of the same approximate size.

## Practice Notes

- Synchronize your breath and movement. Inhale as you press into the belt or block, and exhale as you release pressure. If this doesn't resonate with you, breathe the opposite way.

- Increase or decrease pressure on the belt or block gradually, slowly, and smoothly. Start with minimum pressure and build to a maximum 20 percent effort. Less is more!

- Initiate movement from your center.

- Before you press outward (abduction), anchor the big toe ball joint firmly into the ground. Before you press inward (adduction) anchor the little toe ball joint firmly. This counterbalances outward or inward knee movement and activates core muscles.

- Repeat the movements three times in each position.

## Instructions

- In supine, bend your knees with the inner feet and ankle bones touching at the midline.

### Pressing Out (Abduction and External Rotation)

- Loop the yoga belt around your thighs halfway between the knees and groin, tightening it to hold your knees together firmly but comfortably. Place the clasp where it's accessible.

- On an inhalation, press your big toe ball joints into the floor, maintaining this anchor as you gently press into the belt. As you exhale, gradually release the pressure. Repeat this pressure/release twice more, anchoring the big toe before each movement.

- Loosen the belt and walk your feet approximately 13–18 cm (5–7 in.) apart to align the feet, knees, and hip sockets. Repeat the movements.

- Loosen the belt and repeat the movements with your feet slightly wider than hips.

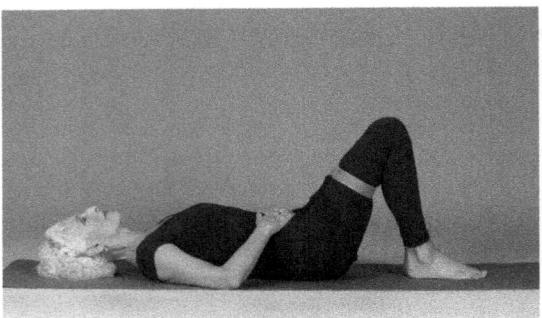

### Pressing In (Adduction and Internal Rotation)

- Place the wide edge of the yoga block between your knees.

- On an inhalation, anchor the little toe ball joints into the floor as you gently press into the block. Gradually release the pressure on an exhalation. Repeat twice more.

- Reposition the block and repeat the movements with the middle edge between your knees, feet adjusted to align with knees.

- Reposition the block and repeat the movements with the narrowest edge between your knees, feet adjusted to align with the knees.

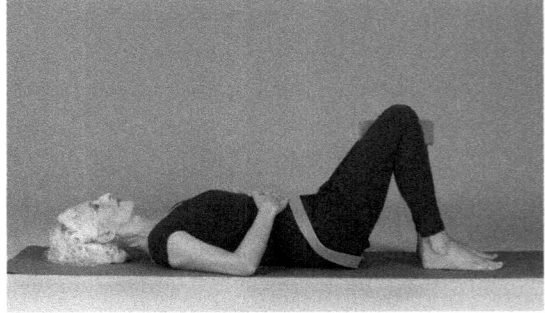

### *Alternate Abduction and Adduction*

- Place either the narrow or middle edge of the block between your knees, whichever feels most comfortable. Tighten the belt to hold the block in place.

- On an inhalation, anchor the big toe ball joints and gently press out into the belt. Exhale and release the pressure.

- On the next inhalation, anchor the little toe ball joints and gently press into the block. Exhale and release the pressure.

- Alternate outward and inward pressure for two more cycles, ending with pressing into the block.

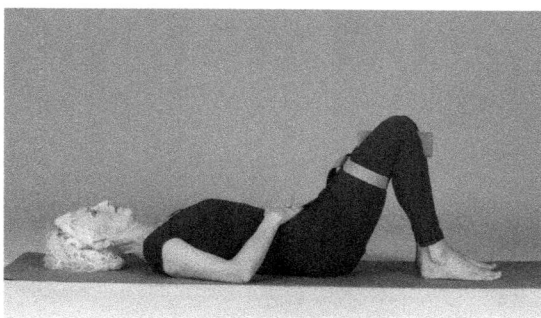

## DYNAMIC BRIDGE POSE (SETU BANDHA SARVANGASANA)

To integrate the pelvic reset, move into dynamic Bridge pose a few times with the props in place to maintain harmonious alignment between the pelvis and legs.

### Instructions

- Remain in the same position with arms alongside your body.

- Press into your feet to lift your pelvis a comfortable distance off the floor on one breath phase, then return to the floor on the other phase. Move in and out of the posture several times, coordinating breath and movement.

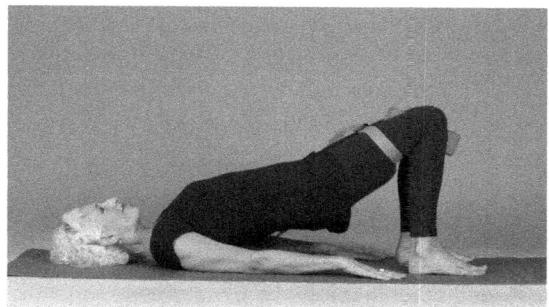

- Remove the props and do several repetitions while maintaining balanced **Foot Triangles**.

- Lie on your back with straight legs and pause to notice any effects. Stand and walk a little.

  - *What's different in your sacroiliac joints and lower back?*
  - *Do you notice changes in stability, physical balance, or how you are standing or walking?*
  - *What else do you notice?*

> When I stood up after doing the pelvic reset, I had a clear sense of having a pelvic bowl holding my organs. I live with anorexia, so it was a whole new perspective in feeling instead of my usual hyperawareness of a rounded, negative-feeling abdomen.
>
> *Iona*

## REPATTERNING PELVIC MOVEMENT IN THREE PLANES

The pelvis is designed to tilt anteriorly and posteriorly side bend, and twist in the three cardinal planes, and move in curved movements across planes. Sometimes, one or more of these movements are absent or compromised through developmental habitual, or adaptive, compensatory patterning. In the following explorations, movement is first explored in a non-weight-bearing position to minimize postural muscle activation and simplify sensory information to the nervous system. This creates a foundation to later explore movement in more complex weight-bearing positions. Practicing pelvic movements in varied positions challenges us to expand relationship possibilities between spine, pelvis, and legs. Approaching the same movements from different positions can promote mobility, strength, stability, and integrity of joints and myofascial structures as they adapt to varying vectors of force.

We usually think of moving our legs from the hip joints, but when we shift perspective and visualize the pelvis moving in relation to the legs, sensory input to the nervous system is different. Initiating the same movement from different aspects of pelvic anatomy can deepen repatterning. Shifting awareness between structures can amplify and enrich sensorimotor maps in the nervous system. Each individual focus gives the nervous system a slightly different perspective that results in a clearer picture of the pelvis as a whole.

When awareness of pelvic structures is highlighted, you are more likely to notice unhelpful habitual ways of moving, and to consciously repattern safe and healing movement.

### Learning Objectives

- Explore moving the pelvis in three planes in non-weight-bearing and weight-bearing positions.

- Notice pelvic movement limitations and repattern limited movements.

- Differentiate experience when initiating the same movement from different pelvic structures.

- Track how pelvic position influences relationships with the spine and legs.

### Precautions

- Those with hip prosthesis, recent fracture, or unmanaged hernia should consult their health professional before practicing hip-mobilizing exercises.

- Students with sacroiliac joint or low back pain, or advanced hip arthritis are advised to proceed with care, modifying as necessary.

### Practice Notes

- Repeat each movement for a minute or two, pausing between movements to register any effects.

- Practice shifting your awareness and initiating several movements from each pelvic bone (pubis, ilia, ischium, and sacrum) or **Harasphere**. Touching individual bones will give your nervous system a tactile cue.

- Notice how each pelvic movement (anterior and posterior tilt, side bend, and twist) changes the shape of your spine.

- Do non-weight-bearing movements as preparation for the **Pelvic Reset** or anytime to relieve low back or pelvic tension.

## EXPLORATION: NON-WEIGHT-BEARING PELVIC MOVEMENT

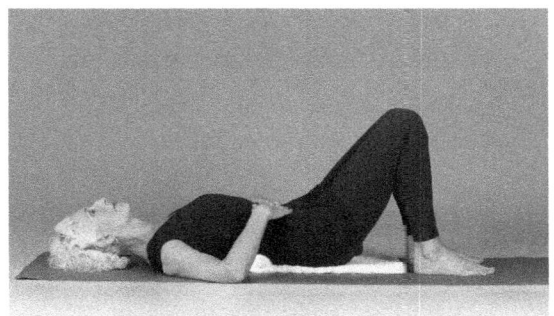

### Props

- A blanket (or towel) rolled to a diameter that will support, but not exaggerate, your natural lumbar curve

### Instructions

- Take a baseline in supine, noticing how your pelvis presses into the floor.

- Bend both knees with feet flat on the floor hip width apart. Place the rolled blanket under your low back to maintain the lumbar curve during movement. Adjust the diameter for comfort.

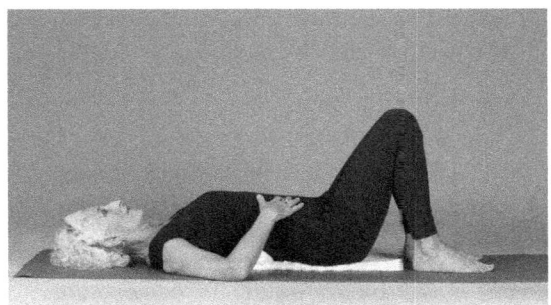

### *Anterior and Posterior Tilt*

- Imagine a central line dividing the triangle of your sacrum in half from tip to base.

- On an inhalation, gently press the midline of the sacrum into the floor starting at the base. Roll point by point to the tip, tilting the pelvis anteriorly and creating a gentle arch in your lumbar spine.

- On the exhalation, reverse directions and gently press point by point up the midline from tip to base, posteriorly rotating the pelvis and flexing the lumbar spine. Isolate this rocking movement in your sacrum without pressing the lumbar spine into the floor.

- Rock back and forth several times, coordinating movement with breath.

- Explore initiating these movements from other pelvic structures and the Harasphere.

- Pause to register sensations.

### *Side Bend*

- Palpate your sitting bones to place them in your awareness. Imagine a line from each sitting bone to corresponding heel.

- On an exhalation, move your right sitting bone down the imaginary line toward the right heel, laterally tilting your pelvis.

- Inhale as you return the pelvis to neutral. Your pelvis remains on the floor throughout the movements.

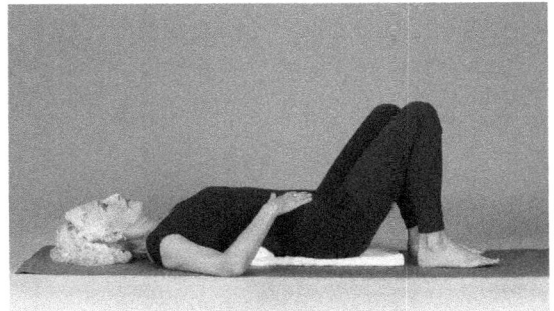

- Repeat several times on one side, then the other side, then alternating sides.

- Explore initiating these movements from other pelvic structures and the Harasphere.

- Pause to register sensations.

### Twist

- Place your feet wider than your hips. Changing the distance between your heels and sitting bones or the width between the feet will vary your experience.

- On each exhalation, initiate movement from your right sitting bone to gently move the right knee in a comfortable controlled diagonal arc across the midline of your body toward the left toes.

- Initiating from the sitting bone, move the knee back to neutral on each inhalation.

- Repeat several times on each side, then alternate sides.

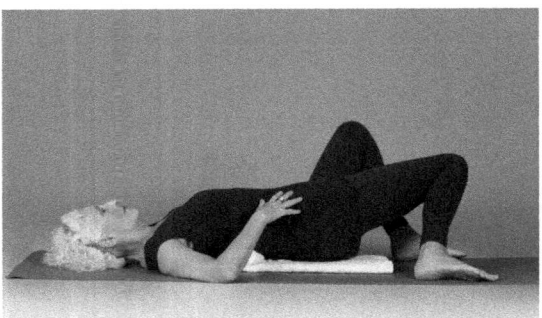

- Explore these movements from other pelvic structures and the Harasphere.

- Pause to register sensations, then stand and walk to notice any effects.

  - *Does one pelvic half have greater range or move more easily?*
  - *How does quality of movement change as you initiate from different places?*

  - *Do you prefer moving from a specific pelvic bone or the Harasphere?*
  - *What is felt sense of your pelvis now?*
  - *How is your standing and walking different?*

## EXPLORATION: SEATED PELVIC MOVEMENT

### Instructions

- Sit in a comfortable cross-legged position with enough support under your pelvis to easily maintain an erect spine. Alternatively, sit in a chair. Rest your hands on your knees. Balance your weight laterally between sitting bones, and front and back between the pubic bone and coccyx.

- Place your awareness on your sitting bones, the "feet" of the pelvis, and slowly roll them backward until your spine rounds.

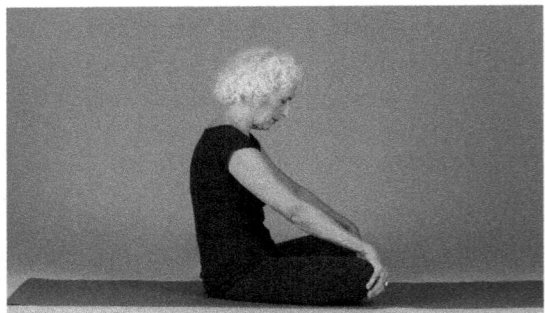

- Slowly roll forward on the sitting bones until your spine arches.

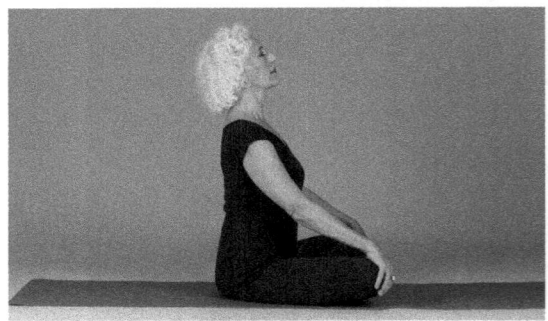

- Alternate rocking backward on exhalations, tilting the pelvis posteriorly and rounding the spine, then forward on inhalations, tilting the pelvis anteriorly and arching the spine. The spine remains vertically oriented as you move, not leaning forward or backward in space. You might imagine balancing a book atop your head.

- Track each point along the arc of movement from posterior to anterior sitting bones.

- Note the corresponding wave of spinal movement from your pelvis to head.

- As you rock back and forth, notice where you feel most stable, balanced, and at ease. After several movements, remain in that balanced place.

  - *Can the rest of your body settle into this balanced base of support?*
  - *Is the placement of your sitting bones different from your habitual sitting posture? Can you practice this way of sitting in your daily life?*

- Explore these movements from other pelvic structures and the **Harasphere**.

- Explore these movements in other seated positions to vary neural input.

## EXPLORATION: WEIGHT-BEARING PELVIC MOVEMENT

Approaching the same movements from different angles can promote mobility, strength, stability, and integrity of joints and myofascia. As structures adapt to changing vectors of force, the nervous system receives varied neural input that can deepen and reinforce neural repatterning.

## Bridge Pose (Setu Bandha Sarvangasana) Variations 📹
### Practice Notes

- Practice each of the following movements several times on one side, then the other, then alternating sides.

- Move in a gentle, controlled way with a small range of motion.

- Place both hands on your pelvis to guide movement.

- Rest in supine after exploring each variation of movement.

- Explore each movement from individual pelvic bones (ilia, sitting bones, pubic bone, and sacrum) and Harasphere.

### Instructions

- Take a baseline in supine.

  - *How is your pelvis resting on the floor?*

- Bend your knees with feet parallel and hip width apart.

- Press into your feet to lift your pelvis 10–12 cm (4–5 in.) off the floor. Maintain equal distance between your knees by pressing your big toe ball joints into the floor to activate inner thigh muscles; balance weight equally on the **Foot Triangle** points.

- Repeat each of the following movements several times in Bridge pose.

### Anterior and Posterior Tilt

- On inhalations, roll the sitting bones toward the floor to anteriorly tilt the pelvis and arch the lumbar spine.

- On exhalations, roll the sitting bones toward the ceiling to posteriorly tilt the pelvis and round the lumbar spine. As you repeat the movement several times, notice when you pass through neutral pelvic position.

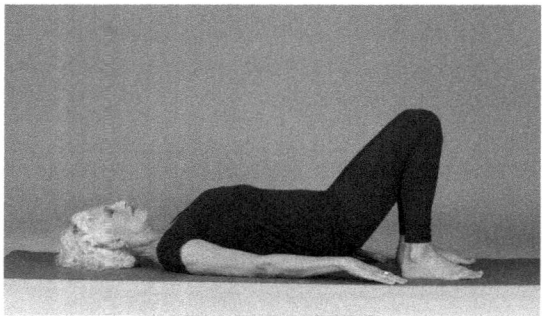

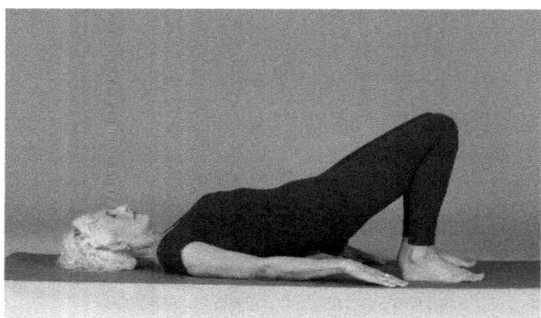

*Side Bend*

- On exhalations, move your right ilium away from your right shoulder, elongating the right side of your torso.

- On inhalations, return to neutral bridge position. Repeat the side bend several times on the right, then the left, then alternating sides.

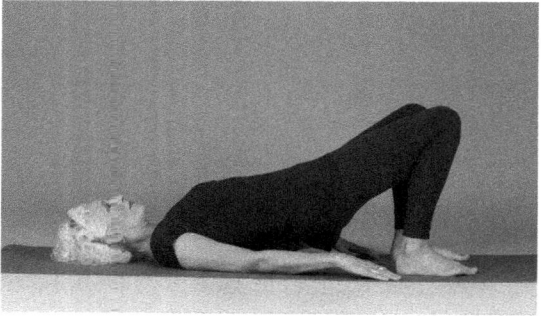

*Twist*

- On exhalations, slowly lower the right pubic bone toward the floor.

- On inhalations, return the pubic bone to horizontal. Repeat the twist several times on the right, then the left, then alternating sides.

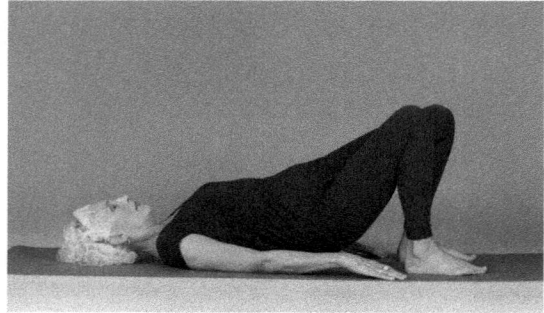

- Pause in supine to notice any effects, then stand and walk around.

  - *What do you notice?*

## Mountain Pose (Tadasana): Finding Neutral in Mountain Pose (Tadasana) 🔊

A neutral pelvic position supports a gentle lumbar curve, optimizing spinal stability, movement, and myofascial efficiency and resilience. This position results when the pelvis is slightly anteriorly rotated, although the degree of rotation varies between genders and individuals. As you vary pelvic position you may sense subtle changes in other koshic dimensions in addition to obvious physical effects on weight distribution through the feet and position and carriage of the spine.

### Learning Objectives

- Explore how pelvic position influences alignment and movement in the upper and lower body.

- Refine felt sense of neutral pelvic position.

## Instructions

- Stand comfortably with feet hip width apart.

- Track changes in weight distribution in your **Foot Triangles** as you slowly and mindfully alternate between posteriorly and anteriorly tilting your pelvis (tucking and lifting your tail). Maintain verticality in your spine. You can imagine balancing a book atop your head.

    - *Which pelvic position feels most familiar?*
    - *Where do you feel most steady?*
    - *How is your breath affected?*

- Shift your awareness to track changes in lumbar lordosis as you continue the pelvic movements.

    - *How do different pelvic positions affect the shape of your spine, orientation of your head, position of your ribcage and shoulders?*
    - *Can you track the wave of movement up your spine?*

- Remain in posterior pelvic tilt for up to one minute (if not too uncomfortable). Imagine this is your "normal" posture.

    - *Where do you feel tension or compression?*
    - *How is your breath affected?*
    - *If your pelvic circle was a headlight, where would it shine?*
    - *How would you perceive and interact with the world if you lived in this posture?*
    - *What message would this posture convey to others?*

- Reflect on the same questions as you remain in anterior pelvic tilt for a minute.

- Return to alternating slow, mindful anterior and posterior pelvic tilt. As you traverse the arc of movement, notice when you pass through the balance point where your weight is equally distributed in the foot triangles.

- Gradually, narrow the range of movement until you oscillate around the balance point.

- Rest in the balance point.

    - *Is neutral pelvic position familiar to you?*
    - *How do you habitually carry your wholeness?*
    - *Do you let it shine into the world, suppress it, or...?*

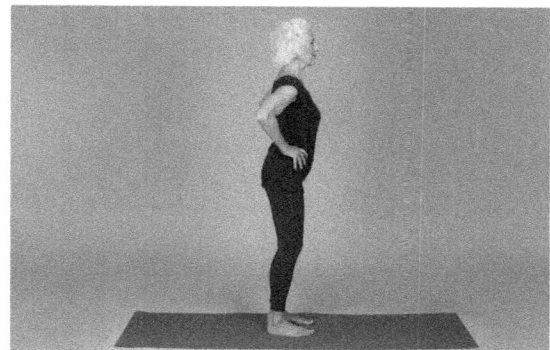

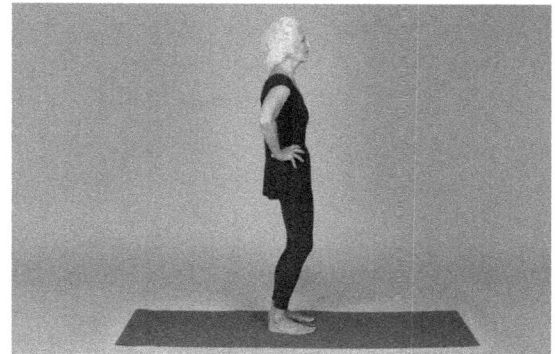

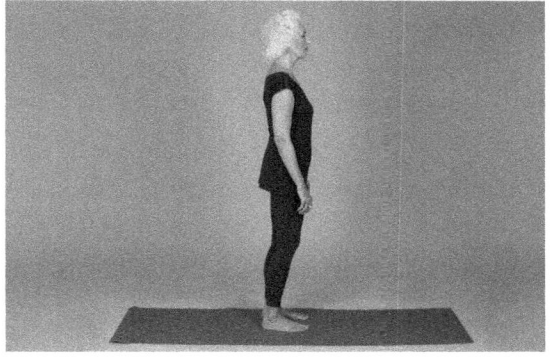

### Warrior I Pose (Virabhadrasana I)

The three planes of pelvic movement can be explored within any standing pose to free restricted joints, clarify lines of force, or maximize balance and integrity. Initially omitting arm involvement allows you to focus on lower body sensations.

### Learning Objectives

- Explore three planes of pelvic movement in a standing yoga pose.

- Experience initiating pelvic movement from the Harasphere.

### Instructions

- Begin standing comfortably with feet hip width apart.

- Step your right foot backward a comfortable distance and turn it out slightly. A shorter stance puts less load on the sacroiliac joints. Anchor your right **Foot Triangle** into the floor as you bend your left knee to align above the left ankle. Place your hands on your hips and orient your body frontally.

- Explore the pelvic movements one by one (flexion and extension, side bend, twist), initiating from the **Harasphere**. Visualize your Harasphere rolling in each plane to initiate small, easy movements. Repeat each movement slowly several times so you can sense changes in weight distribution in your foot triangles.

    – *Which pelvic position equalizes weight between the front and back foot, gives you maximum balance and stability, establishes a neutral lumbar curve?*

- Once you determine the pelvic position that provides the most stable foundation, move in and out of the pose several times, maintaining that optimal pelvic position.

- Finally, settle into the pose and raise your arms overhead, palms facing inward. Stay in the pose for three breaths, adjusting your pelvic position, as necessary, to reaffirm stability.

- To exit the pose, step forward with your right foot.

- Repeat the exploration on the other side.

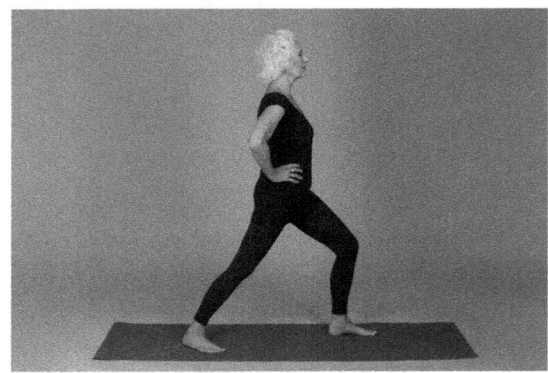

– *What's different when you move from the Harasphere?*
– *Can you feel more core engagement?*
– *Could this awareness help you stay more centered in other movements or daily activities?*

### Walking from the Pelvis

> When I move from my pelvis, my knee pain goes away.
>
> *Sierra*

Evolutionary changes resulted in a human pelvis that traces a three-dimensional figure 8 in space around the center of gravity during walking. This helical movement is necessary for efficient, springy, and graceful walking. Pelvic movement in each plane creates a ripple of movement through the spine and a shift in force transfer through the legs. When one or more of these movements is dysfunctional or absent, imbalanced distribution of ground reaction force can influence structural changes, eventually leading to discomfort and compensatory movement habits.

In this walking exploration, as you initiate movement from the pelvis and exaggerate each movement, you may look a little silly! It can be helpful to play some sexy music (Sade's "Lovers Rock" works well) and slow your walk to a meditative rhythm.

### Learning Objectives

- Isolate pelvic movement in each plane during walking.

- Repattern pelvic movements in walking.

### Instructions

- Take a baseline while walking. Notice the amount of anterior and posterior tilt, side bend, and twist in your pelvis as you walk in your usual way.

- Focus on individual pelvic movements for at least one minute each.

### Side Bend

- During the stance phase of walking (standing on one leg) the pelvis side bends, moving inferiorly on the standing leg. As you walk, track the alternating, rhythmical side bend of your pelvis each time you stand on one leg. Then, exaggerate the movement.

### Twist

- During the swing phase of walking, as one leg swings forward, the same side pelvis follows while the opposite side moves backward. Each time your leg moves

forward, track the alternating, rhythmical twisting movements of the pelvis. Then, exaggerate the pelvic twist and counterrotation of the torso. This version is reminiscent of a model on a fashion runway.

### Anterior and Posterior Tilt

- As you walk, the pelvic halves move in opposite directions. As the right leg swings forward and the heel strikes the ground, the right pelvic half tilts posteriorly. Almost simultaneously, the left pelvic half anteriorly tilts as the left foot pushes off the ground. Since these actions happen in concert, it's less confusing to focus on anterior and posterior tilt separately, or to track both movements on one half of the pelvis at a time.

### Figure 8

- Walk while visualizing a figure 8, tracing multidimensionally in space around your center of gravity. Lightly hold a mental image of the helical movement of the three-dimensional figure 8 resulting from the combination of pelvic movements in three planes. Visualize it curving and diving through and across the planes.

I was walking on a hard-packed beach, and every jarring step exacerbated my chronic back pain. Suddenly, I remembered the three pelvic movements and focused on exaggerating side bending. Immediately, the pain disappeared, and I realized I had been bracing against each heel impact.

*Janet*

- *Which pelvic movements are most obvious in your gait pattern?*

- *Which are lacking?*

- *Which movement creates more ease in walking?*

- *How did walking change as you focused on each pelvic movement?*

- *Was it helpful to initiate movement from a specific pelvic bone?*

## Pelvic Integrity in Movement

The pelvis is designed to move freely through space in three planes in relationship with the spine and hip joints. In gross movement, pelvic and sacral movement usually move together. However, the anatomical structure of the sacroiliac joints permits a few degrees only of intrinsic movement of the sacrum in relation to the pelvis. *Nutation* (from the Latin for *nodding*) describes this minimal forward movement naturally occurring in the sacrum in weight-bearing positions, like standing, or whenever joint loading is anticipated (Willard *et al.*, 2012).

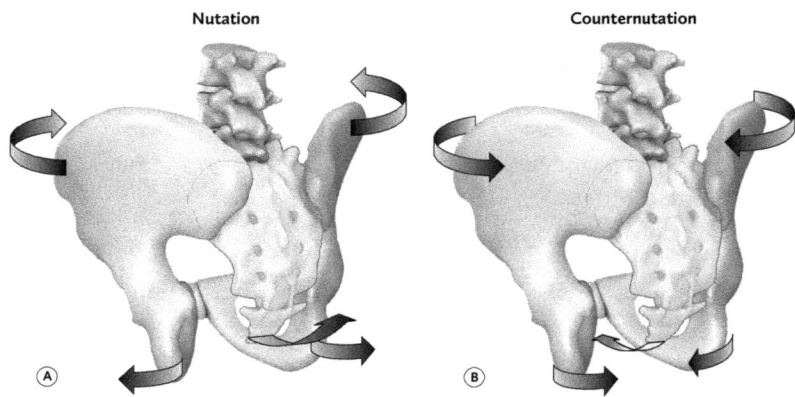

Nutation                                    Counternutation

Ⓐ                                            Ⓑ

The pelvis is more stable when the sacrum is nutated. In supine and seated positions, or when slouching in standing, the sacrum tends to counternutate, or tip backward, which destabilizes the lumbopelvic junction. The sacroiliac joints are diagonally oriented off the sagittal plane, so as the sacrum nods forward in nutation, it wedges the two ilia apart posteriorly, widening the sitting bones while narrowing the ilia anteriorly. Simultaneously, the coccyx is lifted. The ilia do not tip forward in tandem with the sacrum; nutation is a movement of the sacrum within the pelvis. These combined movements of nutation stabilize the pelvis, lumbar vertebrae, and pillars of the legs by engaging core muscles, tensioning sacroiliac ligaments, and increasing compressive forces at the sacroiliac joints (Vleeming *et al.*, 2012). This creates a strong yet resilient foundation. During nutation, multifidis, transversus abdominus, and the anterior pelvic floor activate to stabilize the core body.

The effects of nutation and counternutation also sequence into the spine and legs. As the sacrum nutates, it carries the lumbar spine into subtle extension, without anteriorly tilting the pelvis. Simultaneous nutation movement of the ilia rotates the femurs slightly medially, creating a more stable stance through the hip joint, pelvis, and spine.

Nutation is a subtle micro-movement of the

sacrum. Although usually an automatic, unconscious movement, we can intentionally visualize the sacrum and pelvic bones moving in nutation, and consciously activate associated muscles to encourage pelvic integrity. These intentional acts can alleviate pain and promote safe movement.

For example, students find that in backbends, conscious nutation creates a sense of space and length in the lumbar spine and inhibits unnecessary external rotation of the legs. In forward bends conscious nutation also creates a sense of length in the spine and discourages excessive spinal flexion.

## EXPLORATION: CONSCIOUS NUTATION

When the legs are positioned side by side in standing, simultaneously flexing the hips, knees, and ankles automatically nutates the sacrum. You can enhance the benefits of nutation by visualizing the movements of ischial tuberosities, ilia, and sacrum, or by consciously activating the muscles involved in those movements.

### Learning Objectives

- Differentiate movement of the sacrum in relation to the pelvis from coupled pelvic and sacral movement.

- Discern individual movements of ischial tuberosities, ilia, and sacrum during nutation.

- Explore deliberate initiation of movement from individual pelvic structures.

### Practice Notes

- As you visualize and track movement of the sacrum and pelvic bones, remember that nutation is not a pelvic movement; it's a movement of the sacrum within the pelvis.

- Restrain any tendency to tip your whole pelvis forward; maintain neutral pelvic position as you bend your legs.

- Although movement of the sitting bones is usually more accessible, it's worth tuning into other pelvic bones to deepen awareness.

- This is a very subtle practice. If you don't yet sense individual bone movements of nutation, you can still imagine them!

### Instructions

- Stand with your feet wider than hips and slightly externally rotated.

- Touch both sitting bones lightly with your fingers to highlight them for your nervous system. Slowly, alternate bending and straightening your legs, tracking your knees over your feet. As the legs bend, maintain a neutral pelvic position.

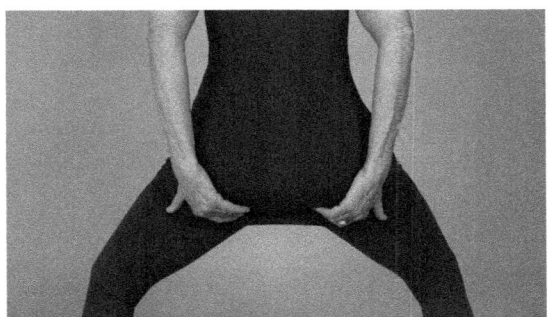

- *Can you detect the ischial tuberosities moving apart as your knees bend, and moving together as your legs straighten?*
- *How does the shape of your pelvic floor change?*
- *Can you sense the anterior pelvic floor condensing?*
- *Can you consciously activate the anterior pelvic floor to support nutation?*

- Continue bending and straightening your legs. Instead of tracking the sitting bones, now actively initiate movement from them.

Deliberately move them apart to initiate knee bending, then move them together to straighten the legs.

- *When you initiate movement from the sitting bones, how does the quality of movement change?*

• Reach behind and place your middle finger vertically on the coccyx. Continue alternately bending and straightening your legs while feeling the subtle sensation of the coccyx pressing into your finger during nutation.

• Shift to initiating movement from the coccyx (or imagining movement), lifting it—as though you have an actual tail—to initiate bending the knees, then lowering it to straighten the legs. The pelvis remains in neutral position.

- *Can you sense the deep paraspinal multifidis muscle activating beneath your fingers as you lift your tail?*
- *Can you consciously activate multifidis to support nutation?*
- *Can you move the coccyx without the pelvis tipping forward?*

• Curl your fingers around the medial edges of the iliac crests superior to the ASIS, fingertips touching abdominal soft tissue. Continue alternately bending and straightening your legs while feeling for movement of the ilia beneath your fingers.

• Shift to actively narrowing the ilia, intending to move them medially as your legs bend, and apart as legs straighten.

- *Can you feel transversus abdominus activate beneath your fingers as you narrow the ilia?*
- *Can you consciously activate transversus abdominus to support nutation?*

• Return upright.

- *Which pelvic bones are most accessible to you?*

• Now take this awareness into yoga poses. Try forward bends, backbends, and other standing poses with a view to discovering what degree of conscious, sacral nutation gives you the most stability and ease in your pelvis, spine, and legs.

## EXPLORATION: RECLINED BIG TOE POSE (SUPTA PADAGUSTASANA)

Awareness of connections between the pelvis and **Foot Triangles** can help balance pelvic and leg myofascia, refine motor control, and hone more efficient movement patterns.

### Learning Objectives

• Establish a mental connection between the pelvis and foot triangles.

• Mobilize the hips while maintaining pelvic integrity.

### Props

• A yoga belt

### Practice Notes

• Deepen felt sense by mentally tracing pathways of force between each pelvic bone and corresponding foot triangle point.

• Visualize "streaming" force from the pelvis to the feet.

• Repeat each variation several times.

- After completing several movements with the leg extended toward the ceiling, experiment with straightening the leg at different angles. If you lose the clear connection between a pelvic bone and foot triangle point, back off to a more accessible angle.

## Instructions

- Lie in supine. Loop the belt around the ball of your right foot, then extend the leg toward the ceiling. Holding the belt in your left hand, place the fingers of your right hand on the right pubic bone as a tactile cue. Alternatively, you can hold the belt with both hands.

- On inhalations, visualize your Harasphere expanding multidirectionally, as in the **Hara Breath**. Simultaneously, slightly bend your right knee.

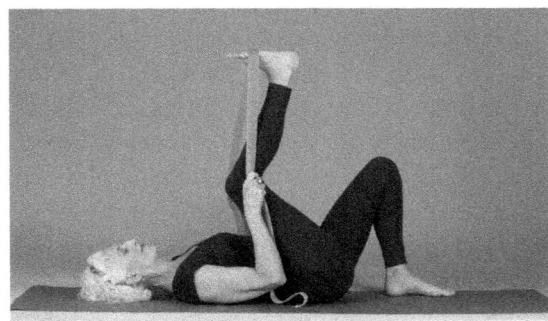

- On exhalations, visualize your breath streaming from the Harasphere, through the pubic bone, and down the volume of the inner leg to your big toe. When the force reaches your foot, press your big toe ball joint into the resistance of the belt, straightening your leg. Mentally trace your breath and the line of force from pubic bone to big toe point.

- As you inhale again, allow your knee to soften and slightly bend as you mentally trace the pathway back to the pelvis.

- Move your right hand onto the right iliac crest. On inhalations, expand your Harasphere while slightly bending your right knee. On exhalations, imagine streaming your breath from the Harasphere, through the iliac crest, and down the volume of the lateral leg to your little toe. When the force reaches your foot, press the little toe ball joint into the belt, straightening your leg. Mentally trace your breath and the line of force from the ilium to little toe, sensing the connection between them.

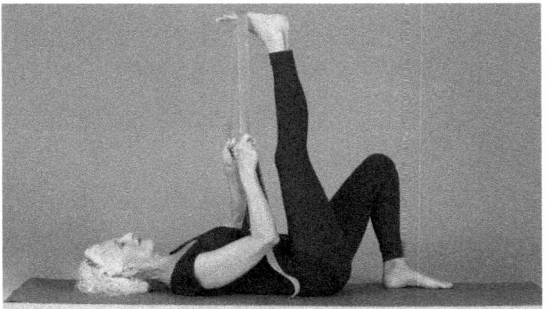

- As you inhale again, allow your knee to soften and slightly bend as you trace the pathway back to the pelvis.

- Move the belt onto your right heel. Touch your right sitting bone with your right fingers. On inhalations expand your Harasphere while slightly bending your right knee. On exhalations, imagine streaming your breath from the Harasphere, into the sitting bone, and down the volume of the posterior leg to the heel. When the force reaches your foot, press the heel into the belt, straightening your leg. Mentally trace the line of force from the sitting bone to the heel, sensing the connection between them.

- As you inhale again, allow your knee to soften and slightly bend as you trace the pathway back to the pelvis.

- Move the belt to the arch of your right foot, holding the ends in each hand. On inhalations, expand the Harasphere while slight y bending your right knee. On exhalations, imagine streaming your breath from the Harasphere through all three pelvic bones and down the volume of your leg to the foot. When the force reaches your foot, activate all three foot triangle points and press your arch into the belt, straightening your leg. Try to equalize transmission of force between each pelvic bone and corresponding foot triangle point, sensing connections between the whole leg and foot.

- As you inhale again, allow your knee to

soften and slightly bend as you trace the pathway back to the pelvis.

- Remove the belt, pause in supine, and notice any effects.

  - *What's different between the two legs?*

- Repeat this exploration with the belt on the left foot.

- Pause to register changes in sensation, then stand and walk around.

  - *What feels different?*
  - *Do your pelvis and feet feel more connected?*

## THERAPEUTIC APPLICATIONS

As the hub of the wheel, the state of the pelvis influences visceral physiology and health, stability, and mobility of both upper and lower body structures  The pelvis, spine, arms, legs, and head are functionally interrelated through myofascial continuities, and the spine and pelvis operate as an integrated, interdependent unit (Vleeming *et al.*, 2012). Pelvic position in standing, sitting, and movement influences spinal position and the efficient (or inefficient) transmission of weight from above and force from below.

A vicious cycle of pain and dysfunction can perpetuate when pelvic integrity is compromised through injury, overuse, or maladaptive alignment and movement patterns, especially when pelvic tissues become sensitized. Without a stable, resilient, and well-organized pelvis, the spine is less robust, load transfer is inefficient, and whole-body movement becomes effortful and uncoordinated. This may contribute to dysfunction and pain within the pelvis itself *and* in distal structures, especially when other koshic factors are present, such as high stress levels or trauma history.

Dysfunction can manifest in pathologies

including pelvic floor complaints, sacroiliac joint dysfunction and ligamentous changes, arthritis, piriformis syndrome, and labral tears. Imbalanced load and force transfer within and distal to the pelvis can compromise dynamic stability and undermine skeletal, myofascial, and neurovascular health distally in both upper and lower limbs. For example, arthritic changes may develop as hip joint spaces narrow from imbalanced pelvic tension and compression forces, or a previously sprained ankle may predispose to successive sprains. Even upper limb pathologies can develop when lack of pelvic integrity impacts the fascially connected shoulder girdle and causes excessive tension or compression in joints and on neurovascular and myofascial structures.

Lack of pelvic integrity can also affect physiology of pelvic viscera. The reproductive, urinary, and digestive organ systems may be subjected to detrimental weight-bearing imbalances and asymmetrical tension and compression forces within the pelvis (Schamberger 2002). Cardiovascular and lymphatic circulation may also be compromised.

As a therapist cognizant of multidimensional influences of the pelvis, addressing pelvic integrity is a primary consideration in my therapeutic plan for most clients, regardless of whether they present with pelvic or back pain or conditions affecting distal structures. Although it makes intuitive sense that pelvic misalignment contributes to low back pain and other spinal pathologies because of the functional interrelationship between spine and pelvis, research is inconclusive. Although pelvic misalignment has been associated with chronic low back pain (Yu *et al.*, 2020) and lumbopelvic pain and pelvic floor dysfunction have been highly correlated (Dufour *et al.*, 2018), it's more likely that lack of pelvic integrity is one of many factors contributing to back pain. Viewing pelvic dysfunction from the koshic perspective, factors including stressful life events, relationship challenges, and personal beliefs may be as relevant as pelvic misalignment or movement dysfunction. Significant reductions in pelvic pain and dysfunction have been seen when people alter their beliefs and develop higher self-efficacy and trust in the strength and capacity of their bodies (Beales *et al.*, 2020).

Clinically, I have found that EA practices that reestablish pelvic integrity and balance associated myofascial structures can reliably decrease pain and restore optimal structural and physiological function globally. The fluid stability resulting from pelvic integrity allows appropriate shock absorption and efficient load transfer, and promotes power and grace in movement. Pelvic and abdominal organs benefit from having adequate support and space to function. Ultimately, dynamic integrity of the physical pelvis provides the foundation for steadiness of mind and emotions. We feel more centered in ourselves and respond to the world with steadfastness. As the container of our wholeness, developing felt sense of the pelvis and initiating movement from it can help us establish the steadiness to proclaim, *This is me, and this is how I stand in the world.*

## KOSHIC CONTEMPLATIONS

### Annamaya Kosha

- *What is your habitual pelvic position?*
- *Have you made any connections between your pelvic position and overall alignment?*
- *Has felt sense of ease and stability in your pelvis, or other structures, changed after doing practices in this chapter?*
- *Has developing felt sense of your pelvis affected your alignment, movement, or tension and pain patterns?*
- *How have you incorporated pelvic awareness into your movement practice and daily activities?*

### Pranamaya Kosha

- *Have you discovered a relationship between your habitual pelvic position and breath?*
- *Has your energy level changed as you establish greater pelvic integrity?*
- *Have you noticed any changes in physiological functions like digestion, urination, or menstruation?*

### Manomaya Kosha

- *How accessible is felt sense of your pelvis?*
- *Have you experienced changes in emotional stability as you establish greater pelvic integrity?*
- *Has your mind settled?*

## Vijnanamaya Kosha

- *How does your habitual pelvic position reflect or influence your psychological stance and the way you interact with the world?*
- *Have you noticed any changes as you establish greater pelvic integrity?*

## Anandamaya Kosha

- *Has working with the Harasphere influenced the way you connect with your inherent wholeness?*
- *Do you feel more seated in your authentic Self?*

## KEY CONCEPTS

- Evolution of the pelvis enabled us to leave the sea to walk and eventually stand erect on land.
- As the foundation for the spine and upper body, the pelvis is key to upright aligned posture, efficient force transmission, and locomotion.
- The pelvis is a movable yet stable structure, constantly shifting and responding to weight and load influences from above and below.
- The pelvis contains the Hara, our energetic center.
- The enteric brain, the seat of gut feelings and primal emotions, is contained in the pelvis.
- Pelvic position and mobility can mirror psychology and conditioning, predisposing us to distinctive ways of perceiving, feeling, and expressing.
- The pelvis can be viewed as the container of our wholeness.
- The three paired pelvic bones are separate cartilaginous structures at birth.
- The pelvic reset is an osteopathic self-help technique using rhythmical isometric activation to stabilize the pelvis.
- Movement potential of the pelvis can be repatterned.
- Conscious nutation stabilizes the pelvis, lumbar vertebrae, and legs.
- Pelvic integrity can provide a foundation for steadiness of mind and emotions.

# The Cosmic Spine

*I've got your back.*
*He's spineless.*
*She has real backbone.*
*Get off my back.*

The flexible, curvaceous spine is the skeleton's central connecting structure. Our head, rib basket, and pelvis balance in gravity by virtue of spinal curves and different shapes and sizes of vertebrae and discs. The respiratory, circulatory, nervous, gastrointestinal, and endocrine systems orient around the midline spine and are affected by its shape and health. Our embryological development reflects the spine's importance; it's the first part of the skeleton to form. The notochord, a flexible longitudinal rod materializing at day 16, is the primary central axis around which we organize ourselves. As adults, we can consciously embody the spine as a central axis to optimize alignment and movement.

From an evolutionary perspective, the spine is the skeletal element we share with early fishy vertebrates. The lateral undulation of ancient fish is echoed in the human spine's ability to side bend. As we emerged from the sea to live on land and navigate variable terrain, vertebrate spines eventually evolved the capacity to move in all three planes. Each individual vertebra is capable of minimal amounts of multiplanar movement, yet collective action of all 24 vertebrae is considerable and allows us to perform intricate, complex movements. According to nuclear physicist Gracevotsky's spinal engine model, the spine generates locomotion, and limbs transfer forces between the body and ground. "Locomotion was first achieved by the motion of the spine. The legs came after as an improvement, not as a substitute" (Gracovetsky 2012). Embodying the spine as the engine for movement can significantly alter the way we move.

Our curvy, bony midline provides verticality and structural integrity for support and stabilization of the body yet allows considerable motion. Contrary to popular narrative, the spine is not a column. Rather, it could be viewed as a tensegrity truss tower that integrates with limbs, head, tail, and visceral system (Levin 2002). As a triangulated system a truss tower transfers and manages tension and compression forces. Vertebrae can be viewed as bony spacers (compression elements) woven together by fascia and maintained in erectness by a tensional network (tension elements). Appropriate tension in the fascial matrix maintains the spaces between the vertebrae, and loading anywhere is distributed throughout the spinal truss as tension or compression.

Spinal curves, intervertebral discs, and elasticity of spinal fascia absorb the impact of movement and distribute forces throughout the spine and surrounding structures, lessening the burden on individual parts. This shock absorbing function protects the delicate brain, spinal cord, and organs. When consciously experienced on a more subtle level, it can strengthen our capacity to absorb and integrate life's emotional shocks.

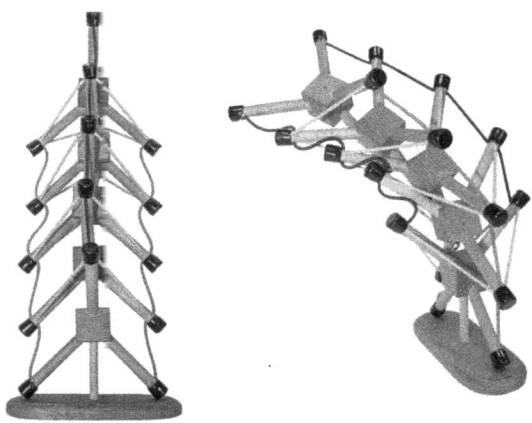

Viewed as a tensegrity truss model, the spine's triangulated structure confers intrinsic stability in any gravitational orientation. Numerous fascial "guywires" applying multidirectional tension stabilize the tower or spinal axis. Further stability is provided by ligaments, aligning, guiding, and limiting movement at over 100 spinal joints. Even vertebral structure contributes to stability. Vertebrae are progressively larger and heavier from top to bottom, forming a long, narrow pyramid to accommodate accumulated body weight.

The spine is designed to move fluidly, dynamically adjusting between dual roles of support and movement. The spine's most mobile areas (cervical and lumbar) are least stable, while the more stable thoracic spine has relatively limited mobility. The shape and orientation of spinous processes, facet joints, and rib connections in the thoracic spine limit movement. Understanding this, we can honor spinal anatomy and avoid forcing mobility in areas structurally designed for stability. Mobile areas, especially transitional vertebrae between zones of relative mobility and stability, require support and strength from surrounding myofascia. Transitional areas—C7–T1, T12–L1, and L5–S1—are more susceptible to overuse, injury, hypermobility, and arthritic changes. Ultimately, a healthy spine has integrity and a functional balance between mobility and stability, and is adaptive and resilient.

> Imagining your spine as central... enables you to have a sense of mobile solidity in your central core as well as to sense volume going into your back space.
>
> *Peggy Hackney (2002)*

Cultivating felt sense of the spine as midline can center us on more subtle energetic, emotional, and mental levels and offers a metaphorical orientation to self. We refer to ourselves by touching the midline of our chest. Without this internal spinal support, we may have compromised ability to self-support, and some of us could be described as "spineless." When we embody and move from the spine, movement is stronger, more integrated, energy efficient, and graceful. As we build connection with our central axis, we may experience a profound sense of moving from our essential Self, easily expressing courage, dignity, and strength of character.

## KOSHIC PERSPECTIVES

In annamaya kosha, we focus on learning about and cultivating felt sense of the spine as the central core, or three-dimensional axis around which movement occurs. From this physical perspective, we explore the spine as an interwoven chain of bones embedded within the fascial matrix, capable of mobility, support, and force transmission. Rather than imposing "correct" or static alignment, we investigate how to balance spinal curves and harness movement potential to discover fluid yet supported verticality. We practice spinal initiation to move with strength and integration. Exploring the spine's physical attributes can reveal new ways of moving that can decrease pain and generate steadiness and ease.

In pranamaya kosha, the spine is viewed as a supersonic core of subtle pranic energies. In the yogic tradition, three intertwining subtle energy channels, or nadis, form the vertical nucleus connecting us to universal energies. *Ida* (lunar, cooling, feminine) and *pingala* (solar, heating, masculine) nadis crisscross the central *sushumna*. Ida and pingala have been compared anatomically to the bilateral autonomic nerve trunks, and functionally to the sympathetic (pingala) and parasympathetic (ida) nervous systems, while shushumna has been correlated with the spinal cord (Khedikar, Erande, and Shukla 2016). Breath and subtle yogic practices can be viewed as ancient methods of up- or downregulating the autonomic nervous system. Subtle energy centers, called chakras, are located at intersections of the nadis, and have been associated anatomically with specific nerve plexi and endocrine glands. The yogic tradition assigns great importance to these main conduits of prana. Many practices are designed to free energy flow through nadis to enhance physical and mental health.

Spinal shape and freedom of movement affects breath and other physiological processes. Chiropractors have mapped associations between spinal nerves and organs and many address specific vertebral segments to treat organ dysfunction. When the spine is "shrink-wrapped" by excessive myofascial tension, rib expansion and fluid spinal movement are limited, the respiratory diaphragm cannot freely descend, and organs and neurovascular structures may be compressed. Consciously moving the spine multidirectionally circulates prana and encourages full breathing, nourishing the spine and organs with both breath and prana.

From the psychological viewpoint of manomaya kosha, the back body represents the unconscious, including unprocessed emotional experience. The spine's shape can reflect this deep-seated emotional patterning and belief systems. For example, one student realized her scoliosis was related to a tendency to "twist" herself around difficult emotions instead of dealing with them directly. She found new emotional courage after discovering that EA practices to balance her spine also unblocked buried emotions to be processed and integrated. In his book *Healing Back Pain*, John Sarno popularized the idea that chronic back pain has a significant emotional component (Sarno 1991). His theory is supported by pain research highlighting associations between back pain and stress, depression, and anxiety (Stubbs *et al.*, 2016). Yogic wisdom has long recognized this intimate body-mind connection.

> When I learned how spines are designed to move with breath, my breath immediately deepened.
>
> *Anne*

In manomaya kosha, we refine sensory awareness by distinguishing sensations of familiar, sometimes maladaptive patterns of spinal alignment, movement, and force transmission from sensory signatures of more functional patterns learned through EA explorations.

Awareness of the spine as a central, resilient, moving structure can catalyze deeper connection with the true Self. Vijnanamaya kosha invites awareness of the spine as a reliable inner support connecting us to our deeper wisdom. As we turn awareness inward, long-standing habits of living a more externally focused life may dissipate. The current epidemic of forward head posture deactivates spinal support and disconnects us from our center, forcing superficial musculature to work overtime to keep us erect—and even encouraging more superficial presence in the world!

Metaphorically, the spine represents courage, resolution, and inner strength. A well-organized and resilient spine can help us embody these qualities. Some people have stiff spines, which may reflect difficulty responding flexibly to life challenges. Others may timidly curve their spines in unconscious attempts to protect tender or fearful hearts. EA practices can help access felt sense of backbone that both supports and helps us respond resiliently to life's complications. We use discerning buddhi mind to understand the uniqueness of our own spine and the ways alignment and movement habits influence our perception and engagement with the world. We can set an intention to explore the spine as an inner resource to remain centered in our essential Self as we interact with the outer world, knowing "*I have my own back.*" During this process, EA practices may prompt content from the unconscious mind to surface in dreams or process work.

Anatomically considered the axis of our physical body the yogic tradition views the spine as the cosmic axis where spirit and matter unite. Like the tree of life, we are rooted in earth and the material world yet simultaneously connected to the Divine. In anandamaya kosha we explore the spine as the conduit for subtle cosmic and earth energies, and consciously connect to this cosmic axis. When the spine is integrated into daily awareness, we can gain a deeper sense of integration on all koshic levels and experience an expanded sense of wholeness. Through EA practices, the spine can become a touchstone for accessing the peace, stillness, and wisdom of our true Self, united with heaven and earth. We start with the physical and ultimately attain the spiritual.

> For a long time now, the universe has been germinating in your spine.
>
> *Hafiz (Ladinski 1999, p. 135)*

## LEARN IT

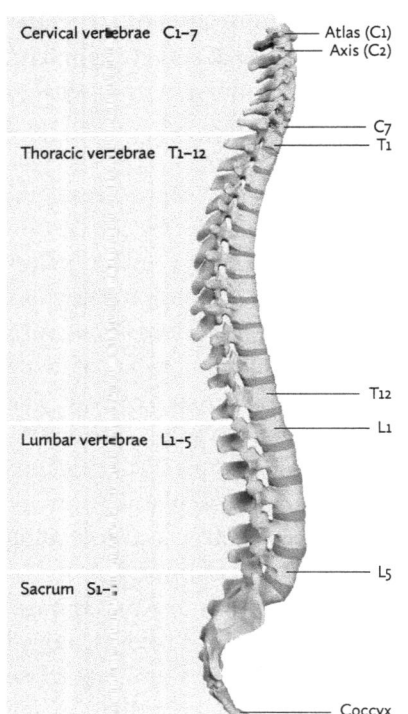

Cervical vertebrae  C1–7

Atlas (C1)
Axis (C2)

C7
T1

Thoracic vertebrae  T1–12

T12
L1

Lumbar vertebrae  L1–5

L5

Sacrum  S1–5

Coccyx

The human spine eventually evolved into an architectural marvel with each anatomical component contributing to coordinated, energy-efficient function. Bones embedded within a tensional fascial network provide supportive and compressive forces. Ligaments knit vertebrae together, providing further skeletal support. Myofascia generates and transfers force to move bones, facilitated by tendons interweaving bones and vertebrae. These components collectively enable spinal stability, three-dimensional mobility, clear force transmission, and elastic resistance to both compression and excessive degrees of movement.

### Vertebrae

Twenty-four spinal vertebrae are embedded in the tensional truss network, forming an articulating chain of three zones with seven cervical, twelve thoracic, and five lumbar vertebrae. Each zone has different movement, weight-bearing, and stability capabilities. Vertebrae in each zone have different shapes and features, yet most share the basic structure of a bony body (*centrum*) and a vertebral arch containing one spinous and two transverse processes. The triad of processes are connected to each other and centrum by pairs of lamina and pedicles forming the protective vertebral canal around the delicate spinal cord. A complex array of tendons and ligaments attach onto each process. Hard cortical bone encases spongy, porous bone marrow of vertebral bodies, an architecture that reflects their role as primary weight-bearing structures.

is always accompanied by a small degree of side bending, and vice versa. Spatial orientation of facet joints in each vertebral zone, and the shape and direction of spinous processes, determine the type and amount of available movement. Lumbar facets orient in the sagittal plane, favoring flexion and extension but limiting rotation. Thoracic facets orient in the coronal plane, permitting side bending and rotation but limiting flexion and extension. This relatively limited movement in the thoracic spine protects the vulnerable heart and lungs. Each thoracic vertebra articulates with its adjacent rib in three places on the vertebral body and transverse process. Cervical facets orient diagonally, allowing the neck to move freely in all three planes. Many movement possibilities!

Spinous process

Transverse process

Lamina

Pedicle

Body

Vertebral foramen

**Superior**

Superior articular process

Transverse process

Pedicle

Inferior articular process

Body

Lamina

Spinous process

**Lateral**

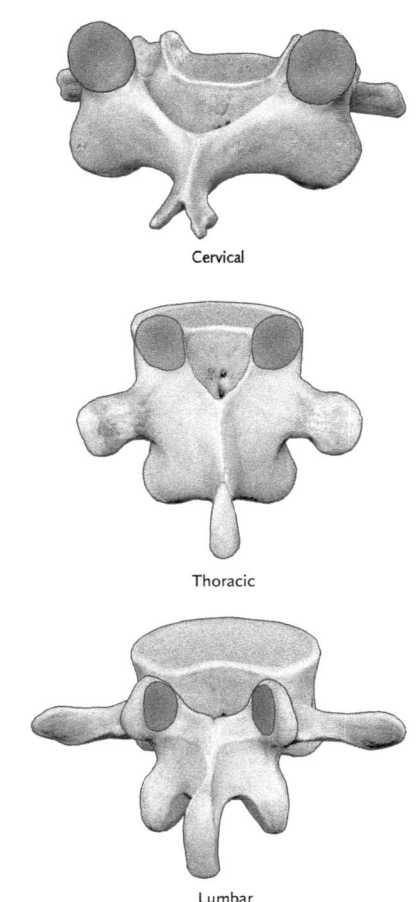

Cervical

Thoracic

Lumbar

Each vertebra contains two pairs of articular facets forming synovial joints with vertebrae above and below. The shape and orientation of facets causes coupled movement in the spine; rotation

## Intervertebral Discs

Spinal discs are remnants of the embryological notochord. They function as fibrocartilaginous "marshmallows" cushioning and separating vertebrae to prevent friction. The tough outer fibrous covering (*annulus fibrosus*) blends into surrounding ligaments and tendons and surrounds the soft, gel-like *nucleus pulposus*. Collagen fibers of the annulus are arranged in concentric layers to distribute compressive forces evenly throughout the disc. Pain neuroscience educators Butler and Moseley aptly describe disc function by renaming discs "living adaptable force transducers" (2003, p. 38). As malleable spacers between vertebrae (except C1 and C2), discs absorb shock and redistribute compression forces in and around intervertebral joints. The springy, resilient design helps maintain spinal curves and promote multidirectional spinal movement. Their relative softness, fluidity (66–88 percent water composition) and size (25 percent of spinal length) add significant movement possibilities to the comparatively rigid bony spine without compromising spinal strength.

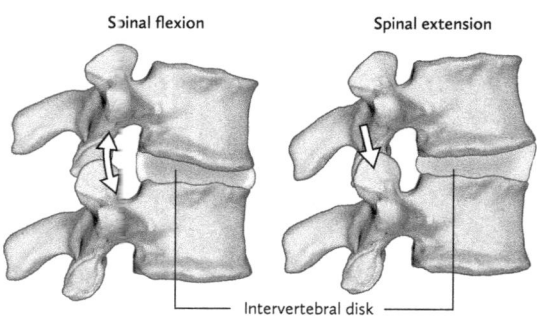

Spinal flexion          Spinal extension

Intervertebral disk

Discs are avascular. Lacking blood supply, the fluid content replenishes through a process of *imbibition*, absorbing fluid through osmosis. Both rest and spinal movement, particularly rhythmical motion, encourage imbibition—a good argument for daily therapeutic practice. We are taller each morning after discs imbibe fluid during rest. Chronic compression of discs lessens hydration and elasticity and can eventually contribute to degeneration, prolapse, or rupture.

Cervical and lumbar discs are thicker anteriorly, which helps to maintain spinal curves. Greater movement potential is available in these two zones, where the ratio of disc to vertebrae is larger. Strong anterior and posterior longitudinal ligaments extending the entire length of the spine stabilize the discs.

## Fascia

Vertical erectness of the spine is maintained partially through a complex, multilayered, overlapping arrangement of myofascial elements weaving into vertebral bodies and posterior arches. Some vertebrae contain over 30 muscular attachments. Four layers of myofascia and the thoracolumbar fascia support, move, and transfer forces to and from the limbs and ground. The myofascial layers are entwined, creating one continuous fabric as part of the body-wide fascial network. Layers differ in function yet collectively stabilize the spine, maintain space between vertebrae, and allow segmental movement. The deepest layers and thoracolumbar fascia are richly innervated with sensory nerve endings providing proprioceptive information necessary for refined motor control. The superficial myofascial layer produces larger spinal movements, and in-between layers function primarily as stabilizers and movers of individual joints. The deepest myofascial layer connects adjacent spinal segments while the larger, thicker superficial layer spans multiple segments. This overlapping myofascial arrangement allows collective sequential movement. When one vertebra moves, a corresponding wave of motion undulates through the whole spine. In the absence of excessive tension, misalignment, or injury, this wave action results in fluid, efficient movement.

From head to tail, vertebrae are knitted together and supported by ligaments providing tensional elements to the spinal truss system and stabilizing it by limiting and directing movement of individual vertebrae. Shorter ligaments link processes and facet joints to form a trusswork between vertebrae. The longer anterior longitudinal ligament interlaces anterior vertebral bodies, while the posterior longitudinal ligament and ligamentum flavum line the vertebral canal on posterior vertebral bodies. A layered, overlapping segmental design of fibers gives strength to the long ligaments and limits range of flexion and extension.

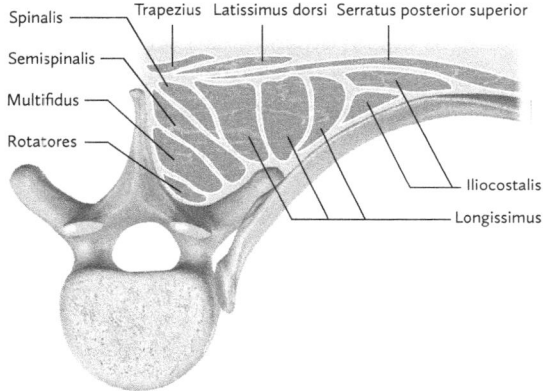

The large, diamond-shaped thoracolumbar fascia (TLF) integrates the spine, pelvis, and rib basket with the upper and lower limbs. It wraps around the posterior body, supporting the spine and transferring forces multidirectionally through the muscles continuous with its multiple fascial planes. It attaches to transverse processes and fascially separates paraspinal muscles from posterior abdominal wall muscles (the abdominals, psoas, and quadratus lumborum). Forces generated by trunk and extremity musculature can alter tension and stiffness of the TLF, influencing its ability to support the spine and pelvis (Vleeming and Willard 2010). Intriguing research suggests the thoracolumbar fascia, a major steward of force transmission through the pelvis, may play a role in generating back pain (Wilke *et al.*, 2017).

## Spinal Curves

In utero and at birth, the spine forms a C-shaped, primary kyphotic curve. The secondary, concave lordotic curves are gradually patterned in the nervous system through developmental movement. Cervical curves evolve as babies lift their heads to look at parents or orient to their environment. Lumbar curves form later as infants lie prone and kick their legs, then push away from the ground to sit, stand, and eventually walk. The convex, primary curve remains in the thoracic spine and sacrum in adulthood. Spiral curves are maintained through the tensegrity truss structure, neuromuscular patterning, and the shape of vertebral discs, which are thicker anteriorly in the cervical and lumbar zones and thicker posteriorly in the thoracic zone.

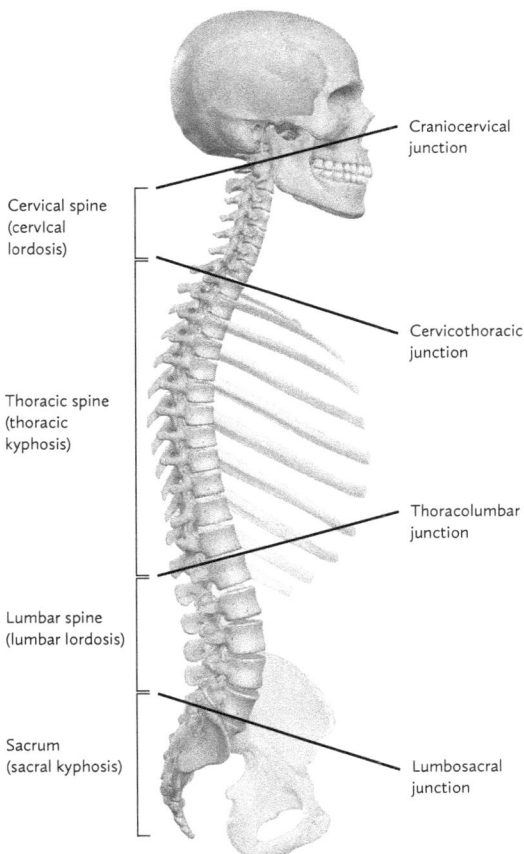

Spinal curves are interdependent. They balance each other, enabling us to stand upright with minimal effort. This balanced arrangement creates a resilient spring-like structure that absorbs shock and distributes weight and force. Imagine how difficult walking and moving would be without spinal curves. We would move robotically and our spines would easily damage with the constant vibration and shock of walking. Gracovetsky's spinal engine model refers to spinal curves as the primary mechanism for controlling force transmission through the body (2012). The undulating movement afforded by spinal curves also maintains spaciousness for the spinal cord and nerve roots and assists disc imbibition. Embodying this springiness can increase spaciousness between vertebrae in spine-lengthening movements. Imbalanced spinal curves can affect alignment and function of all major joints in the body and distort force transmission capacity throughout our structure. Someone who habitually tucks their tail and rounds the lumbar spine will have less ability to absorb and transfer the impact of heel strike during walking and may be more prone to low back pain. As Joseph Pilates reportedly inscribed on his business card: You're only as old as your spine is flexible.

The concept of *neutral spine* describes a state of balanced spinal curves that provide the most energy-efficient position for the body to remain upright in gravity and other extrinsic forces. (Richardson, Hodges, and Hides, 2004). Neutral spine and neutral pelvis are interconnected, each influencing and influenced by the other. In neutral spine, the head, rib basket, and pelvis are aligned in gravity, and joints and surrounding passive tissues are in elastic equilibrium with minimal joint loading (McGill 2007). Like finding neutral pelvis, finding neutral spine is a foundational principle that decreases stress on individual tissues and optimizes motor control, shock absorption, and force transmission. While learning this sensory skill, we can feel differences in weight-bearing, ease of movement, and stability in any gravitational orientation.

## FEEL IT

In these practices, you will use IA to develop felt sense of the size, volume, and central location of the spine. As you begin to sense individual structures through touch and movement, you can consciously organize and integrate fluid movement and stability.

## PARTNER EXPLORATION: DISCOVER YOUR SPINE

### Learning Objective

- Map anatomical features of the spine to deepen felt sense.

### Props

- A yoga bolster and two blankets

### Practice Notes

- Before beginning, establish consent and touch parameters. Communicate with each other during the practice about touch positioning, pressure, and quality of movement.

- While palpating, translate what you are feeling into your own body.

## Instructions

- Place the bolster lengthwise on the floor. Fold one blanket approximately 5 cm (2 in.) thick and 25 cm (10 in.) wide and place it across the middle of the bolster. Fold the other blanket several times and place it on the floor for head support.

- The receiving partner lies prone on the bolster, supported from the pubic bone to sternum. The abdomen is supported by one blanket, the forehead rests on the second blanket, and the arms rest in a comfortable position. Adjust the blankets for comfort. The helper partner sits facing the prone partner's side.

- Observe your partner's lumbar spine moving with breath, then follow any sequential movement into the head and sacrum.

  - *Where does the spine move freely?*
  - *Which vertebrae participate in the breath wave?*
  - *Where is the wave restricted?*
  - *Does breath sequence into the head and limbs?*

### Spinous Processes

- With a soft touch of your finger pads, trace the spinous processes from neck to sacrum. First, slowly stroke from top to bottom several times to get a general sense of different sizes and amount of space between processes.

- Carefully palpate individual spinous processes starting with C7, the most prominent cervical vertebra. Explore the topography of each process using your fingers to distinguish size, shape, and angular differences in the three zones and to contrast distances between processes.

  **Note:** In the cervical spine, spinous processes are shorter and smaller; in the thoracic spine they're longer, narrow, and downward pointing; and in the lumbar spine they're large, hatchet-shaped, and further apart. They may be challenging to access if paraspinal muscles are well developed.

- Form a pincer grasp with thumbs and index fingers and take firm hold of the C7 spinous process. Gently move it back and forth, exploring jiggling movements and slower, more deliberate rocking. Notice how moving one vertebra initiates collective action.

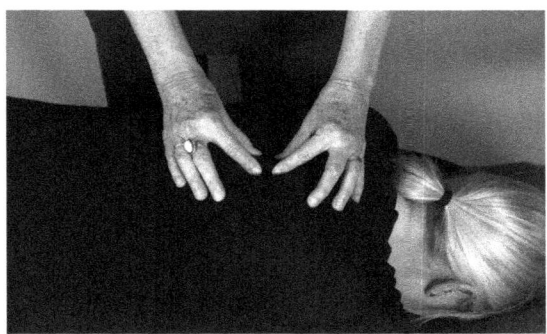

- Move to an upper thoracic spinous process and repeat the movements.

- Explore movement possibilities at intervals in the rest of the spine. Notice the degree of freedom or fixation at each segment.

### Transverse Processes

- Locate an upper thoracic spinous process and place the index- and middle-finger pads of both hands approximately 4 cm (1.5 in.) on either side. Gently, sink your fingers through the myofascia to feel the hard, bony transverse processes, moving your fingers lightly back and forth parallel to the spine to differentiate bone and soft tissue. Once you locate the processes (or think you have), tenderly press into one and feel the opposite side subtly rise into your fingers like a seesaw. Alternate pressure on right and left transverse processes, rocking them back and forth several times.

- Repeat this exploration at several transverse processes in the thoracic and lumbar zones. Notice the degree of freedom or fixation at each segment.

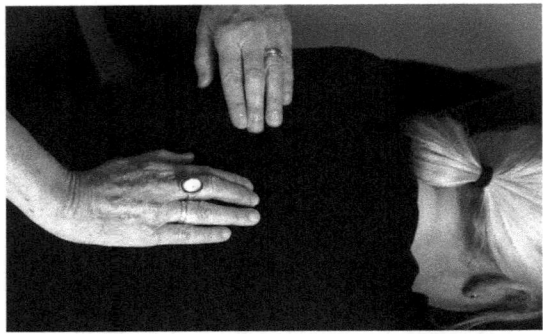

- Soothe the spine by stroking down both sides from top to bottom a few times.

- Once again, observe your partner's spine moving with breath.

  - *Are there changes in freedom of movement?*
  - *Is more of the spine participating in the breath wave now?*
  - *Does the breath wave sequence more clearly into the head, tail, and limbs?*

- The receiving partner moves to a sitting, then standing position to register effects of the practice.

  - *Has felt sense of your spine changed?*
  - *Is your breath different?*
  - *When you move, how is movement different?*

## EXPLORATION: SPINAL BREATHING 🔊

### Learning Objective

- Use breath and visualization to deepen felt sense of the spine, highlighting it for the nervous system.

### Practice Notes

- This exploration can be done seated or standing.

- Breathe a minute or two using each visualization, pausing after each to register sensations.

### Instructions

- To set the baseline, tune into the movement of your spine as you breathe. Remember the fascial connections between the diaphragm and spine.

  - *Where can you sense movement? Lack of movement?*

- Focus on your lumbar spine and notice any breath movement. After several breaths, shift focus, first to the thoracic spine, then to the cervical spine.

  - *Which zone moves the most as you breathe?*

- Visualize the discs sandwiched between vertebrae. Go into a slump, rounding your back and letting your head hang. Visualize the anterior discs compressing. As you inhale, imagine your breath inflating the discs with air, expanding three dimensionally to increase space between vertebrae. Take several breaths to return upright. Repeat several times.

- Focus your attention individually on each zone of the discs for several breaths. With your head erect, imagine the cervical discs inflating elastically and multidimensionally with inhalations, and softening with exhalations. Then, shift your attention to the thoracic and finally to the lumbar discs.

- *Can you sense your spine alternately lengthening and compressing?*
- *What differences do you notice between zones?*

- Now visualize the anterior and posterior longitudinal ligaments on the front and back surfaces of the vertebral bodies. As you inhale, imagine breath flowing up the anterior vertebral bodies from the inner sacrum to the skull, then flowing down the posterior vertebral bodies as you exhale. Create a circuit of breath.

  - *Does your spinal alignment shift as you breathe this way?*
  - *Where are your "blind spots"?*

- Shift your awareness to the subtle spine. As you inhale, imagine earth energy flowing from deep within the earth, up shushumna nadi in the midline to the heart area. Pause for a moment, then as you exhale, imagine this energy flowing out the top of your head into the cosmos like a geyser. For several breaths, imagine inhaling qualities of earth, like strength, stability, and nourishment.

- As you inhale, imagine cosmic energy flowing from the vastness of the universe into the crown of your head and down shushumna to the heart area. Pause for a moment. As you exhale, imagine cosmic energy flowing down your spine and draining into the earth. With each inhalation, imagine receiving qualities of cosmic energy, like pure consciousness, Divine light, and unconditional love.

- Combine these two energies in one breath. As you inhale, imagine earth energy flowing up and cosmic energy flowing down shushumna, meeting at the heart. As you pause, imagine the two energies comingling, then exhale the mixture down into the earth and up into the cosmos. Visualize these energies nourishing, cleansing, and healing you.

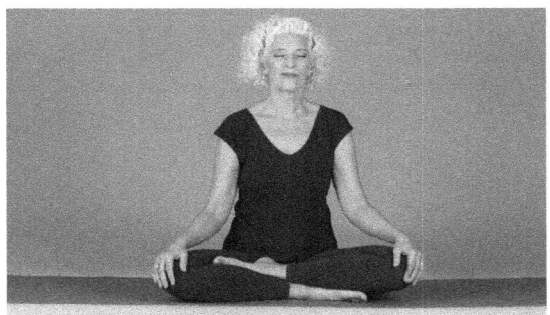

- Release the visualization and breath focus.

  - *Can you sense subtle realignment and lengthening as you visualize streaming these energies up and down your spine?*
  - *What do you notice after the practice?*

## EXPLORATION: SENSING STABILITY

The bodies of vertebrae forming the concave cervical and lumbar curves lie in the midline of the body. When you refine felt sense of your spine as a supportive yet mobile structure in your midline, unnecessary muscular effort can release.

### Learning Objective

- Explore felt sense of central spinal support.

### Instructions

- Set a baseline in standing and visualize the spine as your flexible, curvy axis.

- *What is your felt sense of the position of your spine?*

- Slowly, shift your weight forward and back several times, then pause when you sense maximum weight borne through the vertebral bodies and discs.

- Shift your weight backward until you feel your body weight borne more by the posterior vertebral arches.

- Slowly, shift forward until your body weight is borne slightly anterior to the vertebrae.

- Shift your weight backward again until you sense weight through the vertebral bodies, then the arches.

- Slowly, shift back and forth several times between these three positions, pausing momentarily as your weight is borne centrally through vertebral bodies. Notice changes in weight distribution in your **Foot Triangles** and how your myofascial body adapts and responds to keep you upright.

- Finally, rest in neutral.

  - *Where do you feel most stable, most ease?*
  - *Which position feels most familiar?*
  - *Has felt sense of the central position of your spine changed?*
  - *When you find spinal stability, does muscular tension change?*

> I always thought of my spine as something "back there," but once I sensed my spine in my middle, I felt it giving me inner support.
>
> *Pat*

## HEAL IT

### EXPLORATION: REPATTERNING INDIVIDUAL VERTEBRAL MOVEMENT 🎥

This practice encourages each vertebra to reclaim its ability to move in multiple planes and participate in collective wave-like force transmission. As the nervous system learns to precisely articulate and initiate movement from specific vertebrae, restrictions or "clumps" can be identified and disassembled. Paradoxically, improved vertebral articulation often generates experiences of increased spinal strength and stability. As motor control is refined, right effort emerges, and extraneous peripheral activation is consciously inhibited. Use of a soft foam ball cultivates sensory awareness and can relieve pain by calming the nervous system.

### Learning Objectives

- Initiate movement from individual vertebrae.

- Refine motor control of spinal segments.

### Props

- A 10 cm (4 in.), soft foam ball. A thick, soft kitchen sponge cut into a circle may be used instead

### Practice Notes

- Repeat each subtle movement several times at various vertebral levels. Remain at each level until the movement feels accessible.

- Use fingertip pressure on your sternum to guide vertebral movement. Imagine your fingers sinking into your torso to "steer" the vertebral body or transverse processes.

- Identify and inhibit unnecessary effort and muscular activation. The head, pelvis, shoulders, and feet often habitually preempt spinal movement.

- If you have back pain, do the movements above and below the painful area.

## Instructions

- Take a baseline reading in supine, noticing how your spine rests on the floor.

- Place the foam ball under your upper thoracic vertebrae.

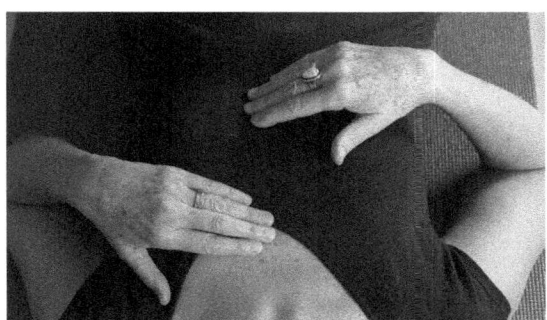

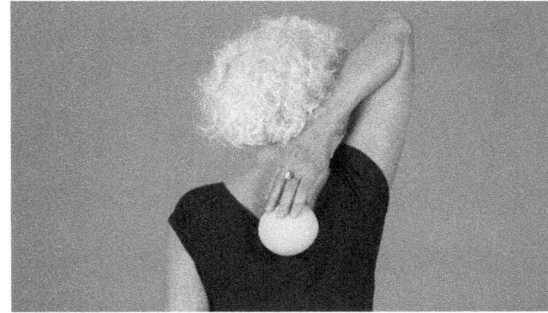

- Position your fingertips on the sternum superficial to the ball. Imagine one specific vertebra centered on the ball. For several breaths, direct inhalations into the vertebra as your body adjusts to the ball, then relax on exhalations.

### Directing Pressure

- For several exhalations, press into your sternum to guide a subtle posterior movement of the vertebrae that slightly flattens the ball. Release the pressure on inhalations.

### Flexion and Extension

- Imagine a tiny seesaw along your spine with the ball as fulcrum and the plank extending just beyond the top and bottom edges of the ball. Place your fingers vertically on the sternum superficial to each end of the imaginary plank.

- On inhalations, use finger pressure to guide the top of the seesaw posteriorly, compressing the upper half of the ball and subtly arching the spine. On exhalations, use finger pressure to guide the bottom of the seesaw posteriorly, compressing the bottom half of the ball and subtly flexing the spine. Move back and forth, initiating flexion and extension from the vertebra centered on the ball.

   – *Can you sense movement sequencing into surrounding vertebrae?*

### Rotation

- Now imagine the seesaw placed horizontally across the individual vertebra. Place your fingers on either side of the sternum superficial to the ends of the imaginary plank.

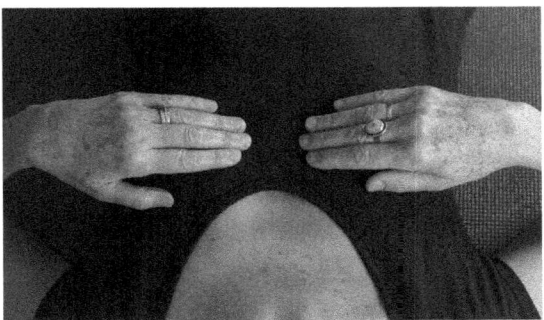

- On exhalations, use finger pressure to guide the right end of the plank posteriorly, compressing the right side of the ball and initiating a subtle spinal twist. Imagine you are steering one transverse process posteriorly and the other anteriorly. On inhalations, steer the transverse process back to neutral position. Alternate sides, initiating a tiny spinal twist from the individual vertebra.

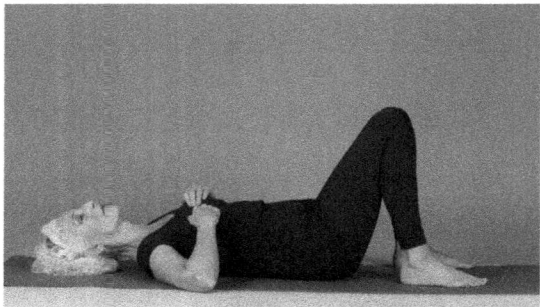

- *Can you sense movement sequencing into surrounding vertebrae?*

### Side Bend

- Maintain the same finger placement on the sternum.

- On exhalations, steer the right transverse process toward the right heel, keeping it parallel to the floor and initiating a subtle vertebral side bend. On inhalations, steer the processes back to neutral position. Alternate sides, coordinating movement with breath.

- *Can you sense movement sequencing into surrounding vertebrae?*

- Repeat the three movements with the ball at different vertebral levels, especially at T12 and the midlumbar areas. Use sensitive, gentle finger pressure on the abdomen. Note that when the ball is placed under the lumbar spine, you will press the bottom of the seesaw posteriorly as you extend the spine on inhalations and the top of the seesaw posteriorly as the spine flexes on exhalations. This change mimics natural pelvic breath movement.

- Remove the ball and pause to register any difference from baseline.

- Stand and walk around.

  - *How does your spinal felt sense differ?*
  - *Is standing or walking different?*
  - *Do you notice any changes in strength, mobility, or stability?*

Practice spinal initiation in your yoga or movement practice and in daily life as you bend, reach, and twist. For example, initiate a shoulder check from your spine when driving and notice how it differs from your habitual way of turning.

## FOUNDATIONAL PRACTICE: INITIATING COLLECTIVE SPINAL MOVEMENT

When I swim from my lumbar transverse processes, I'm stronger and faster!

*Rita*

Once individual vertebral awareness is established in the nervous system, collective movement is more easily initiated from specific anatomical structures. Consciously initiated spinal movement is stronger and more integrated as it emanates from the core. In this practice, as the nervous system receives information from multiple pathways, motor control and sensorimotor maps are refined.

## Learning Objectives

- Explore collective vertebral movement.
- Refine sensorimotor maps.

## Practice Notes

- Repeat each movement several times until it feels accessible.
- Notice how initiating movement in one vertebral zone generates responsive movement in the whole spine.
- Use your fingers and hands to give tactile cues for isolating each movement.
- Identify and inhibit unnecessary effort and extraneous movement. Other parts will want to "help."

## Instructions

- Sit in a comfortable position with your spine effortlessly erect, using support as necessary.
- Establish a baseline by flexing, extending, side bending, and twisting your spine.
  - *Where do you habitually initiate these movements?*
- Begin with the cervical spine. Lightly touch the cervical spinous processes with your three middle fingers. Initiate flexion by visualizing the spinous processes moving apart and minutely spreading your fingers. Initiate extension by visualizing the spinous processes moving together, compacting your fingers.
- Shift your focus to the cervical discs. Now initiate flexion by visualizing the anterior discs compressing and the posterior discs expanding. Initiate extension by visualizing the anterior discs expanding and the posterior discs compressing.

  - *How does the quality of movement change when initiating from bone or disc?*
- Place the three middle fingers of both hands vertically on either side of the neck, lightly touching the skin overlying the cervical transverse processes. Initiate side bending from the transverse processes, visualizing them spreading apart on one side and moving closer together on the other side. Feel your fingers mimicking the movement of the processes. Reverse the movement to return to neutral.
- Initiate a twist by moving the right transverse processes forward and left ones backward. Steer the processes with your fingers.
- Repeat this exploration in the thoracic and lumbar zones. Use your hands to provide tactile guidance and to steer the movement. When exploring these areas, place your finger pads on your chest or abdomen and imagine sinking them through your torso to guide vertebral movement in each zone.
- Contrast spinal-initiated movement with passive-spinal movement initiated from your arms. Raise both arms overhead several times and notice how flexion of the shoulders motivates spinal extension.
- Raise one arm sideways and in an arc overhead to notice how shoulder abduction can initiate spinal side bend.
- To explore twisting, raise one arm in front to shoulder height, then move it laterally in an arc. Notice how horizontal shoulder abduction can initiate spinal twist.
  - *How does the quality of movement differ when vertebrae are moved passively rather than actively?*

## EXPLORATION: REPATTERNING SPINAL CURVES

The fetal C-curve underlies and supports the development of secondary curves. Sensing our original embryological kyphotic curve, then consciously reassembling secondary lordotic curves can be therapeutic, especially when curves are habitually imbalanced. In repatterning explorations, the nervous system draws on early developmental sensorimotor templates of spinal curve patterns and then applies new learning to organize future motor responses.

### Learning Objectives

* Explore spinal curves actively and passively.

* Accentuate spinal curves to refine sensorimotor maps.

### Props

* A blanket or cushion

### Practice Notes

* You will need a trusted partner for the first part of this exploration. Establish permission and parameters of touch.

* Take a baseline reading both seated and standing. Rotate your head side to side a few times to notice range and ease of movement.

### FETAL C-CURVE

### Instructions

* To establish felt sense of the fetal C-curve passively, one partner rests in fetal position with knees and head close together and the head supported on the blanket. The helper places their hands lightly on either side of the lumbar spine, using full palmar contact.

* The receiver focuses on the touch and warmth of the helper's hands on their rounded lumbar spine and directs inhalations into the hands. After several breaths, the receiver experiments with pressing into the helping hands on inhalations, accentuating the C-curve, then releasing pressure on exhalations. After several breaths, the receiver switches to pressing into the helping hands for several exhalations, then continues in the breathing mode that feels most supportive.

* The helper now places both hands across the receiver's lumbar spine and defines the C-curve by slowly stroking one hand up to the base of the skull while the other strokes down to the sacrum. After several strokes, the hands remain on the skull and sacrum. The receiver practices **Back Breathing** into the primary curve of the whole spine.

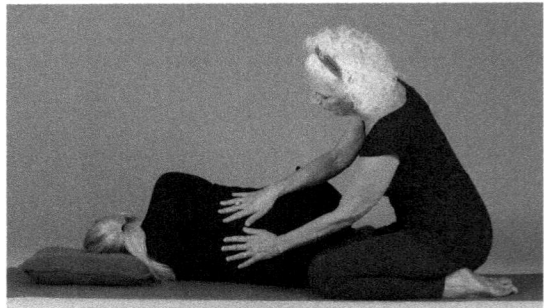

* The receiver moves to a seated position to register the effects of the practice.

  – *What do you notice?*

### SECONDARY CURVE: CERVICAL

### Instructions

* To establish felt sense of the cervical curve *passively*, roll the blanket into an 11 cm (5 in.)

cylinder and place it horizontally on the floor. Lie on your back with knees bent and the roll under your cervical spine filling the space between shoulders and head. Adjust the size of the roll or your head placement to orient your eyes toward the ceiling.

- Rest in this position for a few minutes. With each exhalation, allow the weight of your head and neck to settle into the support of the blanket, shaping and supporting the cervical curve.

- Look at the ceiling. On an exhalation, slowly move your eyes in an arc to look between your knees. Notice how your cervical curve flattens.

- As you inhale, return your eyes to the ceiling and head to starting position. Rest for a few breaths and consciously undo any muscular tension, resting your neck passively on the roll.

- Repeat several times.

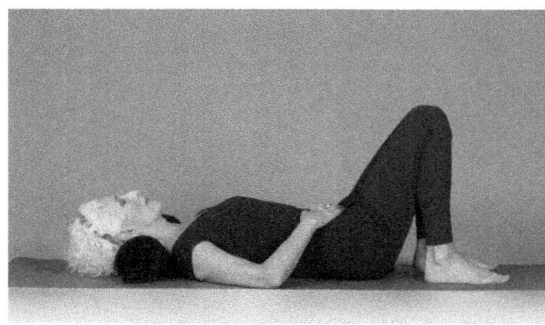

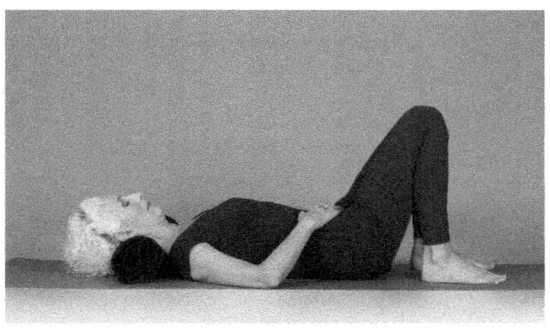

- To actively repattern the cervical curve, lie prone on the bolster, supported from your pubic bone to sternum. Rest your forehead on your hands or the folded blanket.

- As you inhale, move your eyes in an arc from the floor, looking up as though investigating something interesting in the environment. Notice the cervical lordotic curve forming as your head lifts. Slowly, lower your head as you exhale. Sense the organization of your cervical curve as you repeat the lifting movement several times.

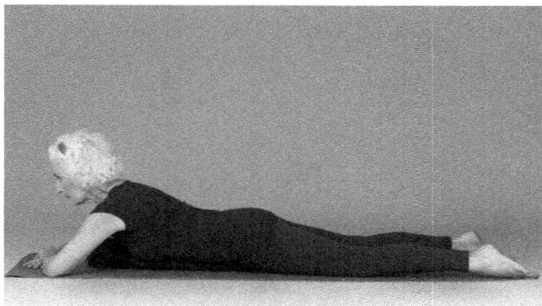

- Sit in a comfortable position to register any effects.

## SECONDARY CURVE: LUMBAR

### Instructions

- To explore the lumbar curve passively in supine position, roll the blanket to a diameter that will support your lumbar arch but not be provocative. Adjust the size of the blanket cylinder for comfort.

- Rest on the rolled blanket for a few minutes. Practice **Back Breathing**, directing your inhalations into the lumbar area. With each exhalation, allow the lumbar curve to soften and settle into the support of the roll. Stay in this passive establishment of the lumbar curve until your low back surrenders and releases.

- On an inhalation, press into your **Foot Triangles** to lift your pelvis off the floor enough to slightly flatten the lumbar curve. As you exhale, slowly lower the pelvis back to the floor and rest your spine on the roll. Sense the organization of your lumbar curve each time you return to the floor.

peel off the floor, arms straighten, and you arrive in Cow pose with an arched lumbar spine.

As you exhale, round your spine into Cat pose and shift your weight backward to return to Child's pose. Sense the organization of the lumbar curve as you repeat the movement several times.

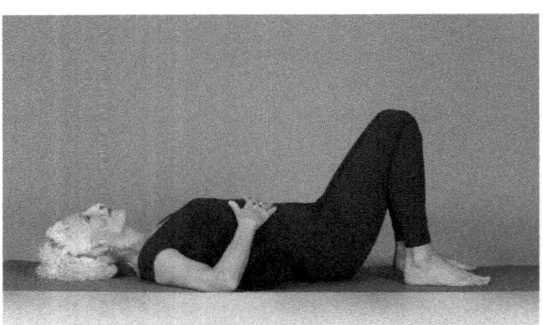

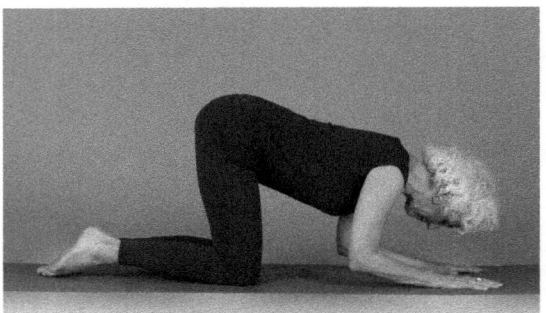

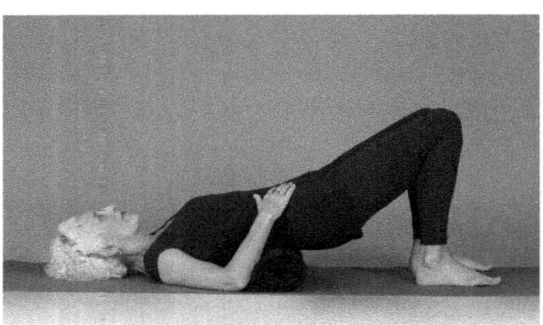

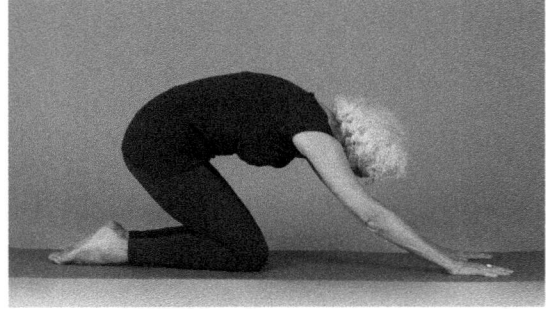

- To actively repattern the lumbar curve, practice a rolling Cat-Cow pose. Begin on all fours with knees directly beneath hips and wrists slightly forward of shoulders.

- Move your pelvis backward into Child's pose (Balasana) (or a comfortable variation) with your elbows and forehead touching the floor. Explore **Back Breathing** as you sense the roundness of your primary curve.

- On an inhalation, incrementally and slowly shift your weight forward until your elbows

- Return to baseline seated and standing positions to register any effects. Rotate your head from side to side a few times.

  - *How is weight distributed on your foot triangles now?*
  - *How do you experience your spinal curves now?*
  - *Is it easier to feel body weight sequencing through your midline and into your legs and feet?*
  - *What's different when you rotate your head?*

## EXPLORATION: REPATTERNING SPINAL WAVE

Once you learn to articulate individual vertebrae and repattern resilient spinal curves, you can explore collective vertebral movement as a wave moving up or down the spine. Movement originating in the head or tail is consciously sequenced vertebra to vertebra, producing a fluid, responsive ripple from one end to the other. Combined movement at facet joints, vertebral segments, and discs undulates the spine in ways that enhance the health of spinal myofascia, joints, and discs.

### Learning Objective

- To incorporate collective vertebral movement into yoga poses.

### SPINE CHAIN IN BRIDGE POSE (SETU BANDHA SARVANGASANA)

### Practice Notes

- Visualize your spine and sacrum as a chain of links or string of pearls to clarify lifting and lowering one vertebra at a time.

- Use specificity and **Right Effort** as you articulate each individual vertebra.

- The greatest benefit lies in returning each vertebra to the floor, as this requires precise motor control.

- Take extra time with clumps of vertebrae or vertebrae that aren't clearly sensed.

### Instructions

- Take a baseline in supine with knees bent, feet hip width apart and arms alongside your body, palms down. Explore **Back Breathing**.

  - *How do your sacrum, spine, and back contact the floor?*

- On an inhalation, press into your **Foot**

**Triangles** and lift the lower half of your sacrum off the floor, creating a posterior pelvic tilt. Imagine lifting one link or pearl. Return the sacrum to the floor as you exhale.

- On the next inhalation, lift the lower, then upper sacrum off the floor. Imagine lifting two links or pearls. Carefully return first the upper, then the lower sacrum to the floor on exhalation.

- Continue in this way, lifting one more vertebra each time. Eventually, the vertebral chain will lift off the floor sequentially until your weight rests on the upper back.

- Once you reach your final position, lower the spine vertebra by vertebra, taking one complete breath to lower each one. Move on exhalations and pause on inhalations. Take as many breaths as required to place each vertebra back on the floor carefully and precisely.

  - *Do your vertebrae move individually or as clumps?*
  - *How fluid is the spinal wave of movement?*

- Pause in supine to register any effects.

  - *Are there changes in the way your back body contacts the floor?*

- Stand and walk around to notice any other effects.

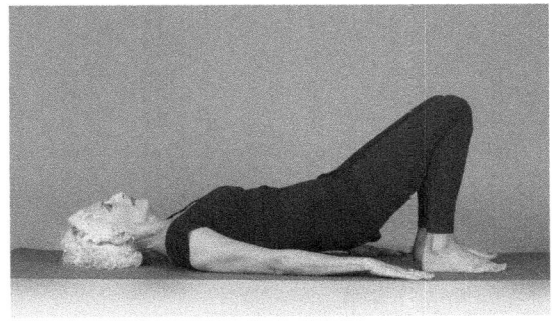

> I diligently practised Spine Chain in Bridge for three weeks and finally ironed out the clumps of vertebrae. It really changed my walking.
>
> *Jennifer*

## STANDING CAT-COW POSE 🎥

### Instructions

- Stand with feet parallel and hip width apart, then bend your knees and place your hands on the lower thighs, fingers pointing inward.

- Initiate an undulating movement by tucking your tail, then sequentially rounding, segment by segment, into the lumbar, thoracic, and cervical vertebral zones. Focus on each vertebra as it sequentially participates in the wave of movement. Inhibit peremptory movement of the head by deliberately waiting until the wave of flexion reaches your neck.

- Once your spine is rounded in Cat pose, reverse the movement by lifting your sacrum and sequentially arching your spine segment by segment to the head. Inhibit peremptory movement of the head by consciously waiting until the wave of extension reaches your neck.

- Repeat the spinal-wave movements several times.

  - *How does your breath instinctively coordinate with the movements?*

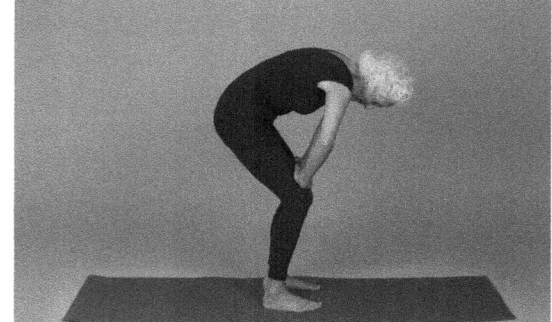

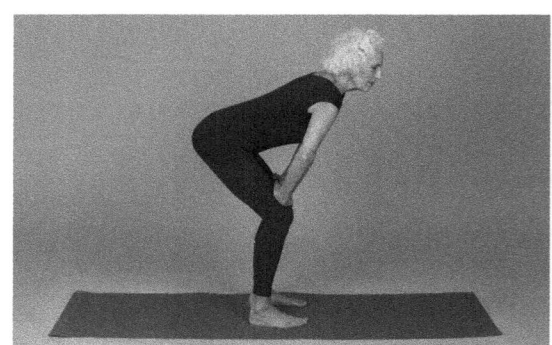

- Stand in Mountain pose and notice effects of the practice.

---

## EXPLORATION: WALKING WITH A SPRINGY SPINE

> While practicing springy spine in walking, I realized I've been bracing against back pain. The pain dramatically decreases when I consciously undulate.
>
> *Marie*

A healthy spine is a springy spine. The tensional truss structure confers elasticity while spinal curves and malleable discs cushion and absorb shock then rebound to provide length. Shock absorption and resilience are more accessible when you sense and visualize these actions while walking. Visualize the graceful, undulating walking rhythm of a Maasai warrior.

## Learning Objective

- Use visualization to alter walking patterns.

## Instructions

- Set a baseline by walking on a flat surface.

  - *How does your spine habitually move as you walk?*

- As you continue walking, feel your spine in your midline.

- Visualize your discs as resilient marshmallows, alternately compressing and rebounding as you walk.

  - *Which parts of the gait cycle compress or release your discs?*

- Shift your focus to the tensegrity truss arrangement of the vertebrae, the long and short ligaments, and extensive surrounding myofascia. Picture the elasticity of ligaments and spinal myofascia as you walk. Imagine them coiling and uncoiling.

- Visualize the psoas muscles and thoracolumbar fascia as industrial-strength springs adding their recoil energy to your walk. Feel the spine alternately compressing and lengthening elastically.

  - *How does your walk change?*

- Shift your focus to the spinal curves. As you walk, track the alternating compression and rebound as the curves adjust to walking forces.

  - *How do the curves change throughout the gait cycle?*

- Let go of visualization and compare your present walk with the baseline.

  - *What's different?*
  - *Which visualization resonates most with you?*

## THERAPEUTIC APPLICATIONS

The spine valiantly attempts to adapt to physical stresses from trauma, disease, or habitual patterns of use or disuse. Koshic factors, including psychological stressors, fear, and embodied archetypes, may also contribute to adaptations resulting in loss of segmental vertebral movement, imbalanced spinal curves, and pain. Tellingly, at least 85 percent of people with back pain don't receive a pathological diagnosis, and poor correlation exists between symptoms and diagnostic findings (Deyo and Weinstein 2001). In my clinical experience, when the primary therapeutic goal is increasing IA and restoring optimal spinal function and integrity through EA practices, back pain commonly reduces significantly regardless of diagnosis. When spinal curves and individual and collective vertebral movement are repatterned to fine-tune motor control and increase proprioception, the tensional fascial network can reconfigure to optimize stability, mobility, and force transmission in the whole body. When the physical body is steady and comfortable, other koshas will benefit.

When the three body weights of head, rib basket, and pelvis are aligned in gravity, less muscular effort is required to maintain lift and verticality and move the spine in integrated ways. Physiological processes also benefit from optimal alignment. The spinal cord and nerves have adequate space for smooth nerve conduction, digestive and other organs can move freely, and blood and fluids can circulate unhindered. The embodied realization that alignment is a dynamic process, and the direct experience of beneficial physiological and psychological effects of resilient uprightness, often motivate students to maintain regular awareness and movement practices. Nonphysical effects inspire practice as students experience the self-support and inner strength provided when the spine is supple and well organized.

Pain and dysfunction in the spine can rarely be viewed in isolation. The spine and pelvis are an integrated, interrelated, functional unit, and pelvic position can alter spinal curves and hamper the spine's ability to absorb shock, transfer load, and sequence movement. As the central connecting structure, the spine also affects and is affected by the pelvis, head, and limbs. If the spine is adapting to consequences of restricted hip or shoulder joints, it's unavailable to effectively participate in collective action or trunk stabilization and may eventually suffer from doing double duty. Alternatively, imbalanced spinal curves can change the orientation of the shoulder and pelvic girdles, affecting head and neck carriage and load transfer through joints. Excessive loading of specific structures ultimately leads to pain and dysfunction. Discs may herniate, joints suffer arthritic changes, and nerves compress as spatial relationships are distorted. Imbalanced spinal curves can also disorganize tension and compression forces acting on vertebrae and disrupt healthy bone density and remodeling. Additionally, spinal function is compromised when excessive myofascial tension or dysfunctional breathing habits restrict rib flexibility and facet, and costovertebral joint movement. The complex structure of the spine can generate diverse types of dysfunctions, making back pain one of the most common reasons for physician visits.

EA practices can catalyze changes on all koshic levels for students with structural and functional spinal hyper- or hypomobility. In my clinical experience, repatterning stability and safe mobility often influences the nervous system to calm the mind, decrease pain output, and increase resilience. Students with hypermobile spines learn to identify areas of spinal rigidity influencing compensatory distal hypermobility. Learning to stabilize hypermobile areas and mobilize rigid areas often brings great relief. Those with hyperkyphosis or scoliosis often experience decreased pain and increased function once optimal vertebral movement is repatterned and the nervous system is reminded of original spinal curves. Although anecdotal, my observations are supported by research highlighting reduction in disability and improvement in quality of life following body-mind rehabilitation utilizing IA and subtle movement (Ahmadi *et al.*, 2020). Gentle movement and active patient involvement has also been associated with improved functional capacity and reduced pain perception (Gonzalez-Medina *et al.*, 2021). EA practices for the spine utilize these therapeutic concepts of IA, gentle movement, and personal agency.

The spine contains an echo of the original central pole around which we self-assembled as an embryo. EA practices can awaken felt sense of the spine and remind us of that innate wisdom and our wondrous ability to continually self-create, self-support, and heal. It may start with a fledgling sense of center, knowing that we have a resilient central structure that supports and propels us, and end with a stronger sense of self as we learn to rely on the spine as a touchstone to inner stability and centeredness.

## KOSHIC CONTEMPLATIONS

### Annamaya Kosha

- *Have you developed felt sense of your spine as a curved flexible axis?*
- *Have you experienced changes in spinal alignment, stability, or ease of movement?*
- *How is the quality of your movement different when you initiate movement from your spine?*
- *How have you incorporated spinal awareness into your movement practice and daily activities?*

### Pranamaya Kosha

- *Does your energy level shift when you consciously access your spine for support and movement initiation?*
- *Have you noticed a relationship between spinal movement and how you breathe?*
- *Has your physiological function improved as you restore optimal movement in your spine?*

### Manomaya Kosha

- *What spinal alignment and movement habits came to light during EA practices?*

- *Have you noticed emotions arising as you consciously move your spine in nonhabitual ways?*

### Vijnanamaya Kosha

- *Does the shape of your spine reflect your personal archetypes or the way you approach life?*
- *After doing these practices, do you feel more connected to your inner support and resources?*

### Anandamaya Kosha

- *Has spinal awareness helped you access your inner stillness?*
- *What is your experience when visualizing your spine as a conduit for cosmic and earth energies?*

> To succeed in life, you need three things: a wishbone, a backbone, and funny bone.
>
> *Reba McEntire*

## KEY CONCEPTS

- The spine is the first bone to form embryologically, reflecting its importance.
- In Gracovetsky's spinal engine model, the spine generates locomotion and limbs transfer forces between the body and ground.
- The spine is not a column; it's a triangular tensegrity truss tower, balancing tension and compression forces to produce stability.
- The spine is designed to move fluidly between dual roles of support and movement.
- Embodying the spine as midline centers us on all koshic levels.
- In the yogic tradition, three intertwining subtle energy channels, or nadis—ida,

pingala, and sushumna—form a spinal nucleus connecting us to universal energies.

- Pain research highlights associations between back pain and stress, depression, and anxiety.
- Metaphorically, the spine represents courage, resolution, and inner strength.
- The spine can be a touchstone for accessing the peace, stillness, and wisdom of our true Self.

- Each vertebra can move in multiple planes and participate in collective wave-like force transmission.
- Sensing the original embryological C-curve and consciously repatterning secondary curves can be therapeutic.
- Gentle movement and active patient engagement can improve function and reduce pain perception.

## CHAPTER 10

# Opening the Gate: The Head and Neck

*Keep a stiff upper lip.*
*Get out of your head.*
*He's a pain in the neck.*
*Hold your head up high.*

The cervical spine developed after vertebrates emerged from the ocean to navigate on land. The evolution of a mobile neck connecting the head and torso gave eyes greater range to negotiate complex earthly terrain, and to scan the environment for food, danger, or potential mates. Upright posture may have stimulated the evolution of larger, more complex human brains in heads that weighed 5–7 kg (12–15 lb.) (Falk *et al.*, 2012). The relative heaviness of the head perched atop a narrow neck subjects it to strong forces, especially gravity. A common response is to meet these forces by unconsciously tensing muscles to hold the head erect. The nervous system "forgets" that myofascial, skeletal, and organ systems, and the earth itself, offer support, and that the head and neck can naturally relax into that support.

Whenever the upper body moves off the vertical axis, the myofascial system adaptively reorganizes to counter gravitational forces acting on the head and neck. This head-righting reflex orchestrates muscular activation to maintain our eyes level with the horizon. In this reflex, stability and head position are adjusted through modifications in muscle tone as visual, vestibular, and somatosensory inputs are processed. Over time, compensatory adaptations to alignment, movement, and breath habits initiated by this postural reflex can cause excessive tension in the upper body that may restrict movement and change cervical curvature. Our habitual use of cell phones and resulting common forward head posture causes compensatory activation of posterior musculature in a valiant effort to prevent our heads from falling forward into gravity. These postural stresses can influence neck and jaw myofascia to respond to lack of stability from the feet with increased tone to stabilize head posture (Rubenstein 2010). It's no wonder that people accept neck pain and tension as "normal."

From a physical perspective, the neck functionally links the head and rest of the body. It's a complex structure supporting the skull and serving as a conduit for fluids and motor and sensory information. On a more subtle level, the neck can be viewed as a multidimensional "gate" between the mind and body, head and heart, and thoughts and emotions. We can blame Descartes for perpetuating valuation of mind and reason over the body and heart wisdom. Neck tension can perpetuate this Cartesian dualism (I think, therefore I am). Feeling sensations or emotions, expressing our truth, or accessing inner wisdom can be difficult if this gate is squeezed by muscular tension.

Over-identification with the head begins in infancy as we discover our mouth as a tool for exploring the world. Everything goes in our mouth! This identification is reinforced as our attention is occupied daily with transmitting, receiving, and processing sensory information. The special senses in the head (eyes, ears, nose, and mouth) receive information from the environment that travels to the brain for processing. The mouth and throat receive nourishment and function as avenues of expression through which thoughts, feelings, and emotions are articulated (or repressed). We may "overeffort," sensing by straining to see or listen, or become overwhelmed by constant sensory bombardment in our hyperactive, information-overloaded world. We may habitually evaluate or judge sensory information, which can generate physical tension and hamper our ability to be present, open, and neutral to incoming data. In Ayurveda, misuse of the senses is considered a main cause of dis-ease.

## KOSHIC PERSPECTIVES

> I have ankylosing spondylosis and normally turn my whole body to look sideways. After articulating each cervical vertebra in class, or at least imagining it, for the first time in years my neck moved independently.
>
> *Derek*

Physical effects of neck and head dysfunction manifest in annamaya as misalignment, pain, tension, and sometimes strange clicking or grinding sounds. On this koshic level, we learn to experience the neck, head, shoulders, and upper torso as a functional unit whose efficient operation depends on support from the feet, pelvis, and spine. When these lower structures are harmoniously organized in gravity, the head is free to find its rightful place resting peacefully atop the spine, naturally relaxed, balanced, and adaptively responsive to movement in the rest of the body. As we explore finding support from below and moving the neck and head in healthier, efficient ways, ease and resilient stability are patterned.

Within pranamaya kosha, we may identify relationships between breathing patterns, energy levels, and habitual neck, jaw, and shoulder tension. After EA practices that release tension and liberate breath, we may experience increased energy levels and sensations of flowing prana between the head and torso. Other physiological functions may improve when constricted neurovascular structures are released by reestablishing structural integrity in the neck and head. Brain function and acuity of the senses can be enhanced as blood circulation to the head is restored. Even stomach symptoms can be relieved by releasing overly tensioned cervical soft tissue compressing the vagus nerve (Ozel Asliyuce, Berberoglu, and Ulger 2020). This relief could reasonably extend to other vagus-innervated organs. Digestion may improve further as myofascial structures involved in chewing and swallowing are rebalanced. On a more subtle level, the upper three chakras (energy centers) are contained in the head and neck, energetically governing communication, clarity of vision, and spiritual connection.

As the primary home of sense organs, the head reflects the sensory aspect of manomaya kosha. Functioning like an airport control tower, the head receives and coordinates responses to incoming sensory data from both inner and outer worlds. Imbalanced tension and compression forces in the head and neck can compress nerve endings and compromise the quality of sensory data received, resulting in faulty proprioception and diminished sensorimotor control.

The emotional aspect of manomaya kosha is reflected in head orientation and facial expressions, which give clear nonverbal messages about emotional states. When we see a contorted face, rigid neck muscles, and aggressive head posture we immediately recognize anger. Excessive neck tension can close the "gate" between the occiput and C1, potentially blocking emotional expression and disrupting our ability to register sensory and emotional messages from the body. This lack of communication between body, heart, and mind may eventually lead to depression, anxiety, dissociative symptoms, and feelings of disconnection.

Our head and neck posture and the way we perceive and present ourselves in the world can be shaped by the content of vijnanamaya kosha—our personalities, personal histories, and metaphors we embody. The reverse is also true. As we reshape posture through EA practices, the way we perceive and respond to the world can change. The wise, discerning Witness consciousness of vijnanamaya kosha helps us develop nonjudgmental awareness and formulate intentions and aspirations according to higher principles. We can clearly see things as they are and not as we wish they would be. We may more easily disidentify with ego attachments and the repetitive content of our mind. Through EA practices, we can establish a reproducible physical "home" for the Witness in the head, where we hear the wisdom of Self more clearly and the airport control tower can wisely coordinate perceptions and responses to inner and outer worlds.

The head carries and protects our precious brain that so brilliantly orchestrates our lives.

Both mundane physical and transcendent spiritual experiences are choreographed and imprinted within its bony dome. In anandamaya kosha, we can intentionally prepare the environment for spiritual experience by seeking out, learning, and committing to spiritual practices. The gift of practice is to experience *ananda*, supreme bliss, the tranquility that gives us inner strength to live an authentic life.

In the yoga tradition, the crown chakra atop the head is our connection to oneness, receiving cosmic energy from the cosmos. This chakra is viewed as the exit portal for the soul at death. If we consider the spine as the axis between heaven and earth, then the head and neck function as floodgates determining how much cosmic and earth energy ultimately flows through the body. If we further consider the spine as an ultrasonic core connecting us to our deepest Self, then freedom of the neck and head determines how much we access that true Self. The control tower of the head and neck can influence, consciously or unconsciously, how much transcendent connection we permit.

> When I intentionally shift my consciousness back in my head, I am more responsive and less reactive interacting with my children.
>
> *Lila*

## LEARN IT

Of all body regions, the neck epitomizes the dichotomy between stability and mobility. Although designed as the most mobile spinal zone, its small and delicate vertebrae must support the moving weight of a bowling ball. Neck stability is required to support the head and protect the delicate spinal cord, nerves, and arteries housed within the cervical spine. The network of surrounding fascia, including joint capsules, ligaments, and muscles, and the shape of articular surfaces collectively contribute to cervical stability. Impressive neck mobility allows subtle balance adaptations and orients our senses in a wide, multidimensional range.

## Bones

The Celestial Design Committee fashioned seven small, delicate cervical vertebrae to optimize range of motion. The first two vertebrae, C1 and C2, have atypical features for support and movement of the skull, while C3 to C6 have more typical structure and functionality. Cervical vertebral bodies are small and oval-shaped, which somewhat restricts side bending movement. The lateral edges have interlocking "lips" at the margins that stabilize yet allow significant mobility. Cervical facet joints are diagonally angled 45 degrees superiorly to the horizontal plane to maximize multiplanar movement. Spinous processes have two branches that increase available surface area for myofascial attachments. Each transverse process contains a triangular passage (the transverse foramen) for the sympathetic nerves and the vertebral artery and vein.

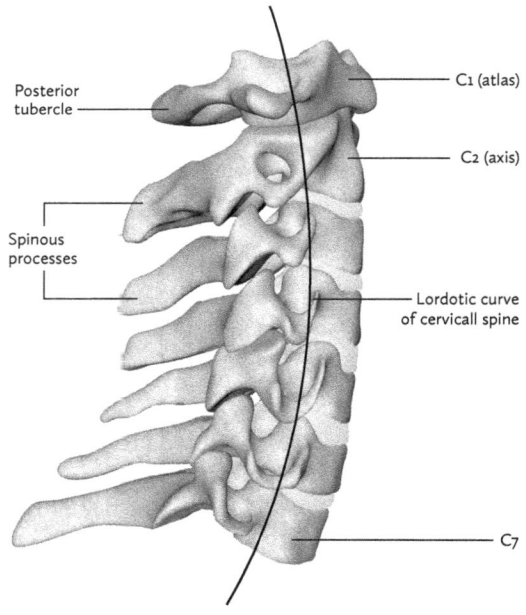

Posterior tubercle

C1 (atlas)

C2 (axis)

Spinous processes

Lordotic curve of cervicall spine

C7

Atlas (C1) supports the considerable weight of the head, like the mythical god Atlas supporting the earth on his shoulders. Shaped like a bony ring without a vertebral body, it has long, easily palpated transverse processes and a rudimentary spinous process. The superior articular facets are concave, kidney-shaped surfaces that permit rocking of the corresponding convex occipital condyles of the skull in tiny nodding and side bending movements. The occipital condyles look like little "feet" of the skull. The second cervical vertebra, C2, is called *axis* because C1 rotates around its dens, a "tooth" projecting superiorly from its vertebral body. As atlas pivots around the dens, it carries the head with it.

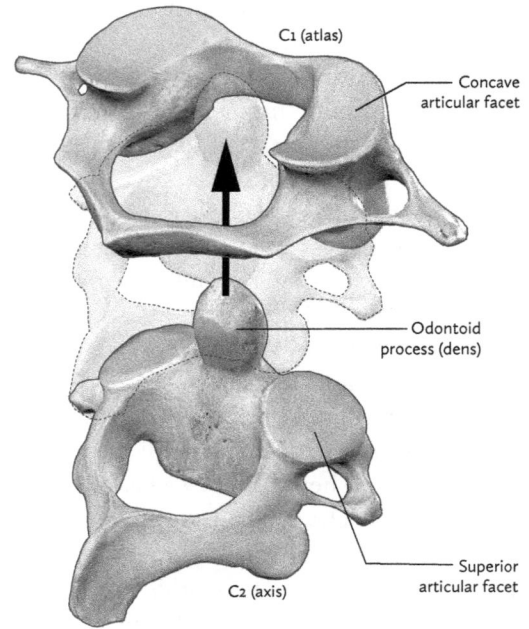

C1 (atlas)

Concave articular facet

Odontoid process (dens)

Superior articular facet

C2 (axis)

The eight cranial and 14 facial bones in the head shape our facial features, contain our special senses, and protect the brain. Eye, ear, nose, and mouth orifices allow sensations and sustenance to enter and waste to leave. The eye sockets are deep, bony cones leading into the center of the head, with optic nerves passing through a tiny hole at the tip to innervate the eyes. The foramen magnum, a large hole at the base of the skull, allows the spinal cord to exit. Fibrous suture joints between cranial bones look like winding rivers and contain connective and ligamentous tissue "knitting" the bones together with varying degrees of mobility. Skilled practitioners of osteopathy and craniosacral therapy can effect significant therapeutic changes through gentle manipulation of cranial bones that impacts fascial membranes and circulation of fluids. The mandible (jawbone) is the only freely movable bone of the face. It forms the temporomandibular joint with the temporal bone, moving multidirectionally as we suck, chew, swallow, and vocalize. This hard-working joint often harbors stress and emotional tension.

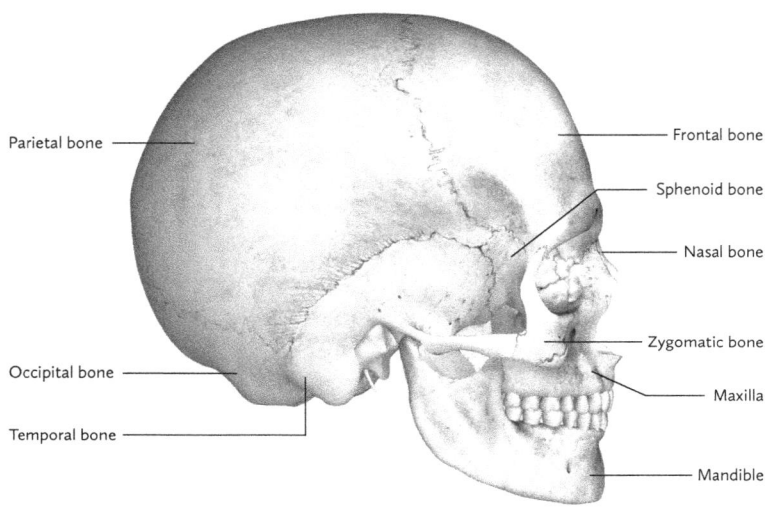

Parietal bone

Frontal bone

Sphenoid bone

Nasal bone

Zygomatic bone

Occipital bone

Maxilla

Temporal bone

Mandible

The hyoid is a U-shaped bone located anterior to the cervical spine at the angle of the jaw. As the only bone in the body that doesn't articulate with another bone (besides sesamoid bones embedded in tendons), the hyoid is suspended in fascia between the skull and sternum. This hyoid complex (the bone and associated myofascia) could be considered the "psoas" of the cervical spine; both structures traverse a diagonal pathway connecting front and back body, and both offer frontal spinal support for upright posture. Like the psoas, the hyoid complex bridges upper and lower body and center to periphery. Spatial relationships of the hyoid are more complex. It connects to the occiput, floor of the mouth, sternum, and scapulae. Both psoas and hyoid complexes are associated with the digestive system. One provides muscular support for digestive organs, while the other forms the base of the tongue, the top end of the digestive tract. Four suprahyoid muscles move the tongue and elevate the hyoid in eating and vocalization.

The position and tone of the hyoid complex can influence tone of the digestive tract and the diameter of the esophagus (Zhang et al., 2021). It makes intuitive sense that anterior hyoid displacement, commonly found in forward head posture, may contribute to laxity in the abdominal wall and digestive organs. (Test this on yourself by slumping while feeling your abdomen.) The hyoid complex also plays a role in breath by maintaining open airways (Cheng et al., 2020). Infrahyoid muscles attach to the larynx, sternum, and scapula and are associated more with vocalization. Imbalance in the hyoid complex may affect head posture, jaw mobility, digestive function, and voice quality.

When the hyoid complex is visualized and engaged in EA practices, it can activate frontal support for the spine and head through muscular engagement and by toning the digestive tract.

When applied to the common forward head posture, hyoid engagement can encourage functional balance between hypotoned anterior and hypertoned posterior neck musculature.

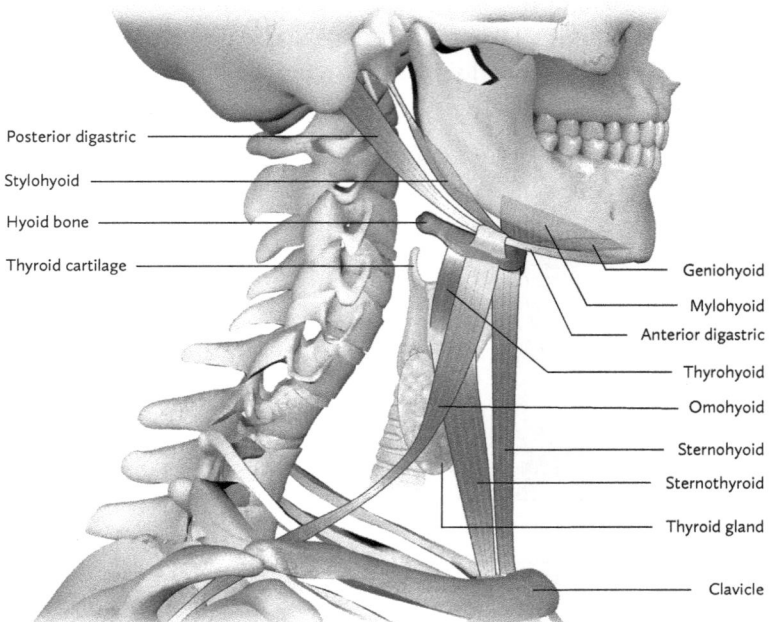

Posterior digastric
Stylohoid
Hyoid bone
Thyroid cartilage
Geniohyoid
Mylohyoid
Anterior digastric
Thyrohyoid
Omohyoid
Sternohyoid
Sternothyroid
Thyroid gland
Clavicle

## Myofascia

Perched atop the spine and subject to strong mechanical forces, the head and neck depend on balanced tension and compression forces throughout the body to maintain a functional cervical curve and efficient upright posture. Like the rest of the spine, the cervical spine is supported and moved by multiple layers of fascial structures. Greater posterior muscular bulk is necessary to counteract the forces of gravity pulling the head forward and down. Some cervical vertebrae contain up to 30 muscles attaching to the body and spinous and transverse processes. Unlike the lumbar and thoracic spines, multiple muscles on the anterior cervical vertebrae contribute frontal support and are activated when we purposely elongate the neck.

Deep cervical musculature is richly endowed with sensory nerve fibers. The head-righting reflex is initiated through interaction of proprioceptive, vestibular, and postural reflex neural pathways that orient the whole body in space (Pettorossi and Schieppati 2014) and adjust head posture to level the eyes with the horizon. Multiple fascial layers on the skull are continuous with myofascia of the cervical spine, jaw, shoulders, and throughout the body. The posterior suboccipital muscles even connect to fascia surrounding the spinal cord (the dura) through a connective tissue bridge (Scali, Marsili, and Pontell 2011). The jaw muscles are apparently so strong they can support the entire body weight of a trapeze artist holding on with their teeth! The talent of wiggling ears requires all four less strong ear muscles. Unsurprisingly, tension in these upper structures can affect distant body parts and vice versa.

We can view cervical myofascia as a multilayered cylinder, supporting and moving the neck and head yet connected to distal structures through the fascial network. In fact, all the main myofascial meridians described by Thomas Myers (in his seminal book *Anatomy Trains*, 2020) pass through the neck. The deeper, more segmental posterior neck muscles are continuous with the spinal musculature extending from the sacrum to occiput. The small suboccipital muscles fine-tune head posture. Leonardo da Vinci apparently first suggested that central neck muscles stabilize the spine, with guywire-like vertebral support provided by more lateral muscles (Crisco and Panjabi 1991). When posterior neck musculature is habitually imbalanced, the head often assumes the notorious forward head posture. As the head projects forward, blood supply to the brain and free flow of cerebrospinal fluid through the dura can be compromised. EA practices can help us find balanced head posture and ease of movement by visualizing support offered directly by the myofascial cylinder and indirectly by distal structures from below.

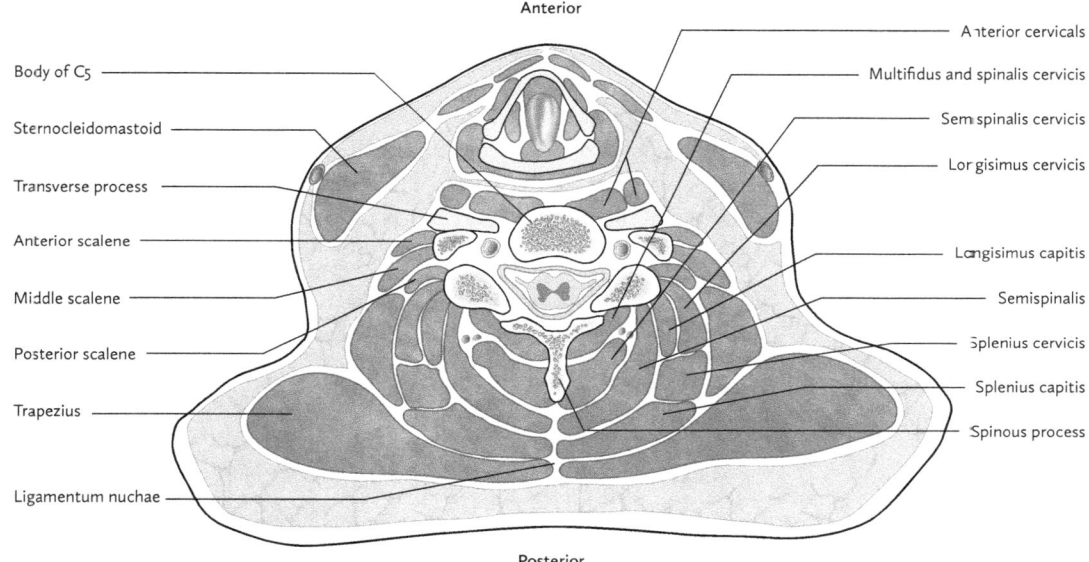

Anterior

Body of C5 — 
Sternocleidomastoid — 
Transverse process — 
Anterior scalene — 
Middle scalene — 
Posterior scalene — 
Trapezius — 
Ligamentum nuchae — 

Anterior cervicals
Multifidus and spinalis cervicis
Semispinalis cervicis
Longisimus cervicis
Longisimus capitis
Semispinalis
Splenius cervicis
Splenius capitis
Spinous process

Posterior

> Just knowing and visualizing that I have muscles supporting the front of my neck helps to balance my head posture.
>
> *Noah*

## Neurovascular Structures

The cervical spine contains important blood vessels and neural structures crucial for sustaining life. The delicate spinal cord is continuous with the brain and exits the skull through the occipital foramen into the protective vertebral canal extending throughout the spine. Felt sense of the spinal cord can promote awareness of continuity between the head, neck, and spine. Cervical structures are innervated by nerves branching off the spinal cord, while 12 pairs of cranial nerves innervate the face, throat, tongue, and sense organs. Cranial nerve ten, the vagus nerve, traverses the neck on its way to the chest and abdominal organs, with branches to the inner ear and face. In addition to its role in autonomic regulation, the vagus nerve is now recognized for its role in trauma, social engagement, and psychological and emotional states. As the nervous system scans the environment for safety or danger cues, the vagus nerve promotes or inhibits physiological processes according to perceived risk.

The precious brain and spinal cord are nourished by the vertebral and carotid arteries.

Vertebral arteries and veins have bony protection within a foramen (hole) in cervical transverse processes. Cervical misalignment or myofascial tension can compromise neurovascular function, causing symptoms including brain fog, headache, altered sensation, pain, and anxiety.

## FEEL IT

Felt sense is deepened when skeletal and soft tissue structures of the head and neck are mapped, enabling you to access support and repattern safe alignment and movement.

## FOUNDATIONAL PRACTICE: CERVICAL VERTEBRAL MOVEMENT 📽

Initiating movement from C1 and C2 activates deep stabilizing musculature and can transform habitual patterns of overusing superficial muscles. It can also be meditative; some students use these movements to settle their mind and establish presence prior to meditation. The atlantooccipital joint can be viewed as a "gate," allowing blood, cerebrospinal fluid, neural impulses, and prana to flow freely. When compressed, it can restrict flow and derail body-mind connection.

### Learning Objectives

- Sense subtle movements at C1 (atlantooccipital) and C2 (atlantoaxial) joints.

- Experience the collective action of the cervical spine.

> When I move from C1 and C2, I feel like I'm moving from my core, a strong inner safe place to move from. No strain and no neck pain.
>
> *Siena*

### PALPATE THE VERTEBRAE

### Instructions

- Sit comfortably in a chair or on the floor.

- Establish a baseline of habitual cervical movement by doing the three movements below a few times each. Register comfortable range of motion, associated sensations, and where you initiate each movement.

  - Flex and extend by moving your chin toward your chest, then toward the ceiling.
  - Side bend by moving each ear toward the shoulder.
  - Rotate by moving your head to each side.

- Use your fingertips to palpate the base of your occiput, starting at the mastoid process behind the ears. Trace along the bone to the midline.

- To palpate the rudimentary spinous process of C1, place one finger gently on the soft tissue inferior to the midoccipital base. Nod your head, slowly, up and down and you will feel the rudimentary C1 spinous process press into your fingertip then recede. Determine the neutral place between nodding up and down.

- Now move into a forward head posture and feel the change in tissue tension. Move back and forth from neutral to forward head posture monitoring tissue tension under your finger.

  - *How does the tissue tension change?*

– Which head position allows the occipital "gate" to remain open and flowing?

- Move your finger slightly inferior to feel the C2 spinous process. Continue palpating each spinous process, ending at the prominent C7.

## Find the Atlantooccipital Joint
### Instructions

- Place one index finger between your eyebrows and the other on the occipital base above C1, then imagine a line between them. Now, place your index fingers behind your earlobes on the mastoid processes and imagine another line between them. Sense the intersection of the two lines and situate your awareness there, deep in your head. This is the approximate location of the atlantooccipital joint between the occiput and C1.

## Atlantooccipital Movement
### Instructions

Repeat the following movements for at least a minute each:

– Visualize the convex occipital condyles resting on the corresponding concave C1 facets—a curve within a curve. Initiate a tiny downward nod of the head from the occipital condyles, visualizing them rolling forward and gliding backward on the C1 facets. Only 5–10 degrees of flexion is available at this joint, which means your nose moves approximately 0.5–1 cm (0.2–0.4 in.). Return your head to neutral, then continue the tiny nod while tracking the rolling and gliding component movements. Visualize slippery synovial fluid providing lubrication for smooth gliding.

– Now, do a tiny extension movement by nodding your head backward. Visualize the occipital condyles rolling backward and gliding forward on the C1 facets. The joint allows 10 degrees of extension, so your nose will move approximately 1 cm (0.4 in.). Continue nodding backward to deepen your felt sense.

- Combine these two mindful movements into a rhythmical tiny nod "yes." Maintain your focus on the rolling and gliding of the occipital condyles on the C1 facets.

– What is your felt sense of component joint movement?

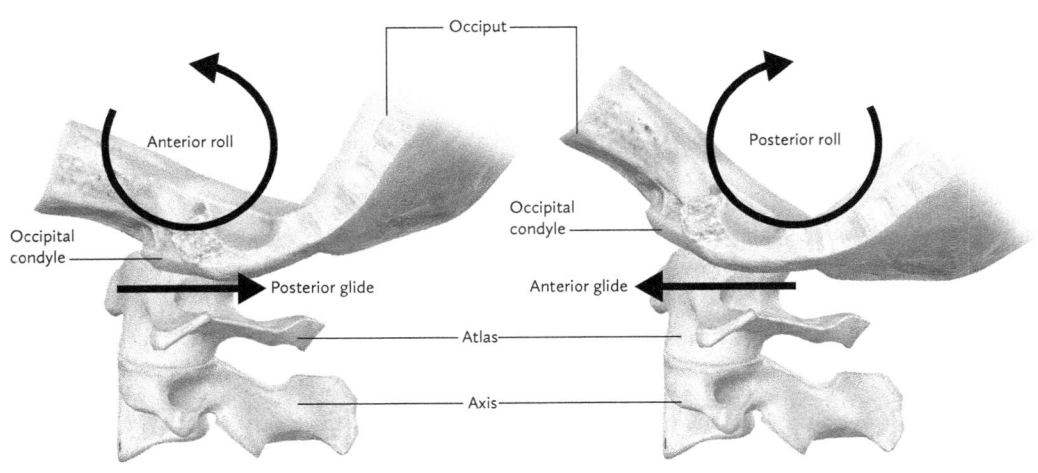

Flexion at atlantooccipital joint

Extension at atlantooccipital joint

- Initiate lateral flexion at the atlantooccipital joint by visualizing the occipital condyles rolling and gliding sideways. Track these component movements as you explore a tiny tilt of your head from side to side (5–7 degrees in each direction). As you right side bend, the occipital condyles roll right and glide left.

- Combine the nodding and lateral flexion movements into a tiny figure 8, tracking the component movements at the joint deep inside your head and the corresponding movement of your nose in space.

  - *Can you visualize these tiny lubricating movements creating ease of movement in the joints?*
  - *Do you notice changes in tension of the suboccipital myofascia?*

- To deepen your sense of these subtle movements, use your hands to move your head passively. Place your hands on either side of your head with the thumbs at the occipital base and fingers holding the lateral skull.

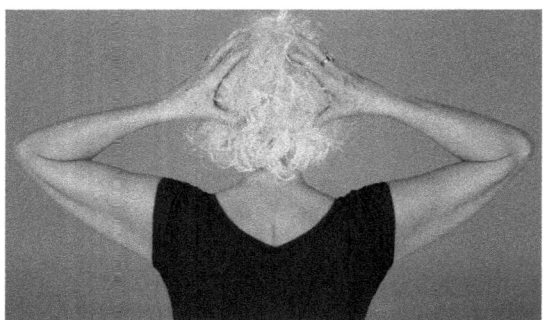

- Use your hands to passively move your head in a tiny "yes" nod while visualizing the rolling and gliding movement of the occipital condyles. Then, use your hands to guide your head in a tiny side bending movement. Release your hands.

- Visualize your head as a bobblehead toy connected to your body by a sturdy spring. "Bobble" your head in random movements.

As you move, keep your occipital gate open and spacious.

## Atlantoaxial Movement
### Instructions

- To help visualize the rotation available between C1 and C2, form a circle with your thumb and index finger, then insert your other index finger into the circle from below. Rotate the circle around your finger to mimic movement at this pivot joint.

- Translate this awareness into your body. Visualize the dens projecting upward from C2 into the bony ring of C1, then imagine it lengthening to the crown of your head. Use your tongue to help you sense the elongation: Slide the tip of your tongue backward on the roof of your mouth and press it into the soft palate near the back of your throat, directing pressure toward the crown of your head.

- Initiate rotation from C1, circling the bony ring around the axis of C2 in a tiny "no" movement.

- Explore the 45-degree range of motion in each direction typically available at this pivot joint (almost half of cervical rotation).

  - *Can you sense how your head is carried by the C1 bony ring?*
  - *Can you visualize spaciousness between the dens and the bony ring?*

- To deepen your sense of these subtle movements, use your hands to rotate your head passively side to side while visualizing the joint movement.

When I visualize fluid movements of C1 and C2, I relax and feel calmer.

*Mitchell*

## Collective Movement
### Instructions

- Explore the additional range of motion available when the whole cervical spine participates.

- Repeat the tiny nodding movement at the atlantooccipital joint, then slowly increase flexion to sense when other vertebrae join the movement.

- Explore flexion, extension, side bending, and rotation, initiating from the occiput or C1 and noticing additional collective movement as you increase range of motion.

- Pause to sense the effects of this practice.

  - *What's different when you initiate movement from the first two cervical joints?*
  - *What happens to your state of mind?*
  - *How could you incorporate this awareness into your daily life?*

## EXPLORATION: THE HYOID BONE

### Learning Objectives

- Develop felt sense of the hyoid bone.

- Explore the role of the hyoid in head and neck posture.

- Experience hyoid influence on abdominal tone.

### Instructions

- To landmark your hyoid bone, touch the top of the superior thyroid cartilage or Adam's apple. Then, form a U-shape with your thumb and index finger and place it on your throat underneath the angle of the jaw and above the thyroid cartilage. Your fingers mimic the shape and angle of the hyoid. Squeeze your fingers slightly together and palpate the area to feel the bony edges of the hyoid.

- Swallow a few times to feel the hyoid moving up and down. Then, make a *la-la-la-la* sound to feel the participation of the hyoid in vocalization.

- Use the pads of your fingers to carefully move the hyoid side to side a few times. Hold it gently to one side for several breaths, then to the other side.

  - *Can you feel a myofascial release in your throat or the floor of your mouth?*

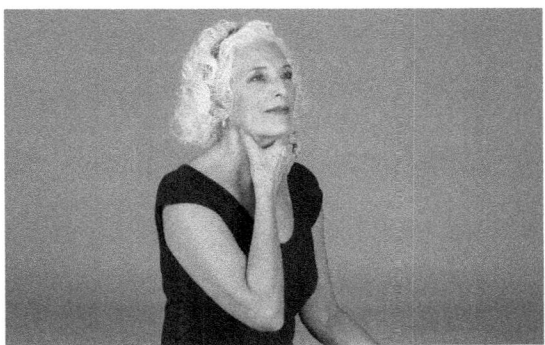

- Lightly hold the hyoid bone steady in its natural placement and slowly rotate your head a little side to side, stopping when you sense dynamic tension in the soft tissue between the stationary hyoid and your moving head. Hold your head in the rotated position for several breaths on each side.

  - *Can you feel a myofascial release in your throat or the floor of your mouth?*

- Release your hold and initiate movement from the hyoid, moving into combinations of cervical flexion and extension, side bend, and twist.

– *How are these movements different when initiated from the hyoid?*

• Pause and attune to the frontal support that the hyoid and other anterior neck muscles provide your cervical spine.

– *What do you notice?*

## HYOID LIFT

### Instructions

• To explore the role of the hyoid complex in head posture, hold the hyoid lightly with one hand. Place the other hand on your abdomen. In this exploration you will guide the hyoid toward the atlantooccipital joint and experience the responsive toning of abdominal muscles and digestive organs.

• Assume a forward head posture, letting your chin jut forward, the sternum drop, and throat and abdomen sag.

– *What do you notice in this posture?*
– *What happens to your suboccipital gate? Your breath?*

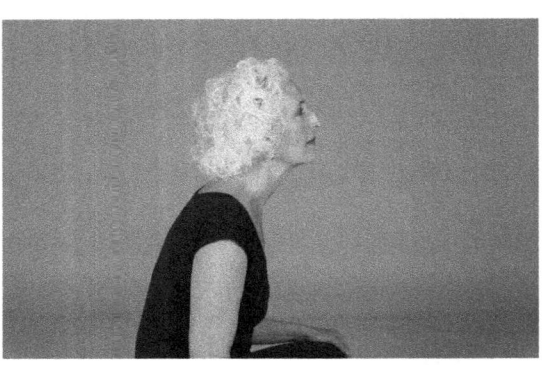

• Gently guide your hyoid diagonally up and back toward the atlantooccipital joint, following the angle of your jaw. As you move the hyoid, notice how the sternum lifts, the chin moves toward the throat and the suboccipital gate opens. Stop when the cervical curve is neutral and the cervical spine feels equally supported anteriorly and posteriorly.

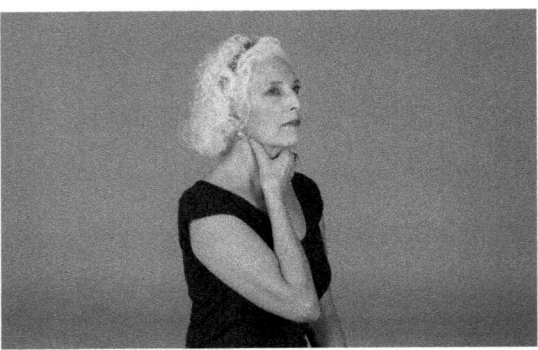

• Go back and forth between the forward head posture and the hyoid lift, tracking the tone of your abdomen.

– *How does your abdominal tone change?*
– *How could this awareness transfer to your daily activities and movement practice?*

• Pause to register sensations in your neck and head.

– *What do you notice?*

## EXPLORATION: CRANIAL FASCIA

If your hair is long enough to grasp between your fingers, you can release cranial fascia by applying traction. It's even better when a friend does it for you. The fascial continuities between the scalp, face, and neck mean that releasing scalp fascia can also relieve neck and jaw tension.

### Learning Objectives

- Sense continuity of cranial fascia with the face and neck.

- Release cranial fascia.

### Instructions

- Either seated or supine, place your fingertips at the front hairline and slide your fingers backward, threading them through the hair as close to the scalp as possible. Gently squeeze your fingers into a fist to lift the hair and cranial fascia off the skull. Hold the fist clenched until the fascia softens and any discomfort recedes, usually within one minute. If you don't feel a release, lighten your pressure.

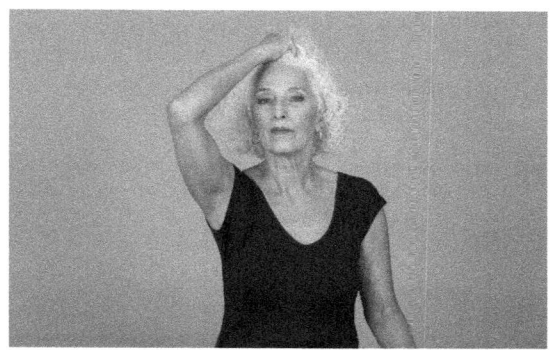

- Duplicate this grasping process at intervals along the hairline and back to the occiput on both sides, then repeat in strips from the forehead to occiput to systematically release cranial fascia.

  - *Can you sense the continuity of the scalp, jaw, and neck fascia?*
  - *Can you feel your jaw, face, or neck releasing?*

## EXPLORATION: HUMMING BEE BREATH (BHRAMARI)

Bhramari is a yogic breath practice traditionally used to calm the mind, reduce blood pressure, and relieve insomnia. Vibration in the throat and ears stimulates the vagus nerve, activating a relaxation response and toning the autonomic nervous system. Bhramari also encourages production of nitric oxide, a vasodilator associated with numerous health benefits (Taneja 2020).

### Learning Objective

- Highlight felt sense of cranial and facial structures through vibration.

### Instructions

- Sit in a comfortable seated position and take a brief breath baseline. Plug your ears with your thumbs, place your palms firmly over your ears, or use earplugs.

- As you exhale, hum gently while extending your exhalation without strain. Relax your facial and jaw muscles, lips gently touching and upper and lower teeth apart. Feel the sound reverberating inside your head. Vary the humming tone, volume, and intensity according to what feels right for you.

- Notice that you can direct vibration into specific areas. "Palpate" different anatomical structures with sound by focusing vibration in different areas of your face and head, especially areas of pain or congestion. Use the humming vibration to "palpate" your cranial and facial bones, the special senses (eyes, ears, nose, and mouth), and different parts of your brain.

- Continue humming for at least six breaths and up to 10 minutes. If your arms tire, rest them while continuing to hum. When you're finished, sit quietly and register the effects.

  - *Are you more aware of your cranial and fascial structures?*
  - *Has your breath changed?*
  - *What is the quality of your mind?*

## HEAL IT

### EXPLORATION: ROOTING THE NECK

When you visualize your neck rooted in lower body structures, you can access support from the rest of the spine, pelvis, and even the ground. The head and neck can release unnecessary tension and settle into this newfound support. Connecting the neck with lower structures also enables the cervical spine and head to fully participate in sequential spinal movement, clarifying structural and fascial continuities that encourage flow between body, mind, and emotions. Awareness of the root of the neck can significantly alter alignment and movement patterns when integrated into movement practices and activities of daily living. It can also encourage a sense of spinal elongation and decrease compression of the atlantooccipital joint and cervical discs. Many students experience improved mental clarity, mood, and emotional expression and more presence as they repattern less than optimal cervical alignment and movement habits.

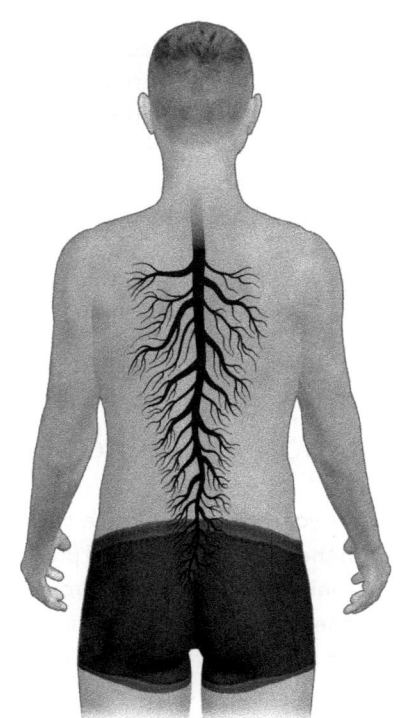

### Learning Objectives

- Access lower body support for the neck and head.

- Encourage sequential spinal movement in the cervical spine.

> When I visualize my neck rooted in my pelvis, movement feels safer and more controlled.
>
> *Gaby*

## Props

- A blanket folded into quarters, then rolled into an 11–15 cm (5–6 in.) cylinder, and a cushion

## Contraindications

- People with osteoporosis, osteoarthritis, neck or upper back injury, or vertigo should exercise caution, although this practice may be helpful in these conditions.

## Practice Notes

- Maintain connection between the anchored and moving ends throughout the movements.

- Sense the dynamic tension between the two ends throughout the movement.

- Maintain spaciousness at the atlantooccipital gate.

- Repeat each movement several times to access fascial continuities.

## SUPINE CURL

## Instructions

- Take a baseline reading in supine, noticing how your head and upper back rest on the floor. Place the blanket cylinder horizontally on the floor, then lie with the roll under your scapulae at the level of the armpits with the knees bent and feet parallel. Support your head with a cushion or decrease the size of the roll for comfort.

- Feel the pressure of the roll and invite your body to surrender and settle into the slight provocation. Do a minute of **Back Breathing**, directing inhalations where your body presses into the blanket, then exhaling and visualize your body draping over it.

- On exhalations, gently press your lower thoracic spine into the space between your pelvis and the roll. Release the pressure on inhalations.

  - *Can you isolate movement in the lower thoracic spine without extraneous movement in the pelvis or neck?*

- Clasp your hands behind your head. On exhalations, first press the lower thoracic spine into the space inferior to the roll, then move your elbows closer together and use your arm strength to lift your head and move it toward your knees, curling your upper spine.

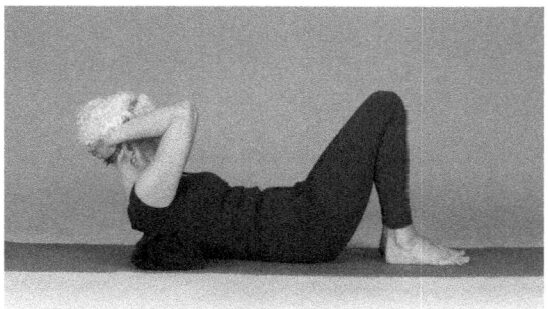

- As you inhale, slowly return to the starting position, reaching through the crown of your head to elongate the spine between the roll and crown. Imagine your neck is rooted into the blanket roll.

  - *Can you flex and extend from this root?*

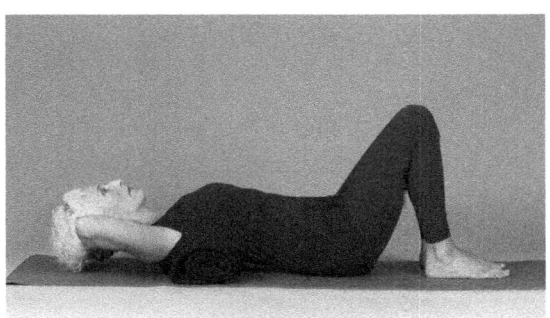

- To initiate cervical rotation from the root of the neck, repeat flexing the upper thoracic spine on an exhalation. From that position, inhale and widen your elbows to slightly extend your thoracic spine. On your next exhalation, rotate to the right, initiating movement from the thoracic root at the blanket roll and tracking the sequential spiralic movement into the head.

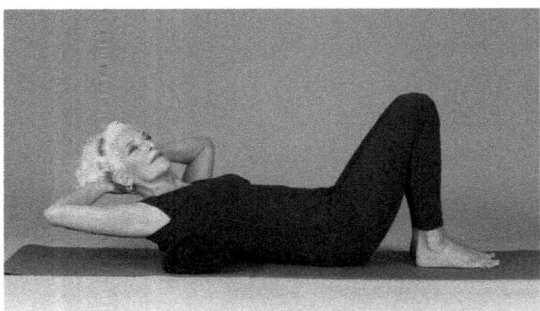

- Inhale and return to center, then repeat to the left before returning to the floor with your next exhalation.

  – *Is one side easier to rotate?*

- Now contrast initiating rotation from higher up at C2. Repeat the cervical rotation practice above but now visualize the bony ring of C1 rotating freely around the axial dens of C2. Track the sequential spiralic movement down to the thoracic root at the blanket roll.

  – *How are the two ways of initiating rotation different?*
  – *Do you have a preference?*
  – *How could you incorporate this awareness into your daily life? Looking at something beside or behind you? Noticing when you are literally headstrong in your movement?*

- Remove the blanket and pause to register any effects.

## COBRA POSE (BHUJANGASANA) 📹

### Instructions

- Unroll the blanket to a diameter that's comfortable when you lie prone with the roll placed across your ribs at the solar plexus. Place your palms on the floor at eye level on either side of your head, elbows tucked into your sides.

- Gently anchor your ribs into the blanket and imagine your neck rooted at the solar plexus. As you inhale, visualize a wave of breath moving from this root to the crown of your head while simultaneously pressing your hands into the floor and lifting your upper body into an easy Cobra pose. Use the breath wave to lengthen your spine and create dynamic tension between the root and crown. You can imagine the breath wave sequencing through the dens of C2.

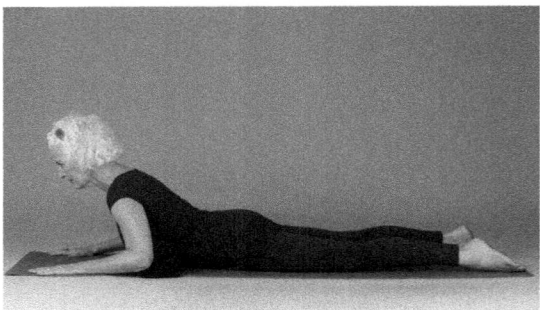

- Exhale and slowly return to the floor while maintaining the dynamic tension, then repeat several times.

- Move the blanket down to your groins. Gently press both pelvic crests into the blanket and imagine your neck is now rooted from your pelvis. As you move into Cobra, visualize a wave of breath sequencing from your pelvis to the crown of your head.

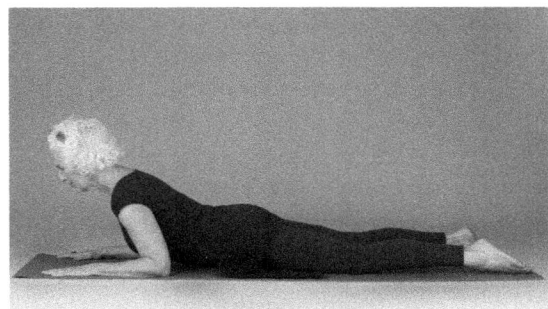

- Use the breath wave to lengthen your spine and create dynamic tension between the pelvis and crown.

- Exhale and slowly return to the floor while maintaining the dynamic tension.

- After several repetitions, remove the blanket.

- In the same starting position, now imagine your head and neck rooted from your feet. On an inhalation, gently press the tops of your feet into the floor. As you move into Cobra, visualize a wave of breath sequencing from your feet to the crown of your head. Use the breath wave visualization to lengthen your spine and create dynamic tension between the feet and crown.

- Turn onto your back to notice any effects, then stand and walk to notice further effects.

  - *What is felt sense of your neck now?*
  - *What else do you notice?*

## EXPLORATION: PASSIVE CERVICAL MOBILITY

In these explorations, you can sense fascial continuities by initiating movement in distal structures to passively move the neck and head. In the first exploration, you will move the pelvis to gently traction the neck. The rolled blanket under the neck "pins" cervical fascia so dynamic fascial tension is created as the pelvis moves in three planes. In the second exploration you will create dynamic tension with the arms.

### Learning Objectives

- Use dynamic tension to develop felt sense of fascial continuities.

- Release neck tension with passive movement.

### Props

- A soft blanket rolled into an 11 cm (5 in.) cylinder

### Practice Notes

- Notice your cervical curve alternately lengthening and compressing during the movements.

- Register dynamic tension between your anchored cervical spine and the moving part.

- Repeat each movement in the practice several times.

### PELVIC MOVEMENT

### Instructions

- Take a baseline in supine, noticing how your back body rests on the floor. Bend both knees with feet flat on the floor hip width apart. Place the rolled blanket behind your neck to support your cervical curve, filling the space from the top of your shoulders to the bottom of the occiput. Adjust the roll diameter so your face is parallel to the floor.

### Flexion and Extension

- On inhalations, gently press the midline of the sacrum into the floor, starting from the wide base at the top and slowly rolling down to the tip, increasing the lumbar curve and creating gentle traction in the neck.

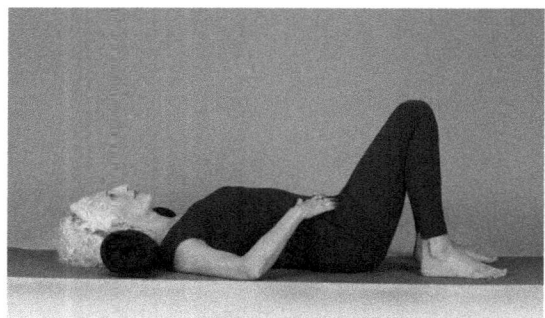

- On exhalations, reverse directions and gently press up the midline from tip to top, decreasing the lumbar curve and lengthening the cervical curve.

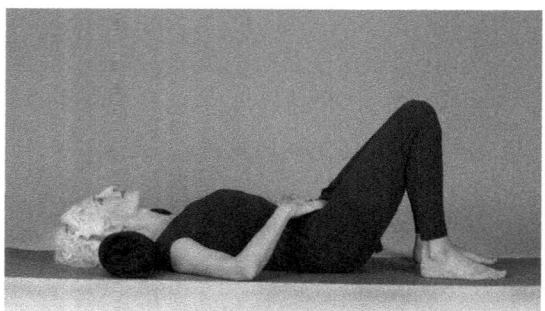

- Slowly rock back and forth several times, then pause to register sensations.

### Side Bend

- Sense your sitting bones and imagine a line from each to the corresponding heel.

- On exhalations, move your right sitting bone down the imaginary line toward the right heel, creating gentle neck traction. Return your sacrum to neutral on inhalations.

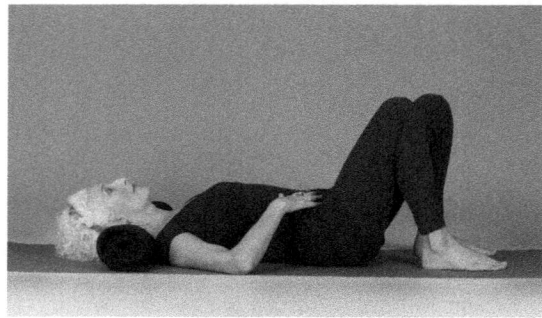

- Repeat several times, alternating sides, then pause to register sensations.

### Rotation

- Move your feet wider apart than your hips.

- On exhalations, move the right knee in a slow, controlled diagonal arc across your midline toward the left toes, creating gentle neck traction. Move to a comfortable range of motion.

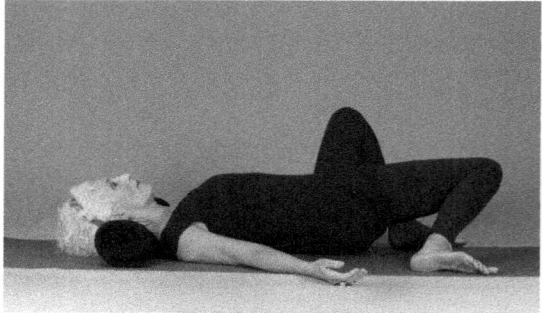

- Move your knee back to neutral position on inhalations.

- Repeat several times, alternating sides.

- Remove the blanket roll to register any differences from your baseline reading.

  - *What do you notice?*

## ARM MOVEMENT

### Instructions

- Still in supine position, move your arms into a T position.

- Slide your right arm further to the right as though you are reaching for something on the floor beyond your fingertips. Allow the movement to sequence into your neck and head, moving them passively. Feel the movement pulling into the root of the neck.

  - *Can you allow your neck and head to be moved passively?*

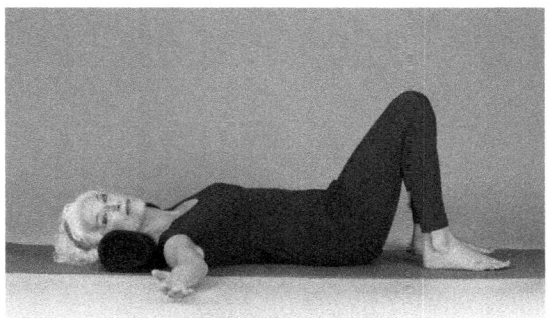

- Reach the left arm along the floor, sliding it sideways until your neck and head are pulled to the left.

- Alternate reaching the arms to each side. Vary the speed; start slowly and, if you can release resistance and allow your neck to be moved with ease, explore faster movement. If it's challenging to let go of control, stay with slower movement.

- Sit or stand to register effects of these movements.

  - *What do you notice?*

## EXPLORATION: HEAD TO KNEE POSE (JANU SIRSASANA), TWO WAYS

### Learning Objective

- Explore different ways of balancing cervical alignment in forward bends.

### Instructions

- Sit on the floor with both legs extended. Bend your left knee and place the sole of your foot comfortably on the right inner leg. Support your pelvis or knee, if necessary, for comfort and alignment. Take a baseline reading of your usual way of doing an easy forward bend.

- Do the following explorations on both sides.

### *Occipital Gate*

- Sitting upright, place one finger on your occipital gate at the **atlantooccipital joint** and find neutral head posture.

- On an exhalation, slowly move your spine forward a short distance, bending from your hip joints without rounding your spine.

- Pause as you inhale, then breath by breath, continue incrementally to move your spine to a comfortable end range. Monitor tissue tension at the occipital gate and stop as soon you feel the gate closing.

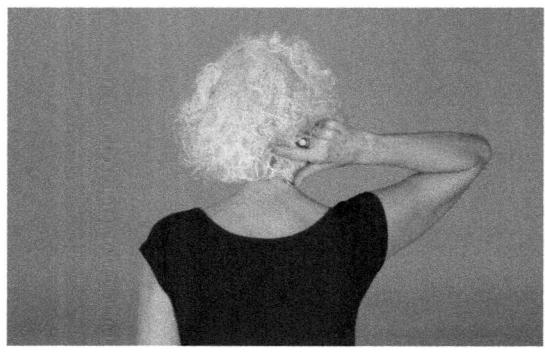

- *How does your range of motion compare to baseline?*

### Hyoid Lift

- Repeat the forward bend using the hyoid lift to elongate the spine and maintain spinal alignment.

- In the starting position, place your thumb and index finger on the hyoid, then allow your body to slump into a forward head posture.

- On an inhalation, gently guide your hyoid diagonally up and back toward the atlanto-occipital joint, following the angle of your jaw. Go back and forth between the forward head posture and the hyoid lift.

  - *Can you feel your spine elongating?*

- On an exhalation, slowly move your spine forward a short distance, bending from your hip joints. Repeat the back and forth forward head posture and hyoid lift in this position.

- Move your spine forward incrementally, pausing in each position to repeat the practice until you reach your comfortable end range.

  - *Which practice for finding cervical alignment is most accessible to you?*

## EXPLORATION: MOVING WITH WEIGHT ON THE HEAD

Most attempts to correct posture are directed toward the spine, shoulders, and pelvis. All are important, but head position takes precedence over all others. The body follows the head. Therefore, the entire body is best aligned by first restoring proper functional alignment to the head.

*Dr. Rene Cailliet and Leonard Gross (1987)*

Visualize the graceful movement and balanced-head posture of indigenous women walking with baskets on their head. Reaching through the crown to carry a weight causes a corresponding lengthening of the spine that can, ironically, decompress spinal discs and optimize head and neck alignment. This posture activates the deep neck flexors that support and stabilize the anterior cervical spine, encouraging superficial muscles to relinquish control.

### Learning Objective

- Find optimal head alignment in standing.

### Props

- A 0.5 kg (1 lb.) bag of grain, beans, or flour tied into a tea towel in a roundish shape

### Instructions

- Stand comfortably upright with the bag at hand. Find a neutral head position by using the **hyoid lift**, **rooting the neck** or **occipital**

**gate** awareness. Balance the bag on top of your head.

- Use your breath to relax any excess tension. Notice what structures you need to activate or inhibit to balance the bag comfortably and with ease.

- Walk around the room.

- Practice a few standing yoga poses like Warrior 1 and 2 (Virabhadrasana 1 and 2) or balance poses like Tree (Vrkasana). Don't worry if the bag falls off!

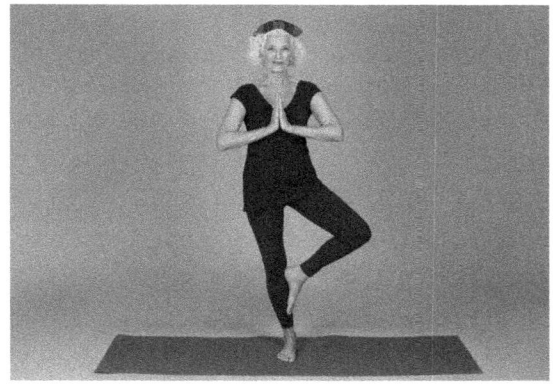

- Remove the bag and notice any effects of the practice.

    - *How are the poses different?*

## FOUNDATIONAL PRACTICE: WITNESS CONSCIOUSNESS ◀))

Forward head posture not only creates muscular imbalance but can shift consciousness into the frontal brain. When you habitually occupy this thinking, judging part of the brain, you tend to be less present, more analytical, or "stuck in your head." It may be challenging to connect with your body sense.

Witness consciousness is a yogic concept describing a sustained state of presence to what is occurring internally and externally, observing compassionately without reactivity or judgment. Practicing Witness consciousness teaches us neutrality and detached awareness of projections and habitual ways of reacting. We can consciously cultivate a state of equanimity, saying, *Isn't that interesting?* to whatever arises. The more we practice, the more we can rest in a state of neutral Witness, abiding in moment-to-moment experience and acknowledging the bigger picture. When life becomes chaotic, the Witness abides in the stillness at the eye of the storm.

The Witness can be accessed by consciously shifting awareness from the busy frontal brain toward the back of the head. The atlantooccipital joint provides a tangible physical location to experience the Witness.

### Learning Objective

- Establish a physical "homebase" for Witness consciousness.

### Instructions

- In a comfortable seated position, spend a few minutes exploring the tiny movements of flexion, extension, side bending, and figure 8 at the atlantooccipital joint. Sense the deep origin of the movements. It may be helpful to place the tip of your tongue on the roof of the soft palate.

- Once again, imagine the lines between your ears, and between eyebrows and occiput. Close your eyes and situate your consciousness at the intersection of these lines deep inside your head. Settle there like you're nestling into a comfortable, familiar easy chair. Some people like visualizing their mind resting into a bowl. Breathe calmly and regularly. With each exhalation, sink your consciousness deeper into the abode of the Witness. Settle into the stillness.

- *What feels different when you situate your awareness here?*
- *How does your state of mind shift?*
- *Does your breath change?*

• Explore some mental "gymnastics" so you can easily replicate the physical location of Witness. Shift your consciousness to the following places, lingering for a few moments to register your feeling and mental state in each place. Return your awareness to the atlantooccipital joint between each mental movement.

• Shift awareness to your forehead, the top of your head, 30 cm (12 in.) in front of your forehead, 30 cm (12 in. above your head, 30

cm (12 in.) behind your head, and back to the atlantooccipital joint. Pause to register any effects of the practice.

- *Which place felt most familiar?*
- *How did your state of mind change in each location? Your breath?*

• To integrate Witness consciousness in your yoga, meditation, or movement practice, purposely situate your consciousness at the atlantooccipital joint. Then, incorporate this perspective in everyday activities like taking walks, preparing a meal, or having a conversation.

- *How do these activities change when you remain in Witness?*
- *How does your perception and response change?*
- *Where else could you practice Witness consciousness?*

## THERAPEUTIC APPLICATIONS

The head neck, and jaw are at the mercy of multidimensional forces extending beyond the usual physical culprits of gravity, injury, and habitual use (or disuse). Trauma, mental health, cultural patterning, and suboptimal breathing can also contribute to postural adaptation, pain, and imbalanced tension and compression forces. These compensations anywhere in the body often have negative repercussions at the top of the kinetic chain (Rubenstein 2010). Finding ease and balance in the head and neck through EA practices addresses these responses and generates positive mind and body-wide outcomes, including modulating excessive tension and shifting mental perspective through sympathetic downregulation and increased vagal tone. Application of the koshic model broadens

the range of potential therapeutic resources by exploring head and neck issues from a whole-body, whole-person perspective.

Chronic neck pain has been associated with an array of conditions, ranging from headaches, decreased cerebral blood flow, compromised breath, and shoulder, upper back, and arm pain. The continuity and interrelationships in the physical body create the possibility of positive change at the top of the kinetic chain by addressing distal structures, and vice versa. Even mouth and jaw dysfunction has been linked to global posture, stability, and physical performance (Moon and Lee 2011). The continuities of kinetic chains are highlighted when interventions such as breath repatterning improve both respiratory and cervical function, suboccipital fascial release improves hamstring flexibility, or lower limb stretching increases cervical range of motion (Harneet and Maman 2019; Joshi, Balthillaya, and Prabhu 2018; Wilke *et al.*, 2017). Further, thoracic spine mobilization was demonstrated to be more effective for neck pain than targeted cervical spine mobilization and stabilization exercises (Cho, Lee, and Lee 2017). Everything is connected.

As the conduit for vital neurovascular structures, head and neck integrity are key to optimal innervation and circulation of multiple anatomical structures and physiological systems. Cervical pain is a risk factor for impaired upper-limb function leading to pain and sensory deficit (Alreni *et al.*, 2017). Even digestion can be affected if mechanical pressure from excessive tension and decreased elasticity in the cervical region compresses the vagus nerve and causes uncomfortable stomach symptoms. Not surprisingly, symptoms can diminish when cervical soft tissue is relaxed (Ozel Asliyuce *et al.*, 2020).

Research correlations between pain and cervical misalignment are variable. Some studies found spinal cord and nerve root tension, pain, disability, poor health, and quality of life associated with neck, jaw, and pelvic misalignment, while others found no association (Grob, Frauenfelder, and Mannion 2007; McAviney *et al.*, 2005). Forward head posture research is also inconclusive. Some research finds no correlation, whereas association has been made in adults but not in children (Correia *et al.*, 2021; Mahmoud *et al.*, 2019). It may be more productive to view neck and head pain or dysfunction as resulting from a constellation of biopsychosocial factors that include stress levels, self-perception, and anxiety or depression (Kim *et al.*, 2018; Parikh and Amarnath 2021).

Rather than imposing concepts of "correct alignment," EA practices give us agency to explore which positions, movements, and mental practices lead to safe, sustainable, and comfortable function. This awareness can be translated into day-to-day activities and ways of being. Habitual ways of taking a drink of water, chopping vegetables, or doing a shoulder check while driving can be transformed into sustainable practices connecting us to the present moment.

## KOSHIC CONTEMPLATIONS

### Annamaya Kosha

- *How has felt sense of your cervical spine changed after doing EA practices?*
- *Have you noticed differences in alignment, stability, or ease in your head and neck?*
- *How does the quality of movement change when you initiate movement from your cervical spine?*
- *How have you incorporated your new awareness into daily activities and physical practice?*

### Pranamaya Kosha

- *How do your breath and energy levels change with optimal neck and head integrity and balance between stability and mobility?*
- *Have other physiological functions improved as you restore integrity to this area—digestion, sleep, nervous system arousal, vocalization?*

### Manomaya Kosha

- *Have you noticed any changes in sensory function?*

- *As you repattern integrity in the cervical spine, have you experienced changes in emotional expression?*
- *Do you feel less stressed?*

## Vijnanamaya Kosha

- *How do your perceptions and responses change when you establish Witness consciousness?*

- *How does your head and neck position reflect your personality and conditioning?*

## Anandamaya Kosha

- *Is it easier to access your inner stillness by situating your consciousness at the atlantooccipital joint?*
- *Have you experienced more flow in your life?*

## KEY CONCEPTS

- The cervical spine developed as vertebrates emerged from the ocean to navigate on land.
- The head-righting reflex activates muscular actions to maintain eyes level with the horizon.
- On a subtle level, the neck is a multidimensional gate between mind and body, head and heart, and thoughts and emotions.
- Habitual neck, jaw, and shoulder tension can affect breathing patterns, energy level, and mental clarity.
- Excessive neck tension can compromise sensory data quality and impair proprioception and motor control.
- The hyoid bone and associated myofascia function in eating, breathing, and vocalization.
- Initiating movement from C1 and C2 activates deep stabilizing musculature and prevents overuse of superficial muscles.
- Visualizing the neck rooted in lower body structures accesses new sources of support and alters alignment and movement patterns.
- The atlantooccipital joint can be viewed as a gate allowing blood, cerebrospinal fluid, neural impulses, and prana to flow freely.
- EA practices can establish a physical "home" for Witness consciousness.

## CHAPTER 11

# The Shoulder and Arm: Giving and Receiving

*It was an empty gesture.*
*He has a cross to bear.*
*She has a chip on her shoulder.*
*I squared my shoulders and carried on.*

The intelligent design of our shoulders and arms allows us to accomplish complex daily tasks and manifest creative intention in the world. On a physical level, the shoulder girdle participates in an integrated system that enables our arms to move in a wide range of motion. Our hands grasp and manipulate objects in the environment to meet basic survival needs—we build homes, perform work, feed ourselves, and tend our children. Once essential survival needs are met, we can create art and music. On more subtle levels, our arms reach out to embrace, push away, give a helping hand, or receive precious gifts. The type and quality of our gestures can sensitively (or aggressively!) communicate intentions and inner processes.

The human shoulder girdle evolved from the pectoral and pelvic fins of primitive fish after emerging from the sea to crawl on land (Cloutier *et al.*, 2020). In their evolution into weight-bearing appendages, fins migrated toward the midline, lifting the torso off the ground and enabling biomechanical efficiency and speedier movement. Eventually semiupright posture liberated the front limbs of our early ancestors from weight-bearing and locomotion functions to enable them to manually interact with the environment. When survival demanded greater range of motion and strength, we evolved the ability to reach overhead to access food and throw weapons to hunt. An opposing thumb developed to give us dexterity for tasks like making tools and picking fruit. Anthropologists speculate that upright posture and using the arms to forage, grasp, and throw objects led to a significant leap in human evolution (Young 2003). As our ancestors stood upright, the clavicles gradually widened and scapulae moved posteriorly, orienting the shoulder joint laterally (Grine, Fleagle, and Leakey 2009). These changes engineered the most mobile joint in the body, enabling an almost complete circular movement. However, increased mobility evolved at the expense of stability; it's not difficult to dislocate the shoulder. Despite an impressive capacity for omnidirectional movement, we tend to gesture and use our arms in limited movement repertoires. EA explorations can repattern comfortable, strong, and integrated shoulder movement that capitalizes on this innate range of motion.

## KOSHIC PERSPECTIVES

In annamaya kosha, we explore the nature and function of the shoulder girdle and upper limb as a functional unit interacting with the spine, rib basket, and pelvis. As a structure suspended within a tensional myofascial network, shoulder girdle orientation is easily compromised by imbalanced tension and compression forces impacting integration of the shoulders with the spine and rib basket. Although the shoulder girdle is usually experienced as a mobile structure, it must have adequate stability for effective motor control and safe sequencing of force and weight. EA explorations utilizing nonhabitual, component, and micro-movements can alter sensorimotor maps to reawaken optimal movement and stability patterns, alignment, and integration of the upper limb and core body.

Working with pranamaya kosha, we explore energetic connections between the lungs, heart, and arms (see Chapter 5) and how to use breath to reinforce arm connections to the midline. We also experience how clear sequencing of force between the torso and arms can minimize excessive compression and maximize strength.

We access manomaya kosha to notice our habitual alignment and movement patterns and how chronic tension causes the shoulders to creep up to our ears. We observe how our shoulders reflect emotional states: curving forward to protect a hurting heart, drooping in defeat, or rigidly communicating aggression. We may discover how chronically unexpressed emotions or impulses to action can translate into restricted movement. We may also experience the physiological relationships between shoulder position, breath, and cardiac function.

The sensory aspect of manomaya kosha is well represented in the upper limb. The hands are one of the most richly innervated parts of the body. They can masterfully yield a surgeon's knife or craft fine art. This dense innervation renders the hands extremely sensitive to tactile stimuli, enabling us to interpret a loving touch or determine the ripeness of fruit.

The shoulders and arms can reflect the content of vijnanamaya kosha. Our history, beliefs, psychological stance, and embodied metaphors may be expressed in shoulder posture and the quality, force, and sensitivity of arm movements. Deeply ingrained habits of giving and receiving can also influence how we hold and use our shoulders and arms. We can easily identify people carrying the weight of the world on their shoulders or recognize confidence and inner strength in those with relaxed shoulders and open, soft chests. Using buddhi mind, we get curious about how our inner world affects our shoulder position, and formulate an intention to explore working with our shoulders from both inside out and outside in. EA explorations can free the natural impulses of the shoulder girdle to appropriately reach out, hold onto, push away, give, take, and receive with ease.

> My frozen shoulder completely resolved after unsuccessful treatments once I realized I didn't want to let go of my precious daughter before she started university.
>
> *Lea*

When working with anandamaya kosha, shoulders and arms can be viewed as means for manifesting spiritual values in the world. One way of describing the relationship between the spiritual and material worlds is the concept of the human cross. The vertical axis represents the "human pole" connecting the cosmos and earth, and the horizontal axis represents interaction with the material world through thoughts, words, and actions, with the heart at their intersection. If we stay connected to the heart through the shoulders and arms as we act in the world, our actions will reflect spiritual values. As we interact with the world, we can practice staying connected to the heart and vertical axis both energetically and physically. Our actions may be more compassionate, and our compassion will be engaged in the wider world.

## LEARN IT

The shoulder girdle is a support structure for the arms formed by bones that encircle yet are detached from the ribs. This upper limb girdle is both suspended and supported. It's suspended from a circle formed by the sternum and first ribs and suspended within a tensional fascial network continuous with the sternum, spine, cranium, and trunk. This top-down suspended arrangement ensures that delicate neurovascular structures and organs are protected from excessive compression or shock. Bottom-up support for the shoulder girdle is provided by the spine, pelvis, organs, and ground. Accessing this support through EA practices can reorient and strengthen shoulder and arm movement efficiency; less physical energy is required with support from below (McMullen and Uhl 2000). Felt sense of upper suspension and lower support can alter habitual alignment and movement patterns and balance dysregulated tension and compression forces that overburden the shoulder joints.

### Bones

The shoulder girdle enables integrated and energy-efficient movement of the arms in the same way the pelvic girdle enables leg movement. The upper girdle consists of two clavicles (collarbones) joined at the sternum and two scapulae (shoulder blades) containing rounded sockets for the ball of the humerus (upper arm bone). These bones form a "yoke" from which the arms hang, reminiscent of shoulder yokes used historically for carrying loads. The upper limb bones also echo the arrangement of the lower limb.

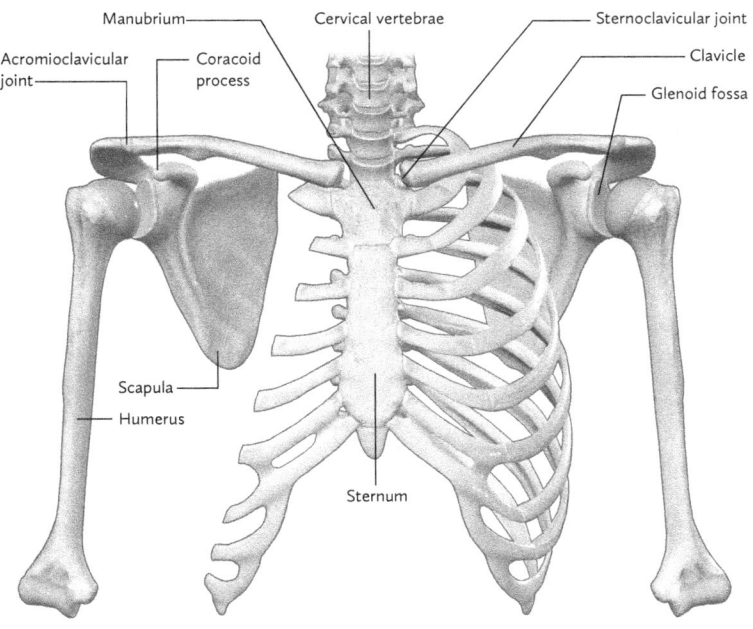

Manubrium — Cervical vertebrae — Sternoclavicular joint

Acromioclavicular joint — Coracoid process — Clavicle

Glenoid fossa

Scapula

Humerus

Sternum

### CLAVICLES

The spiralic, S-shaped clavicles link the sternum and scapulae. Curiously, clavicles are the first bones to begin ossification, normally in the sixth embryonic week, and among the last bones to fully ossify in the 20s (Schwartz 1995). This early ossification may reflect the strong shoulder support required for our ancestors to locomote in trees (Stuart Macadam 2023). Clavicles function as struts, extending the arms laterally and enabling wide and efficient range of movement. This arrangement both stabilizes the shoulders when the arms are moving dynamically and supports the weight of the body when weight-bearing or hanging from the arms. Embodying the width of the clavicles through EA practices can encourage this full and efficient movement.

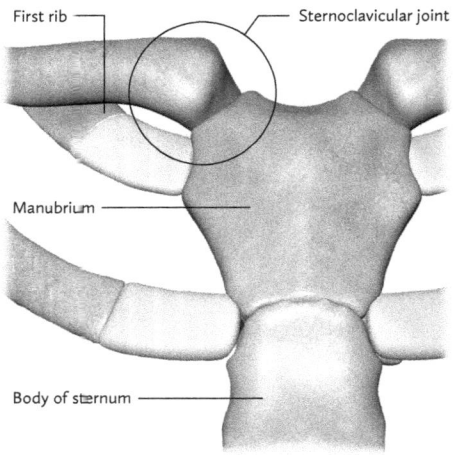

Surprisingly, the only articulation between the arms and the rest of the skeleton is between the clavicle and sternum. To compensate for this singular bony connection, the shoulder girdle is reinforced by an extensive fascial network interweaving the arms and torso. These sternoclavicular joints are synovial, gliding joints between the clavicles, sternum, and first rib cartilage. Their shape permits spiralic clavicular movement, enabling greater arm movement range. The cartilaginous discs in the joints absorb force when the arms bear weight. Awareness of these joints gained through EA explorations can significantly alter how we sense and move our arms and shoulders. Gestures and other arm movements are freer, stronger, and more integrated when initiated from the sternoclavicular joint at the midline.

### STERNUM

See Chapter 3 for the structure and function of the sternum.

### SCAPULAE

The complex three-dimensional scapulae form shallow sockets for each humeral head and provide a protective overhang for the shoulder joints. As the link between the arms and torso, the scapulae play significant dual roles in shoulder stabilization and movement. The large flattish triangular bones conform to the roundness of the ribs, then flare and thicken superiorly to form three-dimensional structures: a scapular spine, a bony trough (superspinatus fossa), and the acromion and coracoid processes. The acromion is the bony shelf on the lateral scapular spine, joining the clavicle at the acromioclavicular joint, a synovial, gliding joint with a cartilaginous disc. The coracoid process projects forward from the bony trough like a crow's beak, emerging inferior to the clavicle to anchor muscle attachments.

The shoulder sockets are formed by the scapulae. The principal joints of the shoulder girdle, the glenohumeral joints are ball and socket joints formed by the half sphere of each humerus and the shallow socket of each scapula. Although capable of wide ranges of movement, these joints are inherently unstable due to the shallow vertical socket. Stability is significantly increased by surrounding ligaments, myofascia, and the ring-shaped fibrocartilage disc of the labrum deepening the sockets. Upper limb mobility and flexibility triumph over stability in contrast to the lower limbs, where stability prevails.

Each scapula is designed to slide freely over the ribs to assist arm mobility. Although no bony connection exists between the scapulae and ribs, this functional articulation is described as the scapulothoracic joint. Orthopedic surgeon and biotensegrity authority Stephen Levin describes the scapula as a "sesamoid bone" floating on the chest wall in a tensional meshwork of shoulder girdle myofascia. He suggests that forces are transferred between the arms and axial skeleton through myofascia attached to the scapulae rather than through bone (Levin 1997).

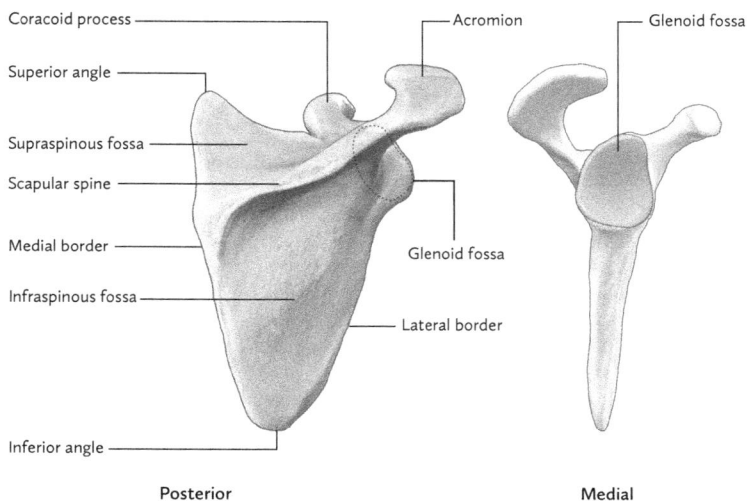

Coracoid process
Superior angle
Supraspinous fossa
Scapular spine
Medial border
Infraspinous fossa
Inferior angle
Acromion
Glenoid fossa
Glenoid fossa
Lateral border

Posterior                              Medial

### ARM AND HAND BONES

Our arms and hands evolved from fins and paws and from primarily weight-bearing appendages to ones capable of highly refined dexterity. The humerus, ulna, and radius reflect this evolutionary development of structures highly specialized for manipulation and fine coordination. The humerus is the longest bone of the upper limb and forms joints at the shoulder and elbow. The forearm bones, the radius on thumb side and ulna on little finger side, articulate with each other at both ends, with the humerus at the elbow and with delicate carpal bones at the wrist. The radius and ulna are linked by a fibrous interosseous membrane that increases surface area available for numerous forearm muscles and stabilizes and transfers force between the two bones. The ulna is larger and more functional at the elbow joint, while the radius is larger at the wrist joint. The radius moves around the ulna in spiralic movements of supination and pronation.

The eight irregularly shaped carpal bones glide over each other to enable multidimensional wrist mobility. They form the carpal tunnel, a bony arch containing and protecting tendons, nerves, and blood vessels. Multiple joints between the carpal bones, five metacarpal bones, and 14 phalanges allow intricate and finely coordinated hand movements.

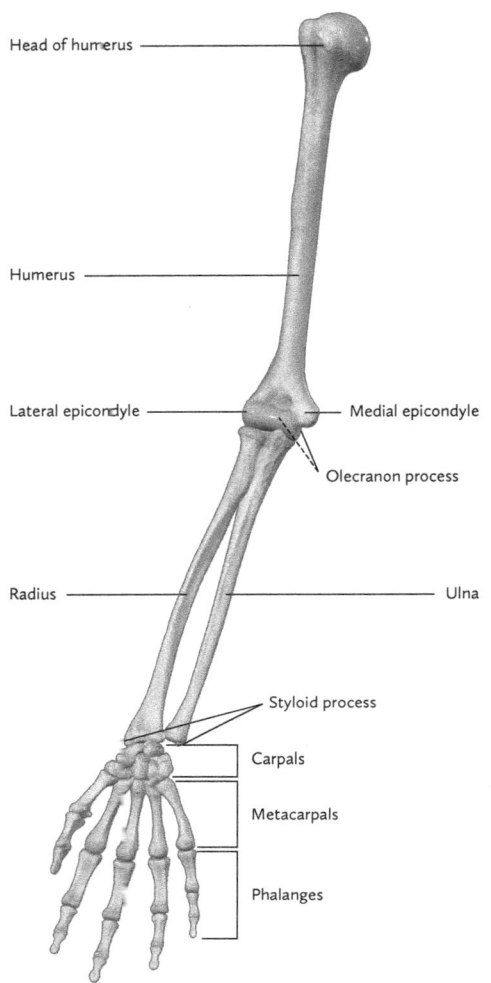

Head of humerus

Humerus

Lateral epicondyle — Medial epicondyle

Olecranon process

Radius — Ulna

Styloid process

Carpals

Metacarpals

Phalanges

arrangement of approximately 50 muscles (!) in each upper limb orchestrates stability, motor control, and range of motion (Sweigard 1974). In movement repatterning, it's helpful to differentiate myofascia that stabilizes the humerus in the glenohumeral joint from myofascia that moves the shoulder and that moves the scapula. This extensive myofascial network interweaves with the forearm and hand, enabling extraordinary manual dexterity and delicate motor control.

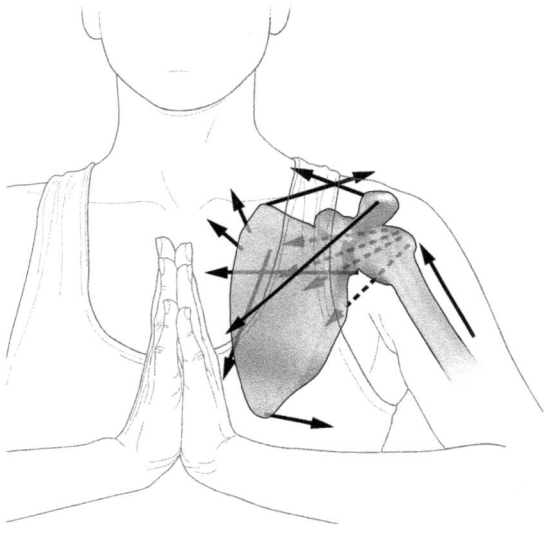

The presence of abundant myofascia with competing directional pulls contributes to the rarity of balanced shoulder alignment. The scapulae floating in the tensional myofascial mesh are the main determinants of shoulder position. Fascial imbalances pull them in the direction of greatest tension, changing glenohumeral joint orientation and setting the stage for restricted movement and injury. This forces other structures to "shoulder" the burden. Shoulder function can be further compromised by emotional tension and other stressors, including distal misalignment patterns, repetitive movements, and faulty biomechanics. The common forward head posture is one example. As shoulders elevate and anteriorly rotate, the chest collapses and the shoulder sockets are

## Myofascia

The shoulder girdle interweaves with the trunk and midline through an array of myofascia, enabling the arm to move with delicacy or strength and to absorb strong forces before they sequence into the trunk and its delicate organ contents. Diagonal myofascial continuities, termed *functional lines*, link arms to legs both anteriorly and posteriorly, conferring greater stability and power to arm movements (Myers 2009).

As an inherently unstable joint, the shoulder relies on surrounding ligaments and myofascia to provide stability and protection. A complex reoriented, compromising arm movement, stability, and strength. As the shoulder girdle loses its suspensory support and collapses onto the ribs, neurovascular structures are compressed, and rib movement and breath are restricted. Supple and balanced myofascia allows the shoulders to move freely and absorb and transmit appropriate force and energy so we can breathe fully and express ourselves effectively in the world.

## Movement

The remarkable mobility of the glenohumeral joint is enabled by its shape, orientation, and support along with the coordination of other shoulder girdle joints. These include the "true" sternoclavicular and acromioclavicular joints and the functional scapulothoracic joints. "True" joints are surrounded by joint capsules and numerous ligaments that stabilize, create integrity, guide, and limit movement. Without the scapulae sliding on the ribs or gliding clavicular movements at the sternum and acromion, complete range of motion at the glenohumeral joints would be impossible. Range of motion is optimized by component rolling and gliding joint movements.

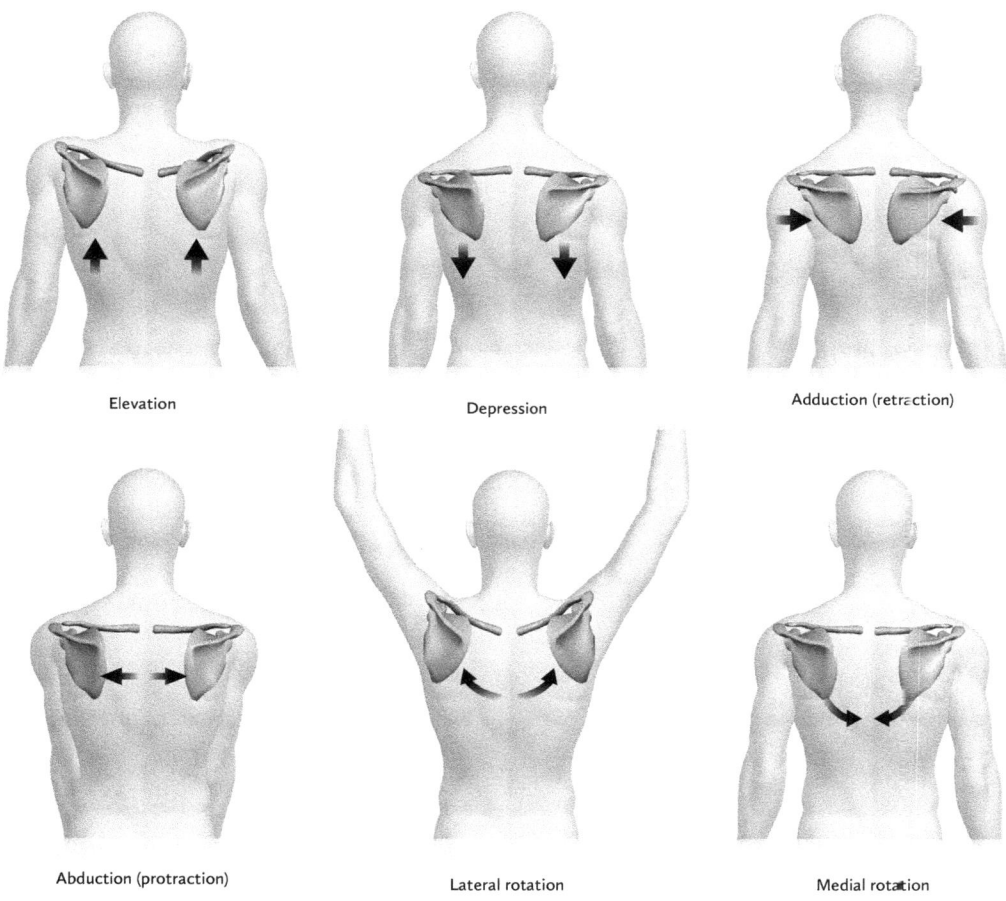

Elevation

Depression

Adduction (retraction)

Abduction (protraction)

Lateral rotation

Medial rotation

Differentiating movement of the clavicle, scapula, and humerus has therapeutic benefits, particularly when students habitually move the shoulder complex as an undifferentiated "clump" or have been given misleading movement cues. Optimal upper limb function can be repatterned through EA practices when each structure is distinguished and students explore moving from individual bones.

Coordinated movement of the shoulder girdle joints efficiently positions and orients the sockets for maximum stability and movement range. The functional scapulothoracic joints enable scapulohumeral rhythm, which is coupled scapular and arm movement that enables 180 degrees of arm elevation. For every two degrees of elevation at the glenohumeral joint, the scapulae laterally rotate and slide on the ribs approximately one degree (with some individual variation). Scapulohumeral rhythm may be distorted by myofascial imbalances or structural changes in the spine, ribs, and shoulder girdle

joints. For example, excessive thoracic kyphosis changes the orientation of the glenohumeral joints which compromises shoulder mobility.

The scapulae can move in opposing directions of elevation and depression, protraction and retraction, and lateral (upward) and medial (downward) rotation. Developing felt sense of these movements through EA practices can improve strength, efficiency, and integration in shoulder movements.

Of the primates, humans have the most complex, finely tuned hand and wrist structure, including an opposable thumb. We can dexterously interact with other people and the environment as well as hold and manipulate objects, grasping them in whatever orientation is necessary for finely skilled tasks like threading a needle.

## FEEL IT

### EXPLORATION: DISCOVER YOUR SHOULDER AND ARMS

#### Learning Objectives

- Map anatomical structures in the upper limb.

- Deepen felt sense of the bones and myofascia of the shoulders and arms.

#### Instructions

- In a comfortable seated position, sense your shoulders and arms to establish a baseline reading. Then, place your left fingers on the right sternoclavicular joint.

#### Clavicle

- Explore contours of the protrusion on the clavicular part of the joint. Notice how the clavicle sits atop the sternum.

- With your fingers on the joint, move your shoulder up and down, forward and back,

and in circles. Feel the corresponding hinging movements at the joint.

- Slowly and sensitively explore the curved superior, inferior, anterior, and posterior clavicular surfaces, gradually moving your fingers laterally.

- When you arrive at the lateral end, palpate the protrusion and slight depression indicating the acromioclavicular joint.

- To sense how the clavicles contribute to arm movement, hook your fingers on the superior clavicle and hold it down as you raise your arm a few times. Then, release your grip and raise your arm again, noticing differences in the range of motion and quality of movement.

### Scapula

- Shift your fingers more laterally to feel the flat horizontal surface of the acromion at the shoulder. Palpate its size and shape.

- Find the anterior "ledge" of the acromion and follow its contours posteriorly, moving your fingertips up and down to palpate the sharp edge to the posterior corner where it transitions into the scapular spine. Continue palpating the horizontal spine to its medial edge.

- Press your fingers into the bulky soft tissue filling the superspinatus fossa (bony trough).

- Slide your fingers off the edge of the scapular spine to find the medial border of the scapula. Move your scapula to confirm that you are on the medial border. Follow it inferiorly as far as you can reach.

- Place your hand underneath your armpit to locate the pointed inferior angle of the scapula, then move your fingers back and forth to walk up the lateral border to the armpit. It may be obscured by soft tissue so moving your scapula will again help to locate the edge. Reach further back to place the palm of your hand on the flat surface of the scapula and gently press your fingers through the soft tissue to explore the expanse of bone.

- Place your fingers on the soft "pocket" of tissue in the anterior shoulder below the lateral end of the clavicle. Move your right arm backward in extension to feel the bony coracoid process protrude into your fingers.

### Upper Arm

- Move your fingertips back to the acromion, then slide off the ledge onto the head of the humerus. Raise your arm up and down a few times to feel your fingers being carried by the movement of the humerus. Then, palpate the roundness of the humeral head and differentiate the "guitar strings" of muscle tendons.

- Moving down the arm, palpate through the overlying myofascia to the anterior, posterior, medial, and lateral surfaces of the humeral shaft. You may need to infer the shape through the overlying soft tissue.

- Palpate the shaft inferiorly as it flares into the pointy medial and lateral epicondyles at the elbow. Explore the angular geography of the epicondyles.

### Forearm

- With your right palm facing upward and arm slightly bent, palpate the pointed olecranon process of the ulna at the elbow joint.

- With a pincer grip formed by the left hand, stabilize your right olecranon process. Pronate and supinate your forearm to sense the spiralic movement of the radius around the ulna.

- Slide medially and inferiorly off the olecranon process to locate the sharp edge of the ulna. Move your fingers back and forth across the edge, following the long, straight shaft toward the wrist to the protuberance at the distal end of the ulna, the styloid process.

- Move to the thumb side of the wrist to palpate the angular styloid process of the radius. Follow the shaft of the radius toward the elbow, moving back and forth across the edge. The bulk of myofascia may prevent you from palpating the entire length of the shaft.

- To map the fascial septum between radius and ulna, use a pincer grip above the wrist with the thumb on the inner arm and fingers on the outer arm. Sensitively compress the overlying myofascia between the thumb and fingers and imagine them slowly sinking through the tissue to meet at the septum (remember the **cornstarch play**). Repeat the compressions at several places on the forearm through the increasingly bulkier myofascia.

### Wrist and Hand

- Move your fingers and thumb to palpate the eight irregularly shaped carpal bones distal to the styloid processes. Feel the contours of the two rows of bones that are approximately two finger widths across.

- Hold the carpals lightly and move your wrist multidirectionally. Feel the carpal bones rolling shifting, and gliding against each other.

- To sense how the radius, ulna, and carpals contribute to wrist movement, first move your wrist in all directions. Then, encircle and stabilize the radius and ulna above the wrist with your left hand, then move your wrist again. Finally, stabilize the carpal bones between your thumb and fingers while moving your wrist.

  - *How does the range of movement change?*

- Use your thumb on the palm and fingers on the back of the right hand to palpate the shafts of the metacarpals. Grasp and move each metacarpal back and forth to differentiate it from its neighbours. Then, gently press into the spaces between the metacarpals to feel the myofascia.

- Spend a little time palpating and moving each phalange (three in each finger and two in the thumb) passively in all three planes.

- Pause to notice differences between the two sides, then explore a few arm movements.

  - *What is felt sense of your right shoulder girdle and upper limb after mapping it?*
  - *How does your movement change?*

- Repeat the exploration on the left side.

## EXPLORATION: ARM BONE CORE 📹

I taught bone core to a patient with relentless chronic pain from a broken humerus on top of thoracic outlet syndrome. Her pain decreased 50 percent after one treatment and she slept well for the first time in weeks. The improvement continued with daily self-treatment.

*Bobbie, a chiropractor*

### Learning Objectives

- Differentiate bone from surrounding myofascia and sense continuities between them.

- Deepen and clarify neural maps.

### Instructions

This exploration may be done individually or in partners.

- Sit in a comfortable position with your right hand resting in your lap.

- Encircle your right upper arm firmly with your left hand and visualize the bony "core" of the humerus surrounded by a "sleeve" of soft tissue. A partner would use both hands to encircle the upper arm.

- Use firm pressure to roll the myofascial

sleeve laterally around the bone core. Sensitively move the flesh enough to sense tension spiralling through the fascia from skin into bone (recall **Exploration: Fascial Palpation** in Chapter 4), then release your pressure. Roll the sleeve back and forth several times without moving the humerus.

- Adjust your hand to repeat the exploration, rolling the myofascial sleeve medially.

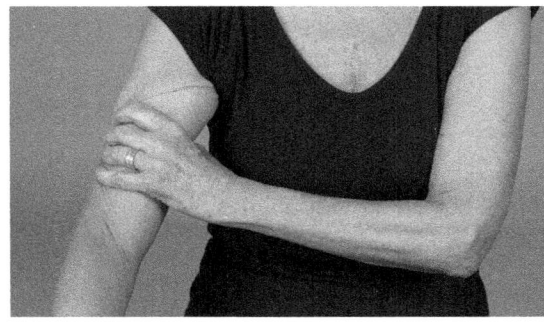

- Roll the myofascial sleeve laterally again, then initiate a subtle, almost imperceptible

movement from the bone core, internally rotating the humerus to create more dynamic tension between the two structures. Hold the tension for a few seconds, then stop the bone movement and check if the myofascial sleeve moves a little more laterally. Take up any available slack in the tissue, and, from this new place of dynamic tension between the structures, repeat the process.

- – *Can you sense the continuity between the bone and myofascia?*
- – *Can you feel a myofascial release as you hold the tension?*

- Repeat the process, rolling the myofascial sleeve medially and the bone core laterally.

- Repeat the process on additional places on the upper arm and forearm.

- Pause to notice any differences between the two arms.

## EXPLORATION: COMPONENT MOVEMENT

As the arm elevates in either flexion or abduction, the humeral head rolls superiorly and glides inferiorly to remain centered in the socket. Visualization and felt sense of these movements can alter maladaptive movement patterns.

### Learning Objective

- Explore component movements of roll and glide during shoulder elevation.

### Instruction

- Either seated or standing, set a baseline by flexing, then abducting both arms a few times.

- Flex your right arm several times while visualizing roll and glide of the humeral head.

- Abduct your right arm several times while visualizing humeral roll and glide.

- Pause to notice any difference between the two sides.

- Repeat with the left arm.

- – *How is movement different when you incorporate this awareness?*
- – *Which way feels more stable? Stronger?*
- – *Which way gives you more range of motion?*
- – *How does the quality of movement change?*

## EXPLORATION: DIFFERENTIATING GLENOHUMERAL AND SCAPULOTHORACIC MOVEMENT

This practice is adapted from a practice taught by Judith Koltai.

### Learning Objectives

- Distinguish movement at the glenohumeral joint and functional scapulothoracic joint.

- Deepen felt sense of the scapulae using a soft foam ball to provide sensory awareness.

### Practice Notes

- Notice and inhibit extraneous movement.

- Be specific and intentional with movement initiation.

- Track the scapulae sliding on the ribs, the clavicles hinging at the sternoclavicular joint, and the relative movements of the scapula and humerus.

- Repeat each movement several times.

- Do all the movements on one side at a time.

### Props

- Two 10 cm (4 in.) soft foam balls or two thick sponges cut into circles. You may also use a soft folded sock.

### Instructions

- Take a baseline reading in supine.

  - *How do your scapulae touch the floor?*
  - *How much of your shoulders touch the floor?*

- Bend your knees with feet hip width apart and parallel. Center a ball under each scapula and arrange your arms comfortably alongside your body. Direct your breath posteriorly to consciously soften and release the scapulae into the support of the balls.

### *Scapulothoracic Movement*

- Shift your attention to the right scapula. With each exhalation, press it gently into the ball. Return your shoulder to neutral position on inhalations.

  - *Can you track your clavicle hinging posteriorly and your scapula moving closer to your spine (retraction)?*

- With each inhalation, lift the scapula off the ball, moving your shoulder toward the ceiling. Return your shoulder to the floor as you exhale.

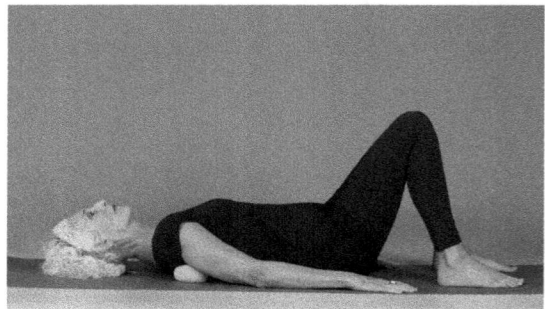

  - *Can you track your clavicle hinging anteriorly and your scapula moving away from your spine (protraction)?*

- Combine these two movements, tracking scapular and clavicular movement while lifting the scapula on inhalations and pressing down on exhalations.

- Slowly raise your right arm toward the ceiling. Find a place where your arm feels effortlessly suspended within the shoulder socket. Move your arm a few degrees in each direction to confirm optimal placement.

- Coordinating movement with breath, on inhalations, lift your scapula off the ball and on exhalations, press into the ball.

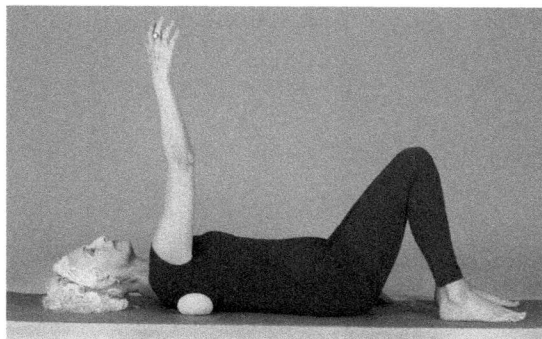

- *Can you sense how the scapula moves the humerus?*

- In baseline position, pause and notice differences between the two sides.

### Glenohumeral Movement

- Raise your right arm toward the ceiling and again find the position of least effort. Imagine your arm "standing" on the support of the scapula like a candle in a candlestick, and that your arm originates from the ball.

- To differentiate glenohumeral movement during this practice, stabilize the scapula by gently pressing into the ball. Restricting scapular movement allows "pure" glenohumeral movement to occur. Maintain gentle backward pressure as you track movement of the head of the humerus in relation to the socket while exploring each of the following movements:

### Compression and Distraction

- Distract the humerus from the socket by reaching your arm toward the ceiling while gently pressing back into the ball. Visualize increased spaciousness between ball and socket.

- Compress the humerus into the socket by plugging the ball deeper into the socket. Imagine pressing the humerus candle into the scapular candlestick.

- Alternate movement several times, coordinating movement and breath.

  - *What changes when you restrain scapular movement?*

### Circling

- Draw slow, tiny circles in the air with your hand. Use minimal muscular effort, as if you could move from the bone. Imagine the round humeral head spinning in the spaciousness of the joint.

- Incrementally increase the size of the circles to a comfortable range, then reverse direction and incrementally return to a tiny circle.

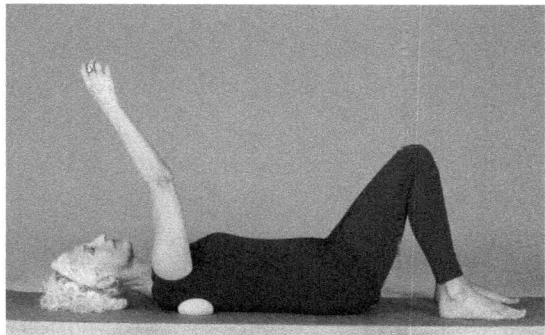

### Other Movements

- Continue to gently press into the ball as you explore other glenohumeral joint movements, visualizing your scapula as the base of support for the moving humerus. Try flexion and extension, abduction, adduction, internal and external rotation, and spiralic multiplanar combinations of movements. Start with small movements.

- Undo the scapular restraint and allow the

scapula to freely participate as you continue to explore movements.

– *How does the movement change?*
– *Can you sense how scapulothoracic movement amplifies arm movement?*

- Lower your arm and pause in baseline to notice differences between the two sides. Move to sitting or standing to explore random arm movements.

  – *How do sensations differ between the two sides?*

- Repeat the exploration with the left arm.

### Bilateral Movement

- Raise both arms toward the ceiling and take a few moments to find the position of greatest ease.

- As you inhale, lift both scapulae off the balls. As you exhale, spread the scapulae apart and place them back on the floor more laterally. The elbows will bend slightly.

- Repeat this movement several times, each time spreading the scapulae further apart and moving the elbows incrementally closer to the floor. When your elbows touch the floor open your arms into a T position.

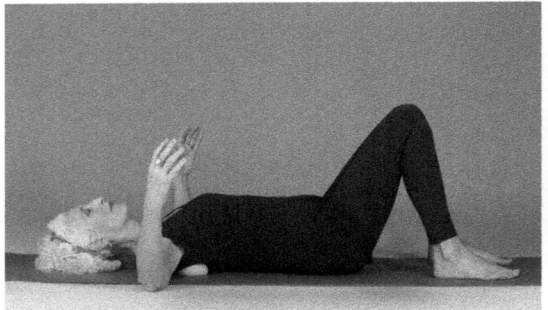

- Rest in baseline and notice how your scapulae and shoulders contact the floor now. Move to a seated position and notice sensation changes in your arms and shoulders. Then, stand and explore moving your arms with this new awareness.

  – *How has felt sense of your arms changed?*
  – *How is your movement different?*

---

## EXPLORATION: CONNECTING ARMS TO SPINE

This practice is adapted from a practice taught by Judith Koltai.

### Learning Objectives

- Deepen felt sense of skeletal and myofascial connections between the arms and spine to access stronger, more efficient, and integrated arm movement.

- Experience spinal support for the arms using a foam ball to awaken sensory awareness of the midthoracic area.

### Props

- One 10 cm (4 in.) soft foam ball or a thick, soft sponge cut into a circle

### Practice Notes

- Move gently and with subtlety.

- Inhibit extraneous muscular activation. The neck, pelvis, shoulders, and other parts of the spine are often unnecessarily involved.

### Instructions

- Take a baseline reading in supine.

- *How do your shoulders and upper back rest on the floor?*

- Place and center the ball between the scapulae at the midthoracic spine. Bend your knees with feet hip width apart. Focus on the interface between the ball and your spine.

- Practice **Back Breathing**, directing inhalations toward the ball, then softening and releasing into the ball on exhalations.

- Position your fingertips on the sternum overlying the ball. For several exhalations, gently press into your sternum to guide a posterior movement that slightly flattens the ball. Release the pressure on inhalations. *Maintain this basic movement throughout the exploration.*

- Arrange your arms at a 45-degree angle to your body, palms down. On either inhalations or exhalations, do the basic backward pressure on the ball and visualize streaming your breath and energy from the ball into the scapulae, middle of the shoulder joint, middle of the elbow joint, middle of the wrist joint, into the fingers, and out into space. As you sequence the movement impulse through each joint, elongate your arm as though someone is gently pulling on your fingers. On the other breath phase, soften and reverse the mental pathway back to the ball.

- Continue with the ball pressure and elongating movement. When your breath, awareness, and movement impulse arrive at the hands, extend your wrists (fingers toward the ceiling), and press the heel of the hand away from you. Again, soften and reverse this mindful pathway on the other phase of breath. Continue for a minute or two.

- Remove the ball and check your baseline.

  - *What's different?*

- In a seated or standing position, do random arm movements initiated from the ball location. Move your arms separately and together.

  - *How does your arm movement change when you initiate from your midline? Is it stronger?*
  - *How could you incorporate this awareness into daily movements?*

## PARTNER EXPLORATION: SENSING CONNECTIONS

During the clavicle class, I discovered a habit of clenching my clavicles (unconsciously protecting my heart?). It makes a huge difference to my shoulder pain when I deliberately maintain width through my clavicles during daily tasks like eating, working at my computer, and lifting my child.

*Rhiannon*

### Learning Objectives

- Deepen felt sense of connections and support available to the arms from the skull, clavicles, scapulae, pelvis, and midline.

- Use these connections to produce stronger, more integrated, and efficient movement.

### Instructions

- Establish touch consent and parameters between partners.

- Start with the giving partner standing a comfortable distance behind the receiving partner, hands resting on their shoulders. Take a minute to pause and attune to each other. Stroke each of the following places several times, covering the entire surface area and varying the intensity and speed of the stroke, as directed by receiver feedback.

- To deepen awareness of myofascial connections between the skull and shoulders, gently and slowly stroke from the occiput, down either side of the cervical spine, then laterally to each acromion.

- To deepen awareness of the myofascial connections between the spine and shoulders, stroke laterally from the upper thoracic spine, across the scapulae, and to the acromion.

- To deepen awareness of the bony and myofascial connections between the sternum and shoulders, stroke laterally from the sternum, along the clavicles, to the acromions, then from the sternum, across the upper chest  and to the acromions.

- To deepen awareness of the myofascial connections between the shoulders and pelvis (mostly the latissimus dorsi), the giver places the palms on the scapulae and drags the tissue diagonally downward to the lumbar spine and pelvis. After several strokes, the receiver abducts both arms as the giver strokes down, relaxing arms between movements.

- To deepen awareness of the contribution of scapulothoracic movement to shoulder movement, the giver immobilizes the receiver's scapula by securing the inferior angle with one hand and pressing down on the scapular spine with the other hand. The receiver abducts the shoulder.

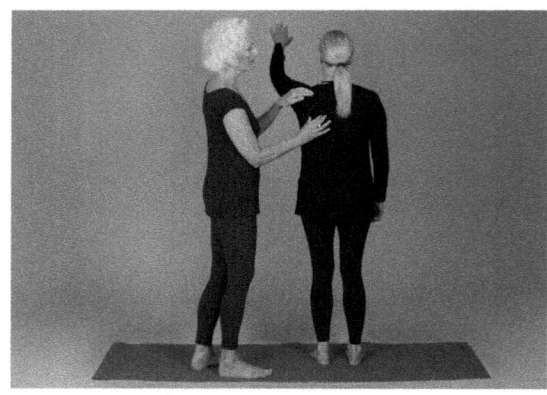

- *How does the range and quality of movement change when scapular movement is restricted?*

- To deepen awareness of the contribution of lateral scapular rotation to arm elevation, the giver places one hand on each scapula. The receiver abducts the arms while the giver follows and exaggerates lateral rotation of the scapulae, swinging the inferior angle of the scapula laterally around the curvature of the ribs.

- To deepen awareness of the shoulder girdle as a suspended structure, the giver moves perpendicular to the receiver and uses the heels of their hands to wedge underneath the clavicle anteriorly and the scapular spine posteriorly. On an exhalation, the receiver actively yields their body weight and sags into gravity, trusting the giver to support the shoulder girdle from below. The rib cage and body weight hang from the shoulder girdle like the clapper of a bell.

- *Can you sense the differentiation of the shoulder girdle from the ribs?*

- Repeat the sagging movements several times dynamically, then remain in the supported position for a few breaths.

- Repeat on the other side.

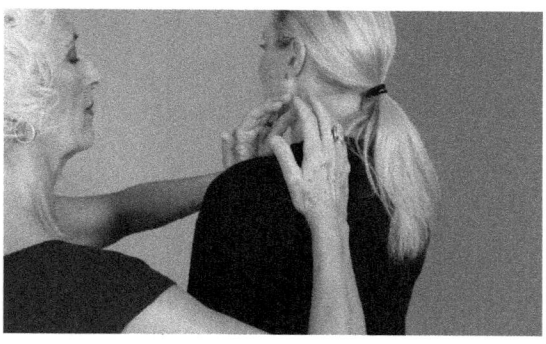

- Pause to allow the receiver to register sensations in stillness, then while moving their arms in random movements.

  - *How does this new awareness change your movement?*
  - *Can you sense new support and connections for your arms?*

## HEAL IT

## FOUNDATIONAL PRACTICE: COUPLED SCAPULAR AND CLAVICULAR MOVEMENT

### Learning Objectives

- Practice initiating shoulder movement proximally by establishing connections between the arms and midline.

- Initiate shoulder movement from the clavicles and scapula while imagining that your arms originate from the midline.

### Props

- A pillow

### Practice Notes

- Track your clavicles hinging and widening and your scapulae moving toward and away from the spine.

- As you move your arms, maintain awareness of the myofascial connections to the spine posteriorly and the myofascial and skeletal connections to the midline anteriorly.

- Imagine your arms originating from the midline.

- The form of this practice will be familiar by now from previous chapters. In this exploration, you will consciously register coupled movement between the scapula and clavicle and explore initiating movement from these structures.

### Instructions

- Take a baseline in supine.

  - *Are your scapulae lying on the floor symmetrically?*

- Position yourself in left side lying with your head supported on the pillow. The bottom shoulder and hip are stacked without your body tipping forward or back. Place your palms together with the arms resting on the floor at shoulder height.

- Focus on your right scapula. On exhalations, move it away from the spine so you roll forward toward the front ribs and the top hand slides over the bottom hand. On inhalations, initiate movement from the scapula, moving it closer to the spine so you roll backward. The top hand simultaneously slides up the bottom hand toward the wrist. The arm is moved passively and the elbow remains straight. As you continue these movements, notice the corresponding hinging and widening across the clavicle.

- – *How easily does your scapula slide?*
- – *Can you sense myofascial and bony connections to the midline between the scapula and spine posteriorly, and clavicle anteriorly?*
- – *Does your arm want to activate and "help" the movement?*

• Shift your awareness to the right clavicle. On exhalations, initiate movement from the clavicle to roll your body forward, sliding top hand over bottom hand. On inhalations, initiate clavicular movement to roll your body backward, passively sliding your top hand up the bottom arm. As you continue these movements, notice corresponding scapular movement toward and away from the spine.

• Combine awareness of the right scapula and clavicle and initiate rolling forward and backward as a coupled movement involving both structures. Track the hinging of the clavicle and sliding of the scapula on the ribs.

- – *Can you sense arm connections to the midline across the clavicle and scapula?*

• Contrast initiating the same movements from your hand.

- – *How does movement differ when you initiate proximally and distally?*

• Contrast initiating the same movements organically from your heart and lungs as in the **Rib Rolls: Organic Initiation** practice in Chapter 5.

- – *How does movement differ when you initiate from your organs?*

• Rest in supine and notice any differences between sides.

• Move to a seated or standing position and explore random arm movements with your new awareness.

- – *Does your movement feel easier, stronger, or more integrated?*

• Repeat the practice on the other side.

## EXPLORATION: DYNAMIC THREAD THE NEEDLE POSE (PARSVA BALASANA) 📽️

### Contraindications

• Neck, shoulder, knee, or spine injury or recent surgery.

### Instructions

• Start on all fours with the shoulders and hips positioned directly over hands and knees.

• On inhalations, initiate shoulder movement proximally by sliding the left scapula toward the spine and hinging from the sternoclavicular joint to lift the left elbow toward the ceiling. As you widen across the left clavicle, simultaneously widen across the right clavicle, and slide the right scapula away from the spine to stabilize the right arm and apply equal counterpressure into the floor.

• On exhalations, initiate a downward arm movement by sliding the left scapula away from the spine and hinging the clavicle anteriorly to thread your left hand under your right armpit and reach right.

• Move back and forth between the two positions several times, initiating proximally from your scapula and clavicles.

• Repeat on the right side.

• Pause in sitting to register any effects.

- – *How does movement differ when initiated proximally?*

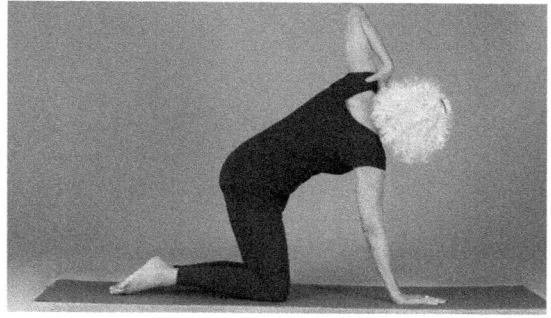

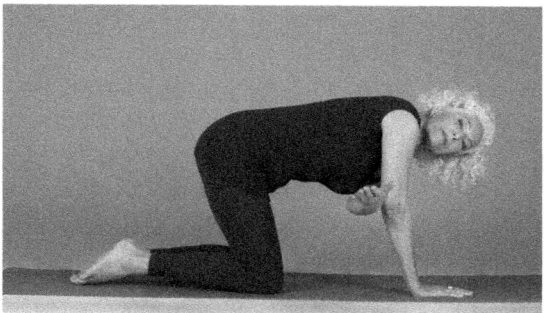

- Work the posture with the breath. On inhalations, "draw the bow" by pressing the left palm away from you and amplifying the movements of both scapulae and clavicles. On exhalations, let the arrow "fly" reversing the scapular and clavicular movements, releasing the mudra, and pressing the right palm forward to align with the left hand. Move back and forth between the two positions.

- After several repetitions, repeat on the other side.

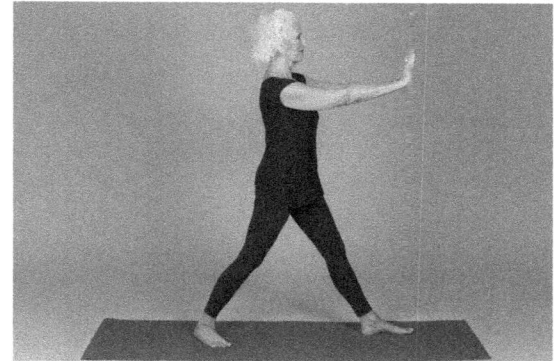

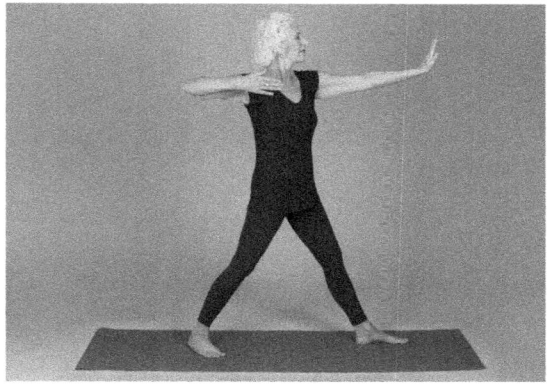

## EXPLORATION: ARCHER POSE (AKARNA DHANURASANA)

### Instructions

- Stand with your feet wider than your shoulders. Turn your left foot 90 degrees and adjust the right heel so your body faces left.

- Raise both arms in front to shoulder height with palms facing forward. Form an arrow mudra with the right hand by pointing the fingers forward, thumb toward the ceiling, second and third fingers extended, and the fourth and fifth fingers bent.

- Initiating shoulder movement proximally, slide the right scapula toward the spine and hinge the clavicle posteriorly, moving the right elbow straight back as though drawing a bow. Simultaneously, slide the left scapula away from the spine and hinge the left clavicle anteriorly to create dynamic tension between the right hand and left elbow.

- *How is movement different when you initiate proximally?*
- *Can you maintain width across your clavicles?*
- *Can you imagine your arms starting at the midline?*

## EXPLORATION: SEQUENCING FORCE IN HALF DOG POSE (ARDHA ADHO MUKHA SVANASANA)

Intention and visualization can affect how force sequences through your body. Through conscious application and direction, mechanical forces may be transmitted through joints and soft tissues in a balanced way, diminishing wear and tear.

### Learning Objectives

- Explore sequencing force through the arms.

- Experience how weight distribution patterns in the hands determine pathways of force transmission through arms and torso.

- Discern which force transmission pathway offers optimal alignment and stability.

### Props

- A chair

### Practice Notes

- As you explore variations, notice how and where force is transmitted and which muscles activate.

- Coordinate your breath and movement, inhaling as you yield and exhaling as you push off. Reverse the breath if it feels more comfortable.

- Repeat each variation several times.

### Instructions

- Place the chairback against a wall and stand facing it.

- Bend forward from your hips and place the heels of your hands shoulder width apart on the front edge of the chair, fingers spread wide. Walk backward until your feet are directly under your hips, arms and legs are straight, and arms, head, and spine are

aligned. Bend your knees slightly so you can focus on your upper body. This is the basic starting position to explore yielding and pushing off different parts of your hands.

- On inhalations, actively yield weight into your hands, bending the elbows to point downward, not laterally. On exhalations, push through the whole palmer surface and slowly and deliberately channel the force through the middle of the wrist joint, elbow joint, shoulder joint, to the scapulae, down either side of the spine, to the sitting bones, and out into space. Visualize force sequencing through the clearly defined pathway from start to finish as you straighten your arms and elongate your spine.

- On inhalations, yield your weight onto the lateral edges of your hands, then push off laterally on exhalations.

  - *Where does force track now?*

- On inhalations, yield your weight onto the medial edges of your hands, then push off medially on exhalations.

  - *Where does force track now?*

- Go back and forth between variations to differentiate force pathways.

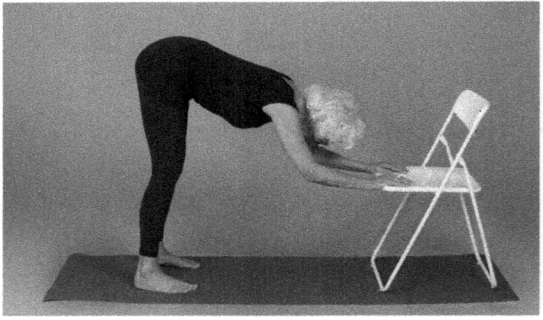

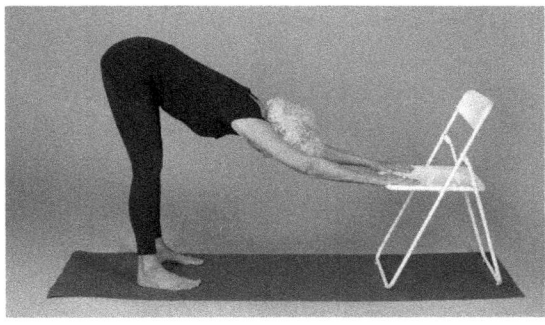

– *Which variation enables you to maintain width across your clavicles?*
– *Which variation feels the safest, most comfortable, and most sustainable?*
– *How could you translate this awareness into other movements?*

## EXPLORATION: WALKING THE ARMS

Swinging the arms when walking is a natural part of the gait pattern. It dissipates energy generated by the torque of the torso and counterbalances the leg swing on the opposite side. This maintains stability of the torso and head and creates energy-efficient, whole-body locomotion (Pontzer *et al.*, 2009). More energy is expended walking without swinging your arms. Normally arm swing is a passive, unconscious function, but, when done consciously, it can have therapeutic benefits.

### Learning Objectives

- Observe habitual patterns of arm swing during walking.

- Explore variations to determine the most functional and efficient arm swing patterns.

### Instructions

- Go for a baseline walk. First, observe the amount of counterrotation in your torso. Then, observe how your arms swing.

- Notice the amplitude of each arm swing, any difference between them, which direction the hands face, whether the arms swing beside your body or across it, and how much the elbows flex.

- Experiment with each of the following variations and notice the effects.

  - Increase the amplitude of arm swing, moving arms equally.
  - Walk with the palms facing your body, facing forward, then backward.
  - Walk while holding your arms at your sides.
  - Walk while imagining your clavicles extend laterally with your arms hanging off the ends (remember the yoke image).
  - Walk while imagining your arms starting at your heart
  - Initiate counterrotation of the torso from your heart.
  - *Which variations feel familiar?*
  - *Which variations do you like? Dislike?*
  - *Which variations give you most ease in walking?*

When I changed my pattern of walking with restricted right arm movement and started to consciously swing my arms equally, my neck pain decreased dramatically.

*Nettie*

## PARTNER EXPLORATION: GIVING AND RECEIVING

### Learning Objectives

- Illuminate (often unconscious) habits of giving and receiving by moving your hands in synchrony with a partner.

- Explore nonhabitual ways of giving and receiving.

### Practice Notes

- Vary speed, direction, shape, intensity, and quality of movement.

- In each variation, notice sensations, memories, and feelings that arise.

- Pause after each variation to register your response and notice habits of giving or receiving.

- Note whether both arms register the same experience.

- Witness yourself nonjudgmentally.

### Instructions

- Establish consent and parameters of touch.

- Stand facing each other with your arms at shoulder height and palms touching. Slow your breath and sense your partner's hands, allowing yourself to touch and be touched.

- Take a few minutes for each of the following explorations.

- To set a baseline, both partners move their hands in tandem through space, noticing preference for leading or following.

- One partner (giver) directs the hand movement and the other (receiver) follows. Then switch roles.

- Both partners try to lead the movement.

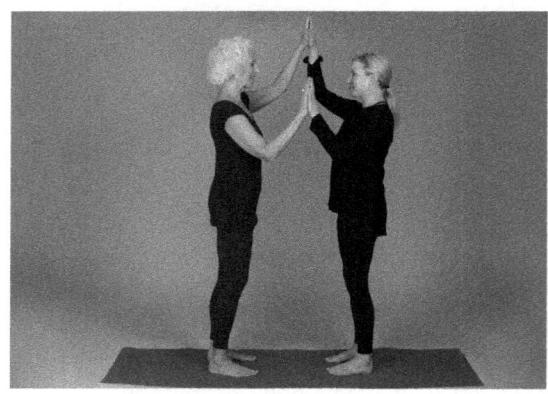

- Both partners try to follow the movement (don't try to figure this out with your mind).

- Both partners cooperate in leading and following, giving and receiving.

- Take a few minutes to share your experience.

  - *How do you habitually express yourself in the world through your arms?*

I realized during the dyad work that I have a strong habit of giving and underdeveloped capacity to receive, and that this imbalance is connected to my chronic shoulder pain.

*Susanne*

## THERAPEUTIC APPLICATIONS

Shoulder tension and pain are common experiences as we shoulder our burdens, hunch over computers, and respond to daily stressors, ranging from rush-hour traffic to information overload and dealing with a post-pandemic world. It doesn't take much for our shoulders to reflexively creep up to our ears. No wonder shoulder pain ranks in the top three musculoskeletal complaints.

Physically, the shoulders, neck, thoracic spine, and pelvis interrelate as parts of a functional unit; all parts affect and are affected by each other. Even the underlying organ body can significantly affect shoulder function. The shoulder girdle is connected skeletally at the sternum only but has fascial continuities with each part of the functional unit and the legs. Healthy shoulder movement is therefore dependent on optimal organization and function of many body parts (Rubin and Kibler 2002). The extreme mobility of the shoulder girdle and its tendency toward myofascial imbalance favors misalignment as the strongest and most tensioned muscles drag the shoulder girdle along their line of pull. A finely tuned interplay between mobility and stability is required for it to remain balanced on the rib basket.

Shoulder girdle positioning can reflect issues within its functional unit or elsewhere in the body. For example, excessive thoracic kyphosis can misalign the shoulder girdle, compromising upper limb circulation and setting the stage for elbow tendinitis or repetitive use injuries; or compensatory consequences of pronated feet may work their way up the kinetic chain to disturb shoulder position. When shoulder movement is restricted, students often compensate by projecting their ribs forward, overarching the lumbar spine, elevating the shoulders, and compressing the posterior neck. EA practices can raise awareness of these common compensations and repattern resilience and more functional habits.

Therapeutic interventions need to consider alignment and function of the entire kinetic chain from spine to fingertips. Solely addressing shoulder dysfunction may overlook significant contributory factors like excessive spinal kyphosis. When arms are experienced as separate units starting at the shoulder, dysfunction and physical injury are more likely. However, as students consciously connect their arms to the midline and to support from below, they consistently experience stronger, more efficient, and integrated movement. Understanding and embodying these functional connections through EA practices can transform movement patterns, motor control, and quality of movement.

On more subtle levels, suboptimal shoulder girdle orientation can reinforce, or catalyze, an emotional or mental stance. For example, it's harder to sustain happiness in the slouched posture that characterizes depression; or someone who "squared" their shoulders to meet challenging circumstances may subconsciously maintain the posture indefinitely. Psychological patterns may be expressed in shoulder girdle orientation, imbalanced tension and compression forces, and compromised movement and function. EA explorations can illuminate subconscious patterns and cultivate the sensory awareness required for self-regulation and healing. Students often comment on how their outlook on life improved as they uncovered embodied metaphors and recognized the interplay between subtle koshas and physical shoulder alignment and movement patterns. Understanding this connection can generate new ways of perceiving, behaving, and interacting in the world. For example, cultivating a connection to the midline can connect us with our deeper Self while "doing" in the world.

Shoulder and arm dysfunction significantly affects work life, leisure activities, and ability to perform daily tasks. A koshic approach to therapy can address diverse factors, including physical components, nervous system responses to pain, and contributing psychosocial factors. Ultimately, the aim of therapy is to empower students and clients to use their shoulders and arms with ease and efficiency in everyday life and to express themselves creatively and in relationships. EA explorations can kindle this by reorganizing upper body structures to improve mobility, efficiency, and force transmission. When supportive anatomical connections are accessed, the arms can truly become the wings of the heart.

## KOSHIC CONTEMPLATIONS

> There are three thermometers: the eyebrow is the thermometer of the mind, the shoulder is the thermometer of the life, and the thumb is the thermometer of the will.
>
> *François Delsarte (Werner 1893)*

### Annamaya Kosha

- *What is your habitual shoulder position?*
- *How does movement change when you initiate arm movement from your midline, scapula, clavicle?*
- *Do neck and shoulder tension patterns change when you visualize your shoulder girdle as a hanging and supported structure?*

### Pranamaya Kosha

- *Have you discovered relationships between your shoulder alignment and breathing or cardiac function?*
- *How does the quality of movement change when you access energetic connections between your lungs, heart, and arms?*
- *When weight-bearing through your arms, what's different when you consciously sequence force from your hands to the pelvis?*

### Manomaya Kosha

- *What have you learned about contributing factors to your habitual shoulder alignment and movement patterns?*
- *Does your shoulder alignment reflect an emotional stance?*

### Vijnanamaya Kosha

- *How does your shoulder carriage reflect a psychological stance or embodied metaphor? Your ability to give and receive?*
- *Have you noticed changes on this level after EA practices?*

### Anandamaya Kosha

- *Does the quality of your manual interactions change when you consciously connect your arms to your heart?*
- *Do your worldly interactions reflect spiritual qualities when you stay connected?*

## KEY CONCEPTS

- The shoulder girdle evolved from pectoral and pelvic fins of primitive fish that emerged from the sea to crawl on land.

- Evolutionary changes engineered the shoulder as the most mobile joint in the body, favouring mobility over stability.
- Dysfunctional movement patterns can be transformed by developing felt sense of the shoulder girdle as a suspended, supported, and connected structure.
- Shoulder carriage can reflect emotional states and psychological stances.
- The only articulation between arms and the larger skeleton is between the clavicle and sternum.
- The scapulae link the arms and torso and play dual roles in shoulder stabilization and movement.

- The shoulder joint is inherently unstable so relies on surrounding ligaments and myofascia for stability.
- Alignment and movement patterns can be altered by differentiating glenohumeral, scapulothoracic, and acromioclavicular joint movement and by sensing connection between the arms and midline.
- Shoulder girdle position may reflect issues elsewhere in the body.

# Practice Summaries

These practice summaries are collections of suggested practices for common conditions. There is no magic to the practices—they have been chosen to demonstrate the multidimensionality of healing and the necessity of considering mind-body interconnectedness and unity. You can do the whole sequence or choose specific practices that may be helpful. Please follow the guidelines in Chapter 2 for safe movement exploration. Begin each practice with a baseline reading in supine and/or standing. End each practice with a few minutes of relaxation lying on your back to register the effects of the practice and any differences in awareness and sensation from your baseline reading.

## FULL-BODY TUNE-UP

### Learning Objective
Rebalance tension and compression forces throughout the body to restore optimal mobility, stability, and force transfer.

- Foundational Practice: The Foot Triangle p.137
- Foundational Practice: Thoraco-Diaphragmatic Breath (Surround Breath) p.78
- Exploration: Pelvic Movement in Three Planes p.166
- Foundational Practice: The Pelvic Reset p.189
- Exploration: Repatterning Spinal Wave p.255
- Rib Rolls: Rib Initiation p.71
- Exploration: Rooting the Neck p.244
- Exploration: Free the Clavicles p.73
- Exploration: Archer Pose (Akarna Dhanurasana) p.273
- Standing Cat-Cow Pose p.226
- Exploration: Legs up the Wall Pose (Viparita Karani) p.148

## FINE-TUNING AWARENESS

### Learning Objective

Deepen interoceptive awareness through physical, breath, and mind practices.

- Setting a Breath Baseline p.61
- Foundational Practice: Heart Hug Breath p.114

- Exploration: Interoceptive Awareness of the Koshas p.33
- Foundational Practice: Right Effort p.38
- Exploration: Sensing Stability p.217
- Foundational Practice: Witness Consciousness p.251

## CALMING ANXIETY

### Learning Objective

Explore physical and breathing practices to decrease body tension and calm the mind.

- Foundational Practice: Spinal Wave p.94
- Setting a Breath Baseline p.61
- Exploration: Humming Bee Breath (Bhramari) p.243
- Exploration: Cranial Fascia p.243
- Exploration: Discover Your Diaphragm p.66

- The Jellyfish Mudra p.67
- Exploration: Discover Your Pelvic Diamond p.69
- Rib Rolls: Organic Initiation p.117
- Exploration: Free the Clavicles p.73
- Exploration: Archer Pose (Akarna Dhanurasana) p.273
- Standing Cat-Cow Pose p.226
- Partner Exploration: Back Breathing p.79
- Foundational Practice: Heart Hug Breath p.114

## HAPPY KNEES SEQUENCE

### Learning Objective

Rebalance and stabilize the functional unit of the pelvis and lower limb to improve force transmission through the knees.

- Foundational Practice: The Foot Triangle p.137
- The Hara Breath p.187
- Exploration: Leg Bone Core p.135
- Foundational Practice: The Pelvic Reset p.189
- Exploration: Defining the Hip Socket p.143

- Exploration: Reclined Big Toe Pose (Supta Padagustasana) p.202
- Exploration: Head to Knee Pose (Janu Sirsasana) p.249
- Mountain Pose (Tadasana): Finding Neutral in Mountain p.196
- Exploration: Yield and Push with Foot Triangles p.145
- Exploration: Roll and Glide in Chair Pose (Utkatasana) p.145
- Exploration: Walking p.150
- Savasana (Corpse Pose)

## PELVIC BALANCE

### Learning Objective
Reconfigure tension and compression forces in the pelvis and legs to restore balanced mobility, stability, and force transmission.

- Foundational Practice: The Foot Triangle p.137
- The Hara Breath p.187
- Exploration: Non-Weight-Bearing Pelvic Movement p.193
- Foundational Practice: The Pelvic Reset p.189
- Exploration: Half Bow Pose (Ardha Dhanurasana) with Isometric Release p.169
- Exploration: Defining the Hip Socket p.143
- Exploration: The Drawbridge p.172
- Exploration: Head to Knee Pose (Janu Sirsasana) p.249
- Exploration: Conscious Nutation p.201
- Warrior I Pose (Virabhadrasana I) p.198
- Exploration: Roll and Glide in Chair Pose (Utkatasana) p.145
- Exploration: Legs up the Wall Pose (Viparita Karani) p.148

## SACROILIAC JOINT AND SCIATICA RELIEF

### Learning Objective
Reconfigure tension and compression forces through the pelvis and legs to decompress and stabilize the sacroiliac, lumbosacral, and femoral joints.

- Foundational Practice: The Foot Triangle p.137
- Exploration: Discover Your Pelvic Diamond p.69
- Foundational Practice: Spinal Wave p.94
- Exploration: Non-Weight-Bearing Pelvic Movement p.193
- Foundational Practice: The Pelvic Reset p.189
- Exploration: Prone Half Butterfly Pose (Ardha Supta Baddhakonasana) p.164
- Exploration: Half Bow Pose (Ardha Dhanurasana) with Isometric Release p.169
- Exploration: Reclined Big Toe Pose (Supta Padagustasana) p.202
- Exploration: Conscious Nutation p.201
- Exploration: Walking with a Springy Spine p.226
- Exploration: Legs up the Wall Pose (Viparita Karani) p.148

## HIP FLEXIBILITY

### Learning Objective

Reconfigure tension and compression forces in the pelvis and legs to decompress the femoral joints and restore optimal range of movement.

- Exploration: Discover Your Pelvic Diamond p.69
- Exploration: Defining the Hip Socket p.143
- Exploration: Pelvic Movement in Three Planes p.166
- Exploration: Half Bow Pose (Ardha Dhanurasana) with Isometric Release p.159

- Bridge Pose (Setu Bandha Sarvangasana) Variations p.195
- Exploration: The Pelvic Dance p.188
- Mountain Pose (Tadasana): Finding Neutral in Mountain p.196
- Exploration: Asymmetrical Forward Bend (Parsvottanasana) p.175
- Warrior I Pose (Virabhadrasana I) p.198
- Exploration: Roll and Glide in Chair Pose (Utkatasana) p.145
- Exploration: Head to Knee Pose (Janu Sirsasana) p.249
- Exploration: Legs up the Wall Pose (Viparita Karani) p.148

## COMPUTER WORK RECOVERY

### Learning Objective

Relieve effects of prolonged seated computer work on the neck, upper back, and shoulders.

- Setting a Breath Baseline p.61
- Foundational Practice: Thoraco-Diaphragmatic Breath (Surround Breath) p.78
- Exploration: Cranial Fascia p.243
- Atlantooccipital Movement p.239
- Atlantoaxial Movement p.240
- Hyoid Lift p.242

- Exploration: Passive Cervical Mobility p.247
- Exploration: Rooting the Neck p.244
- Exploration: Connecting Arms to Spine p.268
- Exploration: Free the Clavicles p.73
- Exploration: Archer Pose (Akarna Dhanurasana) p.273
- Exploration: Moving with Weight on the Head p.250
- Savasana (Corpse Pose)

## SHOULDER COMFORT

### Learning Objective

Reconfigure tension and compression forces in the torso and arms to decrease excessive tension in the shoulders and improve mobility.

- Foundational Practice: Heart Hug Breath p.114

- Exploration: Discover Your Sternum and Clavicles p.62
- Hyoid Lift p.242
- Exploration: Repatterning Spinal Curves – Secondary Curve: Cervical p.222
- Exploration: Arm Bone Core p.264
- Exploration: Connecting Arms to Spine p.268

- Foundational Practice: Initiating Collective Spinal Movement p.220
- Exploration: Free the Clavicles p.73
- Exploration: Sequencing Force in Half Dog Pose (Ardha Adho Mukha Svanasana) p.274

- Exploration: Archer Pose (Akarna Dhanurasana) p.273
- Exploration: Walking the Arms p.275
- Partner Exploration: Giving and Receiving p.276
- Savasana (Corpse Pose)

## WEEKEND WARRIOR ANTIDOTE

### Learning Objective
Decrease whole-body stiffness and soreness caused through overexertion.

- Foundational Practice: Thoraco-Diaphragmatic Breath (Surround Breath) p.78
- Foundational Practice: Spinal Wave p.94
- Exploration: Pelvic Movement in Three Planes p.166
- Foundational Practice: The Pelvic Reset p.189

- Exploration: Prone Half Butterfly Pose (Ardha Supta Baddhakonasana) p.164
- Exploration: Befriend the Psoas p.161
- Exploration: Dynamic Thread the Needle Pose (Parsva Balasana) p.272
- Exploration: Head to Knee Pose (Janu Sirsasana) p.249
- Exploration: Sequencing Force in Half Dog Pose (Ardha Adho Mukha Svanasana) p.274
- Exploration: Legs up the Wall Pose (Viparita Karani) p.148
- Savasana (Corpse Pose)

## LOW BACK PAIN COMFORT I

### Learning Objective
Reconfigure tension and compression forces in the pelvis and spine to decrease pain and restore balanced mobility and stability.

- Foundational Practice: The Foot Triangle p.137
- The Hara Breath p.187
- Foundational Practice: Spinal Wave p.94
- Exploration: Pelvic Movement in Three Planes p.166
- Foundational Practice: The Pelvic Reset p.189

- Exploration: Repatterning Spinal Curves p.222
- Exploration: Prone Half Butterfly Pose (Ardha Supta Baddhakonasana) p.164
- Bridge Pose (Setu Bandha Sarvangasana) Variations p.195
- Exploration: Head to Knee Pose (Janu Sirsasana) p.249
- Exploration: Sequencing Force in Half Dog Pose (Ardha Adho Mukha Svanasana) p.274
- Exploration: Legs up the Wall Pose (Viparita Karani) p.148
- Savasana (Corpse Pose)

## LOW BACK PAIN COMFORT II

### Learning Objective
Reconfigure tension and compression forces in the pelvis and spine to decrease pain and restore balanced mobility and stability.

- Exploration: Spinal Breathing p.
- Exploration: Non-Weight-Bearing Pelvic Movement p.193
- Foundational Practice: The Pelvic Reset p.189
- Exploration: Half Bow Pose (Ardha Dhanurasana) with Isometric Release p.159

- Exploration: Repatterning Individual Vertebral Movement p.218
- Exploration: Locust Pose Variation (Salabhasana) p.98
- Exploration: Reclined Big Toe Pose (Supta Padagustasana) p.202
- Exploration: Mobilize the Spine p.72
- Standing Cat-Cow Pose p.226
- Exploration: Walking with a Springy Spine p.226
- Foundational Practice: Spinal Wave p.94

## DIGESTIVE HEALTH

### Learning Objective
Explore physical and breath practices to increase space for abdominal organs, facilitate organ massage, and stimulate the parasympathetic nervous system to improve digestive physiology.

- Exploration: Discover Your Diaphragm p.66
- The Jellyfish Mudra p.67
- Foundational Practice: Thoraco-Diaphragmatic Breath (Surround Breath) p.78

- Exploration: Discover Your Pelvic Diamond p.69
- Hyoid Lift p.242
- Exploration: Non-Weight-Bearing Pelvic Movement p.193
- Exploration: Befriend the Psoas p.161
- Rib Rolls: Organic Initiation p.117
- Exploration: The Elastic Diaphragm p.74
- Exploration: Legs up the Wall Pose (Viparita Karani) p.148

## ASTHMA PROTOCOL

### Learning Objective
Reconfigure tension and compression forces in the torso to maximize breath capacity and repattern healthy breathing habits.

- Setting a Breath Baseline p.61
- Exploration: Discover Your Diaphragm p.66
- Exploration: Discover Your Ribs p.63

- Exploration: Discover Your Intercostals p.68
- Exploration: Discover Your Costovertebral Joints p.64
- Foundational Practice: Thoraco-Diaphragmatic Breath (Surround Breath) p.78
- Exploration: Lobes of the Lungs p.113
- Rib Rolls: Organic Initiation p.117

- Exploration: Mobilize the Spine p.72
- Exploration: Dynamic Thread the Needle Pose (Parsva Balasana) p.272

- Exploration: Archer Pose (Akarna Dhanurasana) p.273
- Foundational Practice: Spinal Wave p.94

## DEEP SLEEP PRACTICE

### Learning Objective
Explore physical, breath, and mind practices to decrease body tension, calm the mind, and prepare for restorative sleep.

- Foundational Practice: Spinal Wave p.94
- Setting a Breath Baseline p.61
- Exploration: Humming Bee Breath (Bhramari) p.243

- Exploration: Non-Weight-Bearing Pelvic Movement p.193
- Rib Rolls: Organic Initiation p.117
- Exploration: Head to Knee Pose (Janu Sirsasana) p.249
- Exploration: Befriend the Psoas p.161
- Foundational Practice: Witness Consciousness p.251
- Savasana (Corpse Pose)

## MEDITATION PREP

### Learning Objective
Explore physical, breath, and mind practices to decrease body tension, calm the mind, and enter a meditative space.

- Exploration: Discover Your Pelvic Diamond p.69

- Exploration: Seated Pelvic Movement p.194
- Atlantooccipital Movement p.239
- Atlantoaxial Movement p.240
- Foundational Practice: Heart Hug Breath p.114
- Foundational Practice: Witness Consciousness p.251

# Glossary

**Anterior:** A structure positioned in front of another structure.

**Bone core:** A useful anatomical image in which bone is visualized as a solid core surrounded by a malleable sleeve of soft tissue. For example, a cross section of the thigh shows the central femur encircled by thigh myofascia.

**Component joint movements:** Movements between articulating joint surfaces, versus gross movement of body parts moving through space.

**Distal:** Part of a structure positioned distant from the midsection.

**Extension:** Two body parts moving away from each other and increasing the angle between them. In the spine, extension refers to bending backward.

**Flexion:** Two body parts moving closer together and decreasing the angle between them. In the spine, flexion refers to bending forward.

**Force transmission:** Sequencing of muscular and externally generated forces through muscle, bone, and surrounding connective tissue structures.

**Harasphere:** An imaginary sphere visualized in the center of the pelvis to situate awareness for breath and movement practices and to evoke a symbolic representation of wholeness.

**Head-righting reflex:** An automatic postural impulse that orchestrates muscular activation to adjust head position and level eyes with the horizon whenever the upper body moves off the vertical axis.

**Imagery:** Using a mental picture to affect motor control or quality of movement, invoke a state of mind, or create a physiological effect.

**Inferior:** A structure positioned closer to the feet on the vertical axis.

**Interoception:** The perception, processing, and integration of sensations arising from the body that informs perceptual felt sense and emotional feeling states and motivates self-regulatory behavior.

**Kosha:** One of five interpenetrating and inter-dependent sheaths of consciousness covering Atman, the soul. The sheaths are of varying densities and include the densest Annamaya kosha (the physical sheath), Pranamaya kosha (the energy sheath), Manomaya kosha (the mental sheath), Vijnanamaya kosha (the intellectual sheath), and the most subtle Anandamaya kosha (the spiritual sheath).

**Lateral:** A structure positioned further away from the midline than another body structure.

**Mechanotransduction:** Conversion of externally or internally generated physical forces into biochemical responses at the cellular level.

**Medial:** A structure positioned closer to the midline than another body structure.

**Motor control:** The ability to initiate, modulate, and complete a movement with appropriate energy output after nervous system processing and integration of sensory input.

**Neuroplasticity:** The ability of the nervous system to change its structure and function according to thought, experience, and activity.

**Posterior:** A structure positioned behind another body structure.

**Prana:** Life-force energy that animates biological forms.

**Pratyahara:** The fifth limb of yoga, describing deliberate withdrawal of the senses from the outer world and turning them inward.

**Proprioception:** Awareness of body position and movement arising from receptors in fascia, muscles, and joints.

**Proximal:** Part of a structure positioned closer to the midsection.

**Resilience:** The ability to adapt to the consequences of a challenge. In myofascia, resilience is pliability and adaptability. Psychologically, resilience is the ability to cope with and recover from stressful events.

**Sensorimotor:** Integration of sensory stimulation and subsequent appropriate motor responses.

**Somatic:** A reference to lived, direct experience of being and moving in a body.

**Somatosensory:** Sensory information arising from movement, temperature, chemical, and mechanical forces.

**Superior:** A structure positioned closer to the head on the vertical axis.

**Touchstone:** A physical representation serving as a reminder of qualities, inner resources, and states. In experiential anatomy, any anatomical structure can be a touchstone. For example, focusing on the feet can be a reminder to stay grounded.

# Further Reading

Avison, S. (2015) *Yoga, Fascia, Anatomy and Movement.* Handspring Publishing.

Bainbridge Cohen, B. (1993) *Sensing, Feeling, and Action: The Experiential Anatomy of Mind-Body Centering.* Contact Editions.

Bauer, S. (2018) *The Embodied Teen: A Somatic Curriculum for Teaching Body-Mind Awareness, Kinesthetic Intelligence, and Social and Emotional Skills.* North Atlantic Books.

Berland, E. (2017) *Sitting: The Physical Art of Meditation.* Somatic Performer Press, LLC.

Black, M. (2015) *Centered: Organizing the Body through Kinesiology, Movement Theory and Pilates Technique.* Handspring Publishing.

Bond, M. (1993) *Rolfing Movement Integration: A Self-Help Approach to Balancing the Body.* Healing Arts Press.

Bond, M. (2018) *Your Body Mandala: Posture as a Path to Presence.* MCP Books.

Chaitow, L., & Walker Delany, J. (2000) *Clinical Application of Neuromuscular Techniques, Volume 1 The Upper Body.* Churchill Livingstone.

Dowd, I. (1995) *Taking Root to Fly: Articles on Functional Anatomy.* Irene Dowd.

Farhi, D. (1996) *The Breathing Book.* Henry Holt and Company.

Farhi, D., & Stuart, L. (2017) *Pathways to a Centered Body: Gentle Yoga Therapy for Core Stability, Healing Back Pain, and Moving with Ease.* Embodied Wisdom Publishing.

Hackney, P. (2002) *Making Connections: Total Body Integration through Bartenieff Fundamentals.* Routledge.

Hartley, L. (1995) *Wisdom of the Body Moving: An Introduction to Body-Mind Centering.* North Atlantic Books.

Johnson, D. H. (ed.) (1995) *Bone, Breath and Gesture: Practices of Embodiment.* North Atlantic Books.

Kraftsow, G. (2002) *Yoga for Transformation: Ancient Teachings and Practices for Healing the Body, Mind and Heart.* Penguin Compass.

Lesondak, D. (2023) *Fascia: What It Is and Why It Matters.* Handspring Publishing.

Lowe, R., & Laeng-Gilliatt, S. (2007) *Reclaiming Vitality and Presence: Sensory Awareness as a Practice for Life.* North Atlantic Books

Lundgren, M., & Johansson, L. (2020) *Movement Integration: The Systemic Approach to Human.* California, North Atlantic Books.

McClennan, L., & Peck, J. (2020) *Moving from the Inside Out: 7 Principles for Ease and Mastery in Movement.* North Atlantic Books.

Myers, T. (2000) *Body3: A Therapist's Anatomy Reader.* Kinesis Inc.

Olsen, A. (1991) *Bodystories: A Guide to Experiential Anatomy.* Station Hill Press.

Schleip, R. (ed.) (2015) *Fascia in Sport and Movement.* Handspring Publishing.

Sweigard, L. (1974) *Human Movement Potential: Its Ideokinetic Facilitation.* Harper & Row Publishers.

Taylor, M. (2019) *Embody the Skeleton: A Guide for Conscious Movement.* Handspring Publishing.

Timon, T. (2015) *Neurodynamics: The Art of Mindfulness in Action.* North Atlantic Books.

Williams, C. (2022) *Move: The New Science of Body Over Mind.* Profile Books Limited.

# References

## INTRODUCTION

Bertherat, T., & Bernstein, C. (1989) *The Body Has Its Reasons: Self-Awareness through Conscious Movement.* Healing Arts Press.

Chen, J. J. (2006) "Outpatient pain rehabilitation programs." *Iowa Orthopaedic Journal, 26,* 102–106.

Clark, D., Schumann, F., & Mostofsky, S. H. (2015) "Mindful movement and skilled attention." *Frontiers in Human Neuroscience, 9,* 297–297. https://doi.org/10.3389/fnhum.2015.00297

Claxton, G. (2015) *Intelligence in the Flesh: Why Your Mind Needs Your Body Much More than It Thinks.* Yale University Press.

Graham, L. (2018) *Resilience: Powerful Practices for Bouncing Back from Disappointment, Difficulty and Even Disaster.* New World Library.

Hanna, T. (1988) *Somatics: Reawakening the Mind's Control of Movement, Flexibility, and Health.* Addison-Wesley.

Iyer, P. (2014) *The Art of Stillness: Adventures in Going Nowhere.* Simon & Schuster.

Joyce, J. (1914) *Dubliners.* Grant Richards Ltd.

Lephart, S. M., Pincivero, D. M., Giradoi, J. L., & Fu, F. H. (1997) "The role of proprioception in the management and rehabilitation of athletic injuries." *American Journal of Sports Medicine, 25*(1), 130–137. https://doi.org/10.1177/036354659702500126

Or, D. Y. L., Lam, C. S., Chen, P. P., Wong, H. S. S., *et al.* (2021) "Hope in the context of chronic musculoskeletal pain: Relationships of hope to pain and psychological distress." *Pain Reports, 6*(4), e965–e965. https://doi.org/10.1097/PR9.0000000000000965

Osborn, M., & Smith, J. A. (2006) "Living with a body separate from the self, the experience of the body in chronic benign low back pain: An interpretive phenomenological analysis." *Scandinavian Journal of Caring Sciences, 20*(2), 216–222. https://doi.org/10.1111/j.1471-6712.2006.00399.x

Pasqual-Leone, A., Nguyet, D., Cohen, L. G., Brasil-Neto, A., Cammarota, A., & Hallet, M. (1995) "Modulation of muscle responses evoked by transcranial magnetic stimulation during the acquisition of new fine motor skills." *Journal of Neurophysiology, 74*(3), 1037–1045. https://doi.org/10.1152/jn.1995.74.3.1037

Payne, P., Levine, P. A., & Crane-Godreau, M. A. (2015) "Somatic experiencing: Using interoception and proprioception as core elements of trauma therapy." *Frontiers in Psychology, 6.* https://doi.org/10.3389/fpsyg.2015.00093

Small, N., Bower, P., Chew-Graham, C. A., Whalley, D., & Protheroe, J. (2013) "Patient empowerment in long-term conditions: Development and preliminary testing of a new measure." *BMC Health Services Research, 13*(1), 262–263. https://doi.org/10.1186/1472-6963-13-263

van der Wal, J. (2019, July, 28–31) The embryo in us–man as embryo. Workshop presented at the meeting of the Guild for Structural Integration, Salt Lake City, UT, United States.

Weller, F. (2015) *The Wild Edge of Sorrow: Rituals of Renewal and the Sacred Work of Grief.* North Atlantic Books.

## CHAPTER 1

Bushnell, C. M., Čeko, M., & Low, L. A. (2013) "Cognitive and emotional control of pain and its disruption in chronic pain." *Nature Reviews. Neuroscience, 14*(7), 502–511. https://doi.org/10.1038/nrn3516

Butler, D., & Moseley, L. (2013) *Explain Pain* (second edn.). Noigroup Publications.

Cambridge University Press. (n.d.) Gestalt. In Cambridge Dictionary. Retrieved January 14, 2022 from https://dictionary.cambridge.org/us/dictionary/english/gestalt

Chen, W. G., Schloesser, D., Arensdorf, A. M., Simmons, J. M., et al. (2021) "The emerging science of interoception: Sensing, integrating, interpreting and regulating signals within the self." *Trends in Neurosciences, 44*(1), 3–16. https://doi.org/10.1016/j.tins.2020.10.007

Craig, A. D. (2009) "How do you feel now? The anterior insula and human awareness." *Nature Reviews. Neuroscience, 10*(1), 59–70. https://doi.org/10.1038/nrn2555

Di Lernia, D., Lacerenza, M., Ainley, V., & Riva, G. (2020) "Altered interoceptive perception and the effects of interoceptive analgesia in musculoskeletal, primary, and neuropathic chronic pain conditions." *Journal of Personalized Medicine, 10*(4), 201 https://doi.org/10.3390/jpm10040201

Doidge, N. (2007) *The Brain That Changes Itself: Stories of Personal Triumph from the Frontiers of Brain Science.* Penguin Books.

Doidge, N. (2015) *The Brain's Way of Healing.* Penguin Group.

Farb, N., Daubenmier, J., Price, C. J., Gard, T., et al (2015) "Interoception, contemplative practice, and health." *Frontiers in Psychology, 6,* 763–763. https://doi.org/10.3389/fpsyg.2015.00763

Gallagher, L., McAuley, J., & Moseley, G. L. (2013) "A randomized-controlled trial of using a book of metaphors to reconceptualize pain and decrease catastrophizing in people with chronic pain." *Clinical Journal of Pain, 29*(1), 20–25. https://doi.org/10.1097/ajp.0b013e3182465cf7

Gallagher, S. (2000) "Philosophical conceptions of the self: Implications for cognitive science." *Trends in Cognitive Sciences, 4*(1), 14–21. https://doi.org/10.1016/S1364-6613(99)01417-5

Garschagen, A., Steegers, M. A. H., Van Bergen, A. H. M. M., Jochijms, J. A. M. et al. (2015) "Is there a need for including spiritual care in interdisciplinary rehabilitation of chronic pain patients? Investigating an innovative strategy." *Pain Practice, 15*(7), 671–687. https://doi.org/10.1111/papr.12234

Hanh, T. N., & Anh-Huong, N. (2006) *Walking Meditation.* Sounds True.

Harari, Y. (2019) *21 Lessons for the 21st Century.* Random House.

Herbert, B. M., & Pollatos, O. (2012) "The body in the mind: On the relationship between interoception and embodiment." *Topics in Cognitive Science, 4*(4), 692–704. https://doi.org/10.1111/j.1756-8765.2012.01189.x

Hu, X. S., Beard, K., Sherbel, M. C., Nascimento, T. D., et al. (2021) "Brain mechanisms of virtual reality breathing versus traditional mindful breathing in pain modulation: Observational functional near-infrared spectroscopy study." *Journal of Medical Internet Research, 23*(10), e27298–e27298. https://doi.org/10.2196/27298

Khalsa, S. S., Adolphs, R., Cameron, O. G., Critchley, H. D., et al. (2018) "Interoception and mental health: A roadmap." *Biological Psychiatry. Cognitive Neuroscience and Neuroimaging, 3*(6), 501–513. https://doi.org/10.1016/j.bpsc.2017.12.004

Lakoff, G., & Johnson, M. (1980) Conceptual metaphor in everyday language. *Journal of Philosophy, 77*(8), 453–486. https://doi.org/10.2307/2025464

Mansour, A. R., Farmer, M. A., Baliki, M. N., & Apkarian, A. V. (2014) "Chronic pain: The role of learning and brain plasticity." *Restorative Neurology Neuroscience, 32*(1), 129–139. https://doi.org/10.3233/RNN-139003

Mehling, W. E., Gopisetty, V., Daubenmier, J., Price, C. J., Hecht, F. M., & Stewart, A. (2009) "Body awareness: Construct and self-report measures." *PloS One, 4*(5), 5614. https://doi.org/10.1371/journal.pone.0005614

Monti, A., Porciello, G., Panasiti, M. S., & Aglioti, S. M. (2022) "The inside of me: Interoceptive constraints on the concept of self in neuroscience and clinical psychology." *Psychological Research, 86*(8), 2468–2477. https://doi.org/10.1007/s00426-021-01477-7

Moseley, L. (2018, May 5–6) Explain pain [Conference presentation]. Understanding Pain: From Biology to Clinical Care, Vancouver, BC, Canada.

Pinna, T., & Edwards, D. J. (2020) "A systematic review of associations between interoception, vagal tone, and emotional regulation: Potential applications for mental health, wellbeing, psychological flexibility, and chronic conditions." *Frontiers in*

*Psychology, 11*, 1792–1792. https://doi.org/10.3389/fpsyg.2020.01792

Quadt, L., Critchley, H. D., & Garfinkel, S. N. (2018) "The neurobiology of interoception in health and disease." *Annals of the New York Academy of Sciences, 1428*(1), 112–128. https://doi.org/10.1111/nyas.13915

Riegner, G., Posey, G. B., Oliva, V., Jung, Y., Mobley, W., & Zeidan, F. (2022). "Disentangling self from pain: Mindfulness meditation–induced pain relief is driven by thalamic–default mode network decoupling." *Pain, 164*(2), 280–291. https://doi.org/10.1097/j.pain.0000000000002731

Schmitt, C. M., & Schoen, S. (2022) "Interoception: A multi-sensory foundation of participation in daily life." *Frontiers in Neuroscience, 16*, 875200–875200. https://doi.org/10.3389/fnins.2022.875200

Suarez-Rodriguez, V., Fede, C., Pirri, C., Petrelli, L., et al. (2022) "Fascial innervation: A systematic review of the literature." *International Journal of Molecular Sciences, 23*(10), 5674. https://doi.org/10.3390/ijms23105674

Taylor, A. G., Goehler, L. E., Galper, D. I., Innes, K. E., & Bourguignon, C. (2010) "Top-down and bottom-up mechanisms in mind-body medicine: Development of an integrative framework for psychophysiological research." *Explore, 6*(1), 29–41. https://doi.org/10.1016/j.explore.2009.10.004

Todd, M. E. (1937) *The Thinking Body.* Princeton University Press.

Weiner, J. (2022, July 14) Wake Forest University School of Medicine, personal communication.

## CHAPTER 2

Barks, C. (1995) *The Essential Rumi.* HarperCollins.

Doidge, N. (2015) *The Brain's Way of Healing.* Penguin Group.

Farhi, D. (1997) *Yoga Teacher Training Manual* [Unpublished manuscript].

Gendlin, E. (n.d.) "Felt Sense." The Focusing Institute. https://focusing.org/felt-sense/felt-sense

Huijing, P. A. (2007) "Epimuscular myofascial force transmission between antagonistic and synergistic muscles can explain movement limitation in spastic paresis." *Journal of Electromyography and Kinesiology, 17*(6), 708–724. https://doi.org/10.1016/j.jelekin.2007.02.003

Koltai, J. (1999) Embodied Practice Master Class, class notes.

Koltai, J. (2018) Embodied Practice Master Class, class notes.

Markowsky, G. (2023) Information Theory. *Encyclopedia Britannica.* www.britannica.com/science/information-theory

Mezirow, J. (1991) *Transformative Dimensions of Adult Learning* (first edn.). Jossey-Bass.

Munro, M. (2018) "Principles for embodied learning approaches." *South African Theatre Journal, 31*(1), 5–14. https://doi.org/10.1080/10137548.2017.1404435

Palmo, J. T. (2002) Necessary doubt. *Tricycle: The Buddhist Review,* Summer.

Stolz, S. (2015) "Embodied learning." *Educational Philosophy and Theory, 47*(5), 474–487. https://doi.org/10.1080/00131857.2013.879694

## CHAPTER 3

Abidov, A., Rozanski, A., Hachamovitch, R., Hayes, S. W., et al. (2005) "Prognostic significance of dyspnea in patients referred for cardiac stress testing." *New England Journal of Medicine, 353*(18), 1889–1898. https://doi.org/10.1056/NEJMoa042741

Beyer, B., Feipel, V., Sholukha, V., Chèze, L., & Van Sint Jan, S. (2017) "In-vivo analysis of sternal angle, sternal and sternocostal kinematics in supine humans during breathing." *Journal of Biomechanics, 64*, 32–40. https://doi.org/10.1016/j.jbiomech.2017.08.026

Bordoni, B., & Zanier, E. (2013) "Anatomic connections of the diaphragm: Influence of respiration on the body system." *Journal of Multidisciplinary Healthcare, 6*, 281–291. https://doi.org/10.2147/JMDH.S45443

Bordoni, B., & Morabito, B. (2018) "Symptomatology correlations between the diaphragm and irritable bowel syndrome." *Cureus, 10*(7), e3036. https://doi.org/10.7759/cureus.3036

Calais-Germain, B. (2006) *Anatomy of Breathing.* Eastland Press.

Chourpiliadis, C., & Bhardwaj, A. (2022) "Physiology, respiratory rate." In *StatPearls.* StatPearls Publishing. www.ncbi.nlm.nih.gov/books/NBK537306

Gatzoulis, M. A. (2008) "Anatomy of breathing." In S. Standring & N. R. Borley (eds.), *Gray's Anatomy: The Anatomical Basis of Clinical Practice* (fortieth edn., pp. 907–1038). Churchill Livingstone.

Hopper, S. I., Murray, S. L., Ferrara, L. R., & Singleton, J. K. (2019) "Effectiveness of diaphragmatic breathing for reducing physiological and psychological stress in adults: A quantitative systematic review." *JBI Database of Systematic Reviews and Implementation Reports, 17*(9), 1855–1876. https://doi.org/10.11124/jbisrir-2017-003848

Kolar, P., Sulc, J., Kyncl, M., Sanda, J., *et al.* (2012) "Postural function of the diaphragm in persons with and without chronic low back pain." *Journal of Orthopaedic and Sports Physical Therapy, 42*(4), 352–362. https://doi.org/10.2519/jospt.2012.3830

Laffey, J. G. & Kavanagh, B. P. (2002) "Hypocapnia." *New England Journal of Medicine, 347*(1), 43–53. https://doi.org/10.1056/NEJMra012457

Lin, I. M., & Peper, E. (2009) "Psychophysiological patterns during cell phone text messaging: A preliminary study." *Applied Psychophysiology and Biofeedback, 34*(1), 53–57. https://doi.org/10.1007/s10484-009-9078-1

Ljunggren, A. E. (1979) "Clavicular function." *Acta Orthopaedica Scandinavica, 50*(3), 261–268. https://doi.org/10.3109/17453677908989766

Mariotti, A. (2015) "The effects of chronic stress on health: New insights into the molecular mechanisms of brain-body communication." *Future Science OA, 1*(3), FSO23–FSO23. https://doi.org/10.4155/fso.15.21

Merriam-Webster. (n.d.). Inspiration. In Merriam-Webster.com dictionary. Retrieved May 15, 2023, from www.merriam-webster.com/dictionary/inspiration

Perri, M. A., & Halford, E. (2004) "Pain and faulty breathing: A pilot study." *Journal of Bodywork and Movement Therapies, 8*(4), 297–306. https://doi.org/10.1016/s1360-8592(03)00085-8

Philippot, P., Chapelle, G., & Blairy, S. (2002) "Respiratory feedback in the generation of emotion." *Cognition and Emotion, 16*(5), 605–627. https://doi.org/10.1080/02699930143000392

Sammartino, S. (1990) Yoga teacher training class notes.

Smith, M. D., Russell, A., & Hodges, P. W. (2006) "Disorders of breathing and continence have a stronger association with back pain than obesity and physical activity." *Australian Journal of Physiotherapy, 52*(1), 11–16. https://doi.org/10.1016/s0004-9514(06)70057-5

Speads, C. H. (1992) *Ways to Better Breathing.* Healing Arts Press.

Thomas, M., McKinley, R. K., Freeman, E., Foy, C., & Price, D. (2005) "The prevalence of dysfunctional breathing in adults in the community with and without asthma." *Primary Care Respiratory Journal, 14*(2), 78–82. https://doi.org/10.1016/j.pcrj.2004.10.007

Zaccaro, A., Piarulli, A., Laurino, M., Garbella, E., *et al.* (2018) "How breath-control can change your life: A systematic review on psycho-physiological correlates of slow breathing." *Frontiers in Human Neuroscience, 12*, 353–353. https://doi.org/10.3389/fnhum.2018.00353

# CHAPTER 4

Adstrum, S., Hedley, G., Schleip, R., Stecco, C., & Yucesoy, C. A. (2017) "Defining the fascial system." *Journal of Bodywork and Movement Therapies, 21*(1), 173–177. https://doi.org/10.1016/j.jbmt.2016.11.003

Ajimsha, M. S., Shenoy, P. D., & Gampawar, N. (2020). "Role of fascial connectivity in musculoskeletal dysfunctions: A narrative review." *Journal of Bodywork and Movement Therapies, 24*(4), 423–431. https://doi.org/10.1016/j.jbmt.2020.07.020

Bordoni, B., & Zanier, E. (2014) "Clinical and symptomatological reflections: The fascial system." *Journal of Multidisciplinary Healthcare, 7*, 401–411. https://doi.org/10.2147/JMDH.S68308

Bordoni, B., & Marelli, F. (2017) "Emotions in motion: Myofascial interoception." *Complementary Medicine Research, 24*(2), 110–113. https://doi.org/10.1159/000464149

Guimberteau, J. C., Delage, J. P., McGrouther, D. A., & Wong, J. K. (2010). "The microvacuolar system: How connective tissue sliding works." *Journal of Hand Surgery* (European volume), 35*(8), 614–622.

Huston, P. (2022) "A sedentary and unhealthy lifestyle fuels chronic disease progression by changing interstitial cell behaviour: A network analysis." *Frontiers in Physiology, 13.* https://doi.org/10.3389/fphys.2022.90410

Langevin, H. M. (2006) "Connective tissue: A body-wide signaling network." *Medical Hypotheses, 66*(6), 1074–1077. https://doi.org/10.1016/j.mehy.2005.12.032

Langevin, H. M., & Sherman, K. J. (2007) "Pathophysiological model for chronic low back pain integrating connective tissue and nervous system mechanisms." *Medical Hypotheses, 68*(1), 74–80. https://doi.org/10.1016/j.mehy.2006.06.033

Langevin, H. M. (2021) "Fascia mobility, proprioception, and myofascial pain." *Life, 11*(7), 668. https://doi.org/10.3390/life11070668

Langevin, H. M. (2022, September 10–14) Keynote address. Sixth International Fascia Research Congress, Montréal, Quebec, Canada.

Langevin, H. M., Keely, P., Mao, J., Hodge, L. M., *et al.* (2016) "Connecting (t)issues: How research in fascia biology can impact integrative oncology." *Cancer Research, 76*(21), 6159–6162. https://doi.org/10.1158/0008-5472.can-16-0753

Levin, S., & Martin, D. C. (2012) "Biotensegrity: The mechanics of fascia." In L. Chaitow, R. Schleip, P. A. Huijing, & T. W. Findley (eds.), *Fascia: The Tensional Network of the Human Body. The Science and Clinical Applications in Manual and Movement Therapy* (first edn., pp. 137–142). Churchill Livingstone.

Michalak, J., Aranmolate, L., Bonn, A., Grandin, K., *et al.* (2022) "Myofascial tissue and depression." *Cognitive Therapy and Research, 46*(3), 560–572. https://doi.org/10.1007/s10608-021-10282-w

Newton, A. (1995, March) "Basic concepts in the theory of Hubert Godard." *Rolf Lines,* 33–43. https://resourcesinmovement.com/wp-content/uploads/2014/09/basic-conceptsHG-1.pdf

Noda, K., Yoshida, K., Ukichi, T., Furuya, K., *et al.* (2015, September 29) "The fascia is a target organ of inflammation in autoimmune diseases" [Abstract]. *2015 ACR/ARHP Annual Meeting Abstract Supplement, 67.* https://acrabstracts.org/abstract/the-fascia-is-a-target-organ-of-inflammation-in-autoimmune-diseases

Oschman, J. L. (2009) "Charge transfer in the living matrix." *Journal of Bodywork and Movement Therapies, 13*(3), 215–228. https://doi.org/10.1016/j.jbmt.2008.06.005

Park, Y. L., Hunter, J., Sheldon, B. L., Sabourin, S., *et al.* (2021) "Pain and interoceptive awareness outcomes of chronic pain patients with spinal cord stimulation." *Neuromodulation, 24*(8), 1357–1362. https://doi.org/10.1111/ner.13318

Schleip, R. (2005) "Talking to fascia—changing the brain: Explorations of the neuro-myofascial net." *Rolf Lines* 19(2), 18–21.

Schleip, R. (2017) "Fascia as a sensory organ: Clinical applications." *Terra Rosa E-Mag, 20,* 2–7. www.researchgate.net/publication/319182467_FASCIA_AS_A_SENSORY_ORGAN_Clinical_Applications

Schleip, R., & Klingler, W. (2019) "Active contractile properties of fascia." *Clinical Anatomy, 32*(7), 891–895. https://doi.org/10.1002/ca.23391

Schultz, R. L., & Feitis, R. (1996) *The Endless Web, Fascial Anatomy, and Physical Reality.* North Atlantic Books.

Sharkey, J. J. (2021) "Should bone be considered fascia: Proposal for a change in taxonomy of bone—a clinical anatomists view." *International Journal of Biological and Pharmaceutical Sciences Archive, 1*(1), 1–10. https://doi.org/10.30574/ijbpsa.2021.1.1.0001

Stecco, A., Gesi, M., Stecco, C., & Stern, R. (2013) "Fascial components of the myofascial pain syndrome." *Current Pain and Headache Reports, 17*(8), 352–359. https://doi.org/10.1007/s11916-013-0352-9

Stecco, A., Stern, R., Fantoni, I., De Caro, R., & Stecco, C. (2015) "Fascial disorders Implications for treatment." *PM&R, 8*(2), 161–168. https://doi.org/10.1016/j.pmrj.2015.06.006

Stecco, C., Macchi, V., Barbieri, A., Tiengo, C., Porzionato, A., & De Caro, R. (2018) "Hand fasciae innervation: The palmar aponeurosis." *Clinical Anatomy, 31*(5), 677–683. https://doi.org/10.1002/ca.23076

Still, A. T. (1899) *Philosophy of Osteopathy.* A. T. Still.

Suarez-Rodriguez, V., Fede, C., Pirri, C., Petrelli, L., *et al.* (2022) "Fascial innervation: A systematic review of the literature." *International Journal of Molecular Science, 23*(10), 5674. https://doi.org/10.3390/ijms23105674

Tadeo, I., Berbegall, A. P., Escudero, L. M., Alvaro, T., & Noguera, R. (2014) "Biotensegrity of the extracellular matrix: Physiology, dynamic mechanical balance, and implications in oncology and mechanotherapy." *Frontiers in Oncology, 4,* 39–39. https://doi.org/10.3389/fonc.2014.00039

Tozzi, P. (2014) "Does fascia hold memories?" *Journal of Bodywork and Movement Therapies, 18*(2), 259–265. https://doi.org/10.1016/j.jbmt.2013.11.010

Wagh, K., Ishikawa, M., García, D. A., Stavreva, D. A., Upadhyaya, A., & Hager, G. L. (2021) "Mechanical regulation of transcription: Recent advances." *Trends in Cell Biology*, *31*(6), 457–472. https://doi.org/10.1016/j.tcb.2021.02.008

van der Wal, J. (2016) "The fascia as the organ of inner ness: An holistic approach based upon a phenomenological embryology and morphology." In T. Liem, P. Tozzi, & A. G. Chila (eds.), *Fascia in the Osteopathic Field* (pp. 87–100). Handspring Publishing.

Yu, B., Wang, J., Wu, J., Dai, J., *et al.* (2011) "Review of evidence suggesting that the fascia network could be the anatomical basis for acupoints and meridians in the human body." *Evidence-based Complementary and Alternative Medicine*, *2011*, 1–6. https://doi.org/10.1155/2011/260510

## CHAPTER 5

Arrien, A. (1993) *The Four-fold Way: Walking the Paths of the Warrior, Teacher, Healer, and Visionary.* HarperCollins.

Barral, J. P. (2007) *Understanding the Messages of Your Body: How to Interpret Physical and Emotional Signals to Achieve Optimal Health.* North Atlantic Books.

Barral, J. P., & Mercier, P. (1988) *Visceral Manipulation.* Eastland Press.

Bath, M., & Owens, J. (2022) "Physiology, viscerosomatic reflexes." In StatPearls. StatPearls Publishing. www.ncbi.nlm.nih.gov/books/NBK559218

Cohen, B. (1993) *Sensing, Feeling, And Action: The Experiential Anatomy of Body-Mind Centering.* Contact Editions.

Cranz, G., & Chiesi, L. (2014) "Design and somatic experience: Preliminary findings regarding drawing through experiential anatomy." *Journal of Architectural and Planning Research*, *31*(4), 322–339. www.jstor.org/stable/44113090

Goldthwaite, J. E. (1945) *Essentials of Body Mechanics in Health and Disease.* JB Lippincott & Co.

Khalsa, S., Adolphs, R., Cameron, O. G., Critchley, H. D., *et al.* (2018) "Interoception and mental health: A roadmap." *Biological Psychiatry. Cognitive Neuroscience and Neuroimaging*, *3*(6), 501–513. https://doi.org/10.1016/j.bpsc.2017.12.004

Langevin, H. M., Bouffard, N. A., Bader, G. J., Iatridis, J. C., & Howe, A. K. (2005) "Dynamic fibroblast cytoskeletal response to subcutaneous tissue stretch ex vivo and in vivo." *American Journal of Physiology—Cell Physiology*, *288*(3), 747–756. https://doi.org/10.1152/ajpcell.00420.2004

Miller, G. W., Ethridge, P., & Morgan, K. T. (eds.) (2011) *Exploring Body-Mind Centering: An Anthology of Experience and Method.* North Atlantic Books.

Monti, A., Porciello, G., Panasiti, M. S., & Aglioti, S. M. (2021) "Gut markers of bodily self-consiousness." bioRxiv. https://doi.org/10.1101/2021.03.05.434072

Renzaho, A. M., Houng, B., Oldroyd, J., Nicholson, J. M., D'Esposito, F., & Oldenburg, B. (2014). "Stressful life events and the onset of chronic diseases among Australian adults: Findings from a longitudinal survey." *European Journal of Public Health*, *24*(1), 57–62.

Settineri, S., Frisone, F., Alibrandi, A., & Merlo, E. M. (2019) "Emotional supression and oneiric expression in pyschosomatic disorders: Early manifestations in emerging adulthood and young patients." *Frontiers in Psychology*, *10*, 1897–1897. https://doi.org/10.3389/fpsyg.2019.01897

## CHAPTER 6

Barrows, A., and Macy, J. (1996) *Rilke's Book of Hours: Love Poems to God.* Riverhead Books.

Cleary, T. (trans.) (1993) *The Essential Tao.* HarperSanFrancisco Books.

Collinsdictionary.com. (n.d.). Selbststandig. In Collins Dictionary. Retrieved December 27, 2024, from www.collinsdictionary.com/dictionary/german-english/selbststandig

Farhi, D. (1996) *Yoga Teacher Training Manual* [Unpublished manuscript].

Goldberger, A. L., Amaral, L. A. N., Hausdorff, J. M., Ivanov, P. C., Peng, C. K., & Stanley, H. E. (2002) "Fractical dynamics in physiology: Alterations with disease and aging." *Proceedings of the National Academy of Sciences*, *99*(1), 2466-2472. https://doi.org/10.1073/pnas.012579499

Hanh, T. N. (1992) *Peace is Every Step: The Path of Mindfulness in Everyday Life.* Random House.

Huijing, P. A. (2007) "Epimuscular myofascial force transmission between antagonistic and synergistic muscles can explain movement limitation in spastic paresis." *Journal of Electromyography and Kinesiology, 17*(6), 708–724. https://doi.org/10.1016/j.jelekin.2007.02.003

Krause, F., Wilke, J., Vogt, L., & Banzer, W. (2016) "Intramuscular force transmission along myofascial chains." *Journal of Anatomy, 228*(6), 910–918. https://doi.org/10.1111/joa.12464

Marinho, H. V. R., Amaral, G. M., Moreira, B. S., Santos, T. R. T., *et al.* (2017) "Myofascial force transmission in the lower limb: An in vivo experiment." *Journal of Biomechanics, 63*, 55–60. https://doi.org/10.1016/j.jbiomech.2017.07.026

Rolf, I. P. (1989) *Rolfing: Reestablishing the Natural Alignment and Structural Integration of the Human Body for Vitality and Wellbeing.* Healing Arts Press.

Sharkey, J. (2015, December 23) "Biotensegrity:The Fallacy of Biomechanics, Part 2." John Sharkey Events—Biotensegrity, Fasciategrity—Anatomy for the 21st Century. www.johnsharkeyevents.com/research/2015/12/23/biotensegrity-the-fallacy-of-biomechanics-part-2

Shojania, K. M. D. (2010, April 10) Personal communucation.

Viseux, F. (2020) "The sensory role of the sole of the foot: Review and update on clinical perspectives." *Neurophysiologie Clinique, 50*(1), 55–68. https://doi.org/10.1016/j.neucli.2019.12.003

Viseux, F., Lemaire, A., Barbier, F., Charpentier, P., Leterneur, S., & Villeneuve, P. (2019) "How can the stimulation of plantar cutaneous receptors improve postural control?" *Neurophysiologie Clinique, 49*(3), 263–268. https://doi.org/10.1016/j.neucli.2018.12.006

## CHAPTER 7

Anderson, T. E., Lahav, Y., Ellegaard, H., & Manniche, C. (2017) "A randomized controlled trial of brief somatic experiencing for chronic low back pain and comorbid post-traumatic stress disorder symptoms." *European Journal of Psychotraumatology, 8*(1), 1331108–1331109. https://doi.org/10.1080/20008198.2017.1331108

Bogduk, N., Pearcy, M., & Hadfield, G. (1992) "Anatomy and biomechanics of psoas major." *Clinical Biomechanics* (Bristol, Avon), 7(2), 109–119.

Chu, L.-P., Chen, K.-T., Lu, H.-K., Lai, C.-L., Huang, H.-C., & Hsieh, K. C. (2023) "Preliminary study on the application of bioimpedance analysis to measure the psoas major muscle in older adults." *PloS One, 18*(3): e0275884.

Gibbons, S. G. T. (2007) "Assessment and rehabilitation of the stability function of psoas major." *Manuelletherapie, 11*(4), 177–187. https://doi.org/10.1055/s-2007-963466

Michele, A. A. (1962) *Ileopsoas: Development of Anomalies in Man.* Charles C. Thomas Publisher, Ltd.

Rolf, I. P. (1989) *Rolfing: Reestablishing the Natural Alignment and Structural Integration of the Human Body for Vitality and Wellbeing.* Healing Arts Press.

Sanjay, K., Khuba, S., Gautam, S., Agarwal, A., *et al.* (2021) "Association of myofascial pain in patients with thoracolumbar scoliosis, kyphoscoliosis or spinal deformity attending a tertiary care hospital in Uttar Pradesh, India." *Journal of Evidence Based Medicine and Healthcare, 8*(27), 2392–2398. www.jebmh.com/articles/association-of-myofascial-pain-in-patients-with-thoracolumbarscoliosis-kyphoscoliosis-or-spinal-deformity-attending-at-er.pdf.pdf

Siccardi, M. A., Tariq, M. A., & Valle, C. (2023) "Anatomy, body pelvis, and lower limb: Psoas major." In *StatPearls.* StatPearls Publishing. www.ncbi.nlm.nih.gov/books/NBK535418

Todd, M. E. (1937) *The Thinking Body.* Princeton University Press.

Travell, J. G., & Simons, D. G. (1992) *Myofascial Pain and Dysfunction: The Trigger Point Manual,* Volume 2. Lippincott Williams & Wilkins.

Xu, J.-J., Zhu, X.-L., Li, T., Lin, Y., *et al* (2021) "Assessment of the cross-sectional areas of the psoas major in patients with adolescent idiopathic scoliosis before skeletal maturity." *Acta Radiologica, 69*(5), 639–645. https://doi.org/10.1177/0284185120951961

## CHAPTER 8

Albrecht, R., Lüwe, B., Brünahl, C. A., & Riegal, B. (2015) "Chronic pelvic pain syndrome and personality-association of somatic symptoms and psychic structure." *Psychotherapie, Pyschosomatik, medizinische Psychologie, 65*(11), 418–425. https://doi.org/10.1055/s-0035-1554692

ban Breathnach, S. (2016, October 2) "Life's unexpected curtain calls." Sarah ban Breathnach. www.sarahbanbreathnach.com/between-the-lines/2016/10/1/n2eri590mjencz7bzu7mpyaqjpa6ta

Beales, D., Slater, H., Palsson, T., & O'Sullivan, P. (2020) "Understanding and managing pelvic girdle pain from a person-centred biopsychosocial perspective." *Musculoskeletal Science and Practice, 48*, 102152. https://doi.org/10.1016/j.msksp.2020.102152

Brooks, T., Sharp, R., Evans, S., Baranoff, J., & Esterman, A. (2020) "Predictors of depression, anxiety and stress indicators in a cohort of women with chronic pelvic pain." *Journal of Pain Research, 13*, 527–536. https://doi.org/10.2147/JPR.S254120

Damen, L., Buyruk, H. M., Güler-Uysal, F., Lotgering, F. K., Snijders, C. J., & Stam, H. J. (2001) "Pelvic pain during pregnancy is associated with asymmetric laxity of the sacroiliac joints." *Acta Obstetricia et Gynecologica Scandinavica, 80*(11), 1019–1024. https://doi.org/10.1080/obs.80.11.1019.1024

Dufour, S., Vandyken, B., Forget, M.-J., & Vandyken, C. (2018) "Association between lumbopelvic pain and pelvic floor dysfunction in women: A cross sectional study." *Musculoskeletal Science and Practice 34*, 47–53. https://doi.org/10.1016/j.msksp.2017.12.001

Guimond, S. & Massrieh, W. (2012) "Intricate correlation between body posture, personality train, and incidence of body pain: A cross-referential study report." *PloS One, 7*(5), e37450–e3450. https://doi.org/10.1371/journal.pone.0037450

Hogervosrt, T., Bouma, H. W., & de Vos, J. (2009) "Evolution of the hip and pelvis." *Acta Orthopaedica, 80*(s336), 1–39. https://doi.org/10.1080/17453690610046620

Le Page, J., & Aboim, L. (2013) *Mudras for Healing and Transformation* (third edn.). Integrative Yoga Therapy.

Levin, S. (2007) *Movement, Stability andd Lumbopelvic Pain: Integration of Research and Therapy* (second edn.). Churchill Livingstone.

Schamberger, W. (2002) *The Malalignment Syndrome: Implications for Medicine and Sports*. Churchill Livingstone.

Thompson, E. (1995) *The Sense and Sensibility Screenplay and Diaries: Bringing Jane Austen's Novel to Film*. Newmarket Press.

Vleeming, A., Schuenke, M. D., Masi, A. T., Carreiro, J. E., Danneels, L., & Willard, F. H. (2012) "The sacroiliac joint: An overview of its anatomy, function and potential clinical implications." *Journal of Anatomy, 221*(6), 537–567. https://doi.org/10.1111/j.1469-7580.2012.01564.x

Vocabulary.com. (n.d.). Zaftig. In Vocabulary.com dictionary. Retrieved December 1, 2023, from www.vocabulary.com/dictionary/zaftig

Willard, F. H., Vleeming, A., Schuenke, M. D., Daneels, L., & Schleip, R. (2012) "The thoracolumbar fascia: Anatomy, function, and clinical considerations." *Journal of Anatomy, 221*(6), 507–536. https://doi.org/10.1111/j.1469-7580.2012.01511.x

Xiangsheng, T., Long, G., Yingying, S., Xiao, A., Ping, Y., & Mingsheng, T. (2021) "Personality traits predict regression of pelvic girdle pain after pregnancy: A longitudinal follow-up study." *BMC Pregnancy and Childbirth, 21*(1), 1–9. https://doi.org/10.1186/s12884-021-03759-9

Yu, Q., Huang, H., Zhang, Z., Hu, X., *et al.* (2020) "The association between pelvic asymmetry and non-specific chronic low back pain as assessed by the global postural system." *BMC Musculoskeletal Disorder, 21*(1), 1–10. https://doi.org/10.1186/s12891-020-03617-3

## CHAPTER 9

Ahmadi, H., Adib, H., Selk-Ghaffari, M., Shafizad, M., *et al.* (2020) Comparison of the effects of the Feldenkras method versus core stability exercise in the management of chronic low back pain: A randomised control trial. *Clinical Rehabilitation, 34*(12), 1449–1457. https://doi.org/10.1177/0269215520947069

Butler, D., & Moseley, G. L. (2003) *Explain Pain*. Noigroup Publications.

Deyo, R. A., & Weinstein, J. N. (2001) "Low back pain." *New England Journal of Medicine, 344*(5), 363–370. https://doi.org/10.1056/NEJM200102013440508

Gonzalez-Medina, G., Perez-Cabezas, V., Ruiz-Molinero, C., Chamorro-Moriano, G., Jimenez-Rejano, J. J., & Galán-Mercant, A. (2021) "Effectiveness of global postural re-education in chronic non-specific low back pain: A systematic review and meta-analysis." *Journal of Clinical Medicine, 10*(22), 5327–5237. doi.org/10.3390/jcm10225327

Gracovetsky, S. (2012, December 19) Non invasive assessment of spinal function [Video]. YouTube. www.youtube.com/watch?v= EAMK7yR9Rgl

Hackney, P., (2002) *Making Connections: Total Body Integration through Bartenieff Fundamentals.* Routledge.

Hafiz, translated by Ladinski, D. (1999) *The Gift.* Penguin Compass.

Khedikar, S. G., Erande, M. P., & Shukla, D. V. (2016) "Critical comparison of yogic nadi with nervous system." *Joinsysmed, 4*(2), 108–113.

Levin, S. M. (2002) "The tensegrity-truss as a model for spine mechanics: Biotensegrity." *Journal of Mechanics in Medicine and Biology, 2*(3n04), 375–388. https://doi.org/10.1142/S0219519402000472

McGill, S. (2007) "Lumbar spine stability: Mechanism of injury and restabilization." In Liebenson, C.

(ed.), *Rehabilitation of the Spine: A Practitioner's Manual* (pp. 93–111). Lippincott Williams and Wilkins.

Richardson, C., Hodges, P., & Hides, J. (2004) *Therapeutic Exercise for Lumbopelvic Stabilization: A Motor Control Approach for the Treatment and Prevention of Low Back Pain* (second edn.). Churchill Livingstone.

Sarno, J. (1991) *Healing Back Pain: The Mind-Body Connection.* Warner Books.

Stubbs, B., Koyanagi, A., Thompson, T., Veronese, N., *et al.* (2016) "The epidemiology of back pain and its relationship with depression, psychosis, anxiety, sleep disturbances, and stress sensitivity." *General Hospital Psychiatry, 43*, 63–70. https://doi.org/10.1016/j.genhosppsych.2016.09.008

Vleeming, A., & Willard, F. (2010) Foreclosure and optimal stability of the lumbopelvic region [Paper]. Seventh Interdisciplinary World Congress on Low Back & Pelvic Pain, Los Angeles, CA, US www.fasciaresearch.com/literature/wc-low-back-and-pelvic-pain/Vleeming10.pdf

Wilke, J., Schlei, R., Klingler, W., & Stecco, C. (2017) "The lumbodorsal fascia as a potential source of low back pain: A narrative review." *BioMed Research International, 2017*, 1–6. https://doi.org/10.1155/2017/5349620

# CHAPTER 10

Alreni, A. S. E., Harrop, D., Lowe, A., Potia, T., Kilner, K., & McLean, S. M. (2017) "Measures of upper limb function for people with neck pain. A systematic review of measurement and practical properties." *Musculoskeletal Science and Practice, 29*, 155–163. https://doi.org/10.1016/j.msksp.2017.02.004

Cailliet, R., & Gross, L. (1987) *Rejuvenation Strategy: A Medically Approved Fitness Program to Reverse the Effects of Aging.* Doubleday.

Cheng, J.-H., Hsiao, S.-Y., Chen, C.-M., & Hsu, K.-J. (2020) "Relationship between hyoid bone and pharyngeal airway in different skeletal patterns." *Journal of Dental Sciences, 15*(3), 286–293. https://doi.org/10.1016/j.jds.2020.05.012

Cho, J., Lee, E., & Lee, S. (2017) "Upper thoracic spine mobilization and mobility exercise versus upper cervical spine mobilization and stabilization exercise in individuals with forward head posture: A randomized clinical trial." *BMC Musculoskeletal*

*Disorders, 18*(1), 525. https://doi.org/10.1186/s12891-017-1889-2

Correia, I. M. T., Macedo, T., de Sá Ferreira, A., Fernandez, J., *et al.* (2021) "Association between text neck and neck pain in adults." *Spine, 46*(9), 571–578. https://doi.org/10.1097/BRS.0000000000003854

Crisco, J. J., & Panjabi, M. M. (1991) "The intersegmental and multisegmental muscles of the lumbar spine. A biomechanical model comparing lateral stabilizing potential." *Spine, 16*(7), 793–799. https://doi.org/10.1097/00007632-199107000-00018

Falk, D., Zollikofer, C. P., Morimoto, N., & Ponce de León, M. S. (2012) Metopic suture of Taung (Australopithecus africanus) and its implications for hominin brain evolution. *Proceedings of the National Academy of Sciences of the United States of America, 109*(22), 8467–8470.

Grob, D., Frauenfelder, H., & Mannion, A. F. (2007) "The association between cervical spine curvature and neck pain." *European Spine*

*Journal*, *16*(5), 669–678. https://doi.org/10.1007/s00586-006-0254-1

Harneet, K., & Maman, P. (2019) "Chronic neck pain and its influence on respiratory function: A review article." *International Journal of Advanced Science Technology*, *28*(8), 333–342. http://sersc.org/journals/index.php/IJAST/article/view/561

Joshi, D. G., Balthillaya, G., & Prabhu, A. (2018) "Effect of remote myofascial release on hamstring flexibility in asymptomatic individuals—A randomized clinical trial." *Journal of Bodyworks and Movement Therapy*, *22*(3), 832–837. https://doi.org/10.1016/j.jbmt.2018.01.008

Kim, R., Wiest, C., Clark, K., Cook, C., & Horn, M. (2018) "Identifying risk factors for first-episode neck pain: A systematic review." *Musculoskeletal Science and Practice*, *33*, 77–83. https://doi.org/10.1016/j.msksp.2017.11.007

Mahmoud, N. F., Hassan, K. A., Abdelmajeed, S. F., Moustafa. I. M., & Silva, A. G. (2019) "The relationship between forward head posture and neck pain: A systematic review and meta-analysis." *Current Reviews in Musculoskeletal Medicine*, *12*(4), 562–577. https://doi.org/10.1007/s12178-019-09594-y

McAviney, J., Schulz, D., Bock, R., Harrison, D. E., & Holland, B. (2005) "Determining the relationship between cervical lordosis and neck complaints." *Journal of Manipulative and Physiological Therapeutics*, *28*(3), 187–193. https://doi.org/10.1016/j.jmpt.2005.02.015

Moon, H. J., & Lee, Y. K. (2011) "The relationship between dental occlusion/temporomandibular joint status and general body health: Part 1. Dental occlusion and TMJ status exert an influence on general body health." *Journal of Alternative and Complementary Medicine*, *17*(11), 995–1000. https://doi.org/10.1089/acm.2010.0739

Myers T. W. (2020) *Anatomy Trains, Myofascial Meridians for Manual Therapists and Movement Professionals* (4th ed.). Elsevier.

Ozel Asliyuce, Y., Berberoglu, U., & Ulger, O. (2020) "Is cervical region tightness related to vagal function and stomach symptoms?" *Medical Hypotheses*, *142*, 109819. https://doi.org/10.1016/j.mehy.2020.109819

Parikh, P. R., & Amarnath, T. K. (2021) "To study the relationship between neck pain and anxiety, depression in computer works: A correlation study." *International Journal of Health Sciences and Research*, *11*(6), 356–361. https://doi.org/10.52403/ijhsr.20210653

Pettorossi, V. E., & Schieppati, M. (2014) "Neck proprioception shapes body orientation and perception of motion." *Frontiers in Human Neuroscience, 8.* https://doi.org/10.3389/fnhum.2014.00895

Rubenstein, D. (2010) "Kinetic chain from the toes influences the craniofacial region." *Practical Pain Management*, *10*(5). www.practicalpainmanagement.com/pain/maxillofacial/kinetic-chain-toes-influences-craniofacial-region

Scali, F., Marsili, E. S., & Pontell, M. E. (2011) "Anatomical connection between the rectus capitis posterior major and the dura mater." *Spine*, *36*(25), E1612–E1614. https://doi.org/10.1097/BRS.0b013e31821129df

Taneja, M. K. (2020) "Modified Bhramari Pranayama in Covid 19 infection." *Indian Journal of Otolaryngology and Head & Neck Surgery*, *72*(3), 395–397. https://doi.org/10.1007/s12070-020-01883-0

Wilke, J., Vogt, L., Niederer, D., & Banzer, W. (2017) "Is remote stretching based on myofascial chains as effective as local exercise? A randomized-controlled trial." *Journal of Sports Sciences*, *35*(20), 2021–2027. https://doi.org/10.1080/02640414.2016.1251606

Zhang, Z., Kurosu, A., Coyle, J., Perera, S., & Sejdic, E. (2021) A generalized equation approach for hyoid bone displacement and penetration–aspiration scale analysis. *SN Applied Sciences*, *3*(688). https://doi.org/10.1007/s42452-021-04632-2

## CHAPTER 11

Cloutier, R., Clement, A. M., Lee, M. S. Y., Noel, R., *et al.* (2020) "Elpistostege and the origin of the vertebrate hand." *Nature 579*(7800), 549–554. https://doi.org/10.1038/s41586-020-2100-8

Grine, F., Fleagle, J., & Leakey, R. (2009) *The First Humans: Origin and Early Evolution of the Genus Homo*. Springer Publishing.

Levin, S. M. (1997) "Putting the shoulder to the wheel: A new biomechanical model for the shoulder girdle." *Biomedical Sciences Instrumentation*, *33*, 412–417. http://biotensegrity.com/resources/shoulder-to-the-wheel.pdf

McMullen, J., & Uhl, T. L. (2000) "A kinetic chain approach for shoulder rehabilitation." *Journal of*

*Athletic Training*, 35(3), 329–337. www.ncbi.nlm. nih.gov/pmc/articles/PMC1323395/

Myers, T. W. (2009) *Anatomy Trains: Myofascial Meridians for Manual and Movement Therapists* (second edn.). Churchill Livingstone.

Pontzer, H., Holloway, J. H., Raichlen, D. A., & Lieberman, D. E. (2009) "Control and function of arm swing in human walking and running." *Journal of Experimental Biology*, 212(4), 523–534. https://doi.org/10.1242/jeb.024927

Rubin, B. D., & Kibler, W. B. (2002) "Fundamental principles of shoulder rehabilitation: Conservative to postoperative management." *Arthroscopy: Journal of Arthroscopic & Related Surgery*, 18(9), 29–39. https://doi.org/10.1053/jars.2002.36507

Schwartz, J. (1995) *Skeleton Keys: An Introduction to Human Skeletal Morphology, Development, and Analysis*. Oxford University Press.

Stuart Macadam, P. (2023, January 15) Personal communication.

Sweigard, L. E. (1974) *Human Movement Potential: Its Ideokinetic Facilitation*. Harper & Row.

Werner, E. S. (1893) *Delsarte System of Oratory* (fourth edn.). Urbana, IL: Project Gutenberg. Retrieved 1 December 2023 from www.gutenberg.org/files/12200/12200-h/12200-h.htm

Young, R. W. (2003) "Evolution of the human hand: The role of throwing and clubbing." *Journal of Anatomy*, 202(1), 165–174. https://doi.org/10.1046/j.1469-7580.2003.00144.x

# Subject Index

Note: illustrations and references in tables are referenced by page numbers in *italics*

# Author Index